Assistive Technology
for Persons With Disabilities

Assistive Technology for Persons With Disabilities

William C. Mann, PhD, OTR

Professor and Chair,
Department of Occupational Therapy

Director,
Center for Assistive Technology

University at Buffalo

Director,
Rehabilitation Engineering Research Center On
Assistive Technology and Environmental Interventions
For Older Persons With Disabilities

Joseph P. Lane, MBPA

Associate Director,
Center for Assistive Technology

University at Buffalo

Director,
Rehabilitation Engineering Research Center On
Technology Evaluation and Transfer

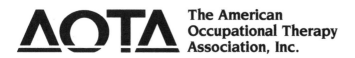

AOTA The American
Occupational Therapy
Association, Inc.

The American Occupational Therapy Association, Inc.
Bethesda, Maryland

For information address: The American Occupational Therapy Association, Inc., 4720 Montgomery Lane, PO Box 31220, Bethesda, MD 20824-1220.

Disclaimers
"This publication is designed to provide accurate and authoritative information in regard to the subject matter covered. It is sold or distributed with the understanding that the publisher is not engaged in rendering legal, accounting, or other professional service. If legal advice or other expert assistance is required, the services of a competent professional person should be sought."
—From the Declaration of Principles jointly adopted by the American Bar Association and a
    Committee of Publishers and Associations.

It is the objective of the American Occupational Therapy Association to be a forum for free expression and interchange of ideas. The opinions expressed by the contributors to this work are their own and not necessarily those of either the editors or the American Occupational Therapy Association.

Cover photo by Lightscapes, copyright © 1995.
Designed by Robert Sacheli

Printed in the United States of America

ISBN: 1-56900-028-X

Contents

Dedication

To Gwen and Jill, our thanks for your encouragement, patience, and love.

Acknowledgments

A book is the product of numerous collaborations from concept to printing. We thank the American Occupational Therapy Association for providing us with the opportunity to compile this book, particularly Executive Director Jeanette Bair, Nonperiodical Publications Director Frances McCarrey, and Carol Gwin, Practice and Technology Program Manager. We also thank Managing Editor Laura Farr Collins at AOTA for her thorough editing. We are grateful to our colleagues at the University at Buffalo support contributions. Our chapter co-authors, Katie Beaver, Jeffrey Higginbotham, Shelly Lane, James Lenker, Susan Mistrett, Susan Nochajski, Christine Oddo, Stephen Sprigle, made this second edition much richer by imparting their practical experience. We are indebted to the professional staff at the Center for Assistive Technology for their unfailing support. Our special thanks go to Robbie Dingle who personally integrated all the materials that transferred the first edition into this second edition. Thanks also to Mark Eberle for the book's layout and graphics work, and to Susan Ertel who kept work flowing around this project. We thank hundreds of researchers, service providers, and other professionals whose preceding work made this compilation possible. Finally, we wish to acknowledge the consumers of assistive technology and services, from whom we learn much about perseverance, motivation, and ingenuity.

Unit I: Introduction to Assistive Technology

Chapter 1:
Technology, Disability, and Professional Services

I. The Human/Technology Interface
- A. Humans as Tool Users
- B. Human Function and Tool Use
    - 1. Tools Extend Human Functions
- C. Tools, Technology, and Assistive Devices
    - 1. Technology as Tool
    - 2. Technology as Assistive Devices

II. Occupational Therapy and Disability
- A. Defining Occupational Therapy
- B. Disability Areas
    - 1. Physical Disabilities
    - 2. Sensory Impairments
    - 3. Cognitive and Speech Disabilities
    - 4. Other Disabilities
    - 5. Multiple Disabilities

III. Variables in the Human/Technology Interface
- A. Human Performance
    - 1. Human Intellect and Motivation
    - 2. Human Motor and Sensory Abilities
    - 3. Human Strength and Endurance
- B. Assistive Device Capabilities
    - 1. Device Functions and Options
    - 2. Device Cost and Availability
    - 3. Device Maintenance and Repair
- C. Functional Tasks
    - 1. Task Type
    - 2. Task Variety
    - 3. Task Attributes
- D. Task Environments
    - 1. Home Environment
    - 2. School and Work
    - 3. Recreation
    - 4. Transportation
    - 5. Support Networks

IV. Professions in Assistive Technology
- A. Architecture
- B. Medicine

4

1.

Technology, Disability, and Professional Services

Joseph P. Lane, MBPA, and William C. Mann, PhD, OTR

The focus of intervention is all too often on limitations, overlooking the fact that persons with disabilities have a diverse range of functional abilities. Combining these diverse abilities with the capabilities of technological tools—assistive devices—to optimize human task performance is a challenge beyond the expertise of any particular person or any one profession. Assessing the functional abilities of people and helping to evaluate device capabilities are essential first steps in providing assistive technology services. Selecting and delivering an appropriate device within an individual's social and environmental context is a "team" process, requiring input from members of multiple professions.

This chapter has six objectives:
1. Describe the human/technology interface.
2. Describe occupational therapy's role in disabilities.
3. Describe occupational therapy's role in technology.
4. Identify the variables in the human/technology interface.
5. Describe the role of each profession in addressing these variables.
6. Discuss the value of transdisciplinary teamwork for assistive devices.

The Human/Technology Interface

Humans as Tool Users

Tool use is a distinguishing characteristic of the human species. The use of physical objects as tools helps archaeologists identify our early ancestors. Other animal species also use objects as tools: Chimpanzees use sticks to retrieve termites from hives; sea otters balance rocks on their bodies as anvils to break open clam shells. However, no other species uses tools as extensively as modern *Homo sapiens.*

Human Function and Tool Use

To appreciate the value of tools, imagine the limits of human functions without them. The limits of physical functions without tools extend to our fingertips and toes; communication functions project to our range of sight, hearing, and voice; and mental functions comprise the thoughts in our heads. Without tools, our labors, mobility, senses, and security—our very survival—are bounded by our muscular strength, intellectual wiles, and endurance.

Tools Extend Human Functions

As tool users, modern humans routinely transcend their physical and mental limitations without thought or effort. Tools augment existing human functions or add new functions. Physical tools include kitchen appliances, workshop power tools, automobiles, and space shuttles. Communication tools include telephones, televisions, fiber-optic networks, and satellites. Computers, tape recorders, books, and pens expand our mental functions. Tool use literally provides humans with the capabilities of Superman—to bend steel, see into space, and fly.

No tool provides unlimited new capabilities. While tool use expands human functions, each tool establishes a new limit. That new limit remains until a more advanced tool further expands human functions. By this definition, devices and processes that help persons with disabilities are considered tools. These devices and processes, which assist in restoring or expanding human functions, are commonly called *assistive devices*.

Tools, Technology, and Assistive Devices

According to Webster's Dictionary (1977), the word *technology,* derived from the Greek words *techne* (meaning an art), and *logos* (meaning word or discourse), is the application of scientific knowledge. Thus, technology is some output or product of scientific advances. Technology has two attributes: tangibility and complexity. Tangibility encompasses hard technology—material objects such as wheelchairs; and soft technology—methods and designs such as making metal alloys and composite materials for high strength and lightweight sport wheelchairs. Complexity includes low technology—simple items with few moving parts, like crutches; and high technology—items with greater complexity in their components or design such as computer-based synthetic speech devices.

These distinctions blur quickly when applied to working devices. For example, it is difficult to categorize computer software on a diskette as either hard technology or soft technology. Likewise, does a walker made of lightweight resin composites represent a low technology or a high technology device? The distinctions are more important to understanding the concept of technology than to categorizing particular devices.

Technology as Tool

Regardless of the finer distinctions between tangibility and complexity, all forms of technology are considered tools. Hard technologies are tool instruments and soft technologies are tool uses. Successive advances in technologies translate into successive improvements in tools and tool use. The varied forms of technology/tools drive the industrial, commercial, agricultural, military, and medical fields. Biotechnology is a newer field spawned by technological advances in multiple scientific disciplines including biology, engineering, and chemistry.

Technology as Assistive Devices

While each scientific discipline holds certain unique forms of technology, most technologies are transferable; they are useful tools from and for more than one discipline or field. As such, new technology tools are often hybrid combinations of advances in established tools from various disciplines. For example, new assistive devices for persons with disabilities are based on technologies from many fields. Computer-based devices (hard technology) come from the electronics industry, while applications (soft technology) come from health and education. Controls, switches, and robotics are based on advances in the industrial and aerospace programs. Commercial and military developments generate new composite materials useful for mobility devices. Advances in biotechnology will generate unimaginable devices and functions for persons with disabilities.

Technological tools that restore or extend human functions are called *assistive devices,* and the field concerned with research, development, and service on assistive devices is called *assistive technology.* As with most new fields, assistive technology is a hybrid combination of advances in established areas. Such new fields defy traditional classifications. Assistive technology is at once the domain of mechanical engineers and physicians working on advanced prosthetics, orthotics, and robotics; of electrical engineers and software developers creating new computer-based applications and environmental control units; of architects and industrial designers modifying environments to accommodate persons with disabilities; and of occupational therapists, physical therapists, and speech/communication therapists working to restore human capabilities and functions through the application of technological devices.

The federal government defined the terminology in the Technology Related Assistance for Individuals with Disabilities Act of 1988 and has used those definitions in all new federal legislation since, including laws covering children, seniors, school, work and civil rights. The definitions are:

- Assistive Technology Device: "Any item, piece of equipment, or product system whether acquired commercially off the shelf, modified or customized, that is used to increase, maintain, or improve functional capabilities of individuals with disabilities."
- Assistive Technology Service: "Any service that directly assists an individual with disability in the selection, acquisition, or use of an assistive technology device...."

Occupational Therapy and Disability

Defining Occupational Therapy

"I understand you are an occupational therapist; what do you do?" Occupational therapists often have difficulty answering this question because of the breadth of their practice. "I work with children with emotional problems" or "I help people with physical disabilities become more independent"—these are common responses to the question.

"Yes, that sounds interesting, but what is occupational therapy?," the inquisitor persists. Occupational therapists help people with disabilities to overcome the limitations presented by the disabilities. There are many kinds of disabilities: blindness, deafness, paralysis, loss of an extremity, inability to speak, emotional illness. The type of disability, the age of the individual with the disability, the interests of the person with the disability—these are just a few of the considerations of an occupational therapist in selecting an appropriate intervention to overcome the effects of disability.

The American Occupational Therapy Association's (AOTA, 1994) definition is:

"Occupational therapy" is the use of purposeful activity or interventions designed to achieve functional outcomes which promote health, prevent injury or disability and which develop, improve, sustain, or restore the highest possible level of independence of any individual who has an injury, illness, cognitive impairment, psychosocial dysfunction, mental illness, developmental or learning disability, physical disability, or other disorder or condition. It includes assessment by means of skilled observation or evaluation through the administration and interpretation of standardized or nonstandardized tests and measurements.

Occupational therapy is indeed a broad field, and occupational therapists work in a wide variety of settings. This book will focus on those areas of the definition in italics: *evaluation, treatment, and consultation relating to designing, fabricating, or applying selected orthotic and prosthetic devices or selective adaptive equipment and adapting environments for the handicapped.*

Disability Areas

The term *disability* is itself continually undergoing revision. It is one term in a series of categories attempting to capture a condition within a particular system's context. The following definitions will also undergo future revisions, but they at least present conditions traditionally grouped under the terms "handicap" or "disability," within a functional context.

- Pathology: Interruption or interference of normal bodily processes or structures. Pathology occurs at level of cells or tissues.
- Impairment: Loss and/or abnormality of mental, emotional, physiological, or anatomical structure or function, to include pain. Impairment occurs at level of organs or organ systems.
- Functional Limitation: Restriction or lack of ability to perform an action or activity in the manner or within the range considered normal resulting from impairment. Functional limitation occurs at level of action or activity performance of organ or organ system.
- Disability: Inability or limitation in performing tasks, activities, and roles to levels expected within physical and social context. Disability occurs at level of task performance by individual in physical and social context.
- Societal Limitation: Restrictions attributed to social policy or barriers (structural or attitudinal), which limit fulfillment of roles or deny access to services and opportunities that are associated with full participation in society (National Institutes of Health, 1993).

We use the term disability in this book because we are most concerned with the value of assistive technology on task performance by people in their physical and social contexts.

Physical Disabilities

Physical disabilities include paralysis, weakness, contractures, amputations, tremors, spasticity, and other limitations related to coordinated movement. A person may have one or more physical disabilities. Physical disabilities are the result of either a disease process or a trauma that includes such things as falls, gunshot wounds, and burns. The physical disability may not remain static. Some physical disabilities may become progressively more severe over time, while others improve. This is an important factor to consider in evaluating and prescribing assistive technology.

The person's needs may change over time, and therefore the assistive device's functions may also need to change. Physical disabilities can be grouped into three major categories that relate to function:

1. Gross Motor Impairments: Illness or trauma can cause damage to the large muscles of the legs, shoulders, and arms; or damage to the nervous system resulting in limitations in strength, coordination, and joint range of motion.
2. Fine Motor Impairments: The precise movements of the wrist and fingers relate to fine motor performance.
3. Mobility Impairments: Injury or disease affecting the musculoskeletal or nervous system of the lower extremities may affect a person's ability to walk.

Sensory Impairments

Sensory impairments fall into four general categories:

1. Visual Impairments: There are several types of visual impairments that can result in partial or total loss of sight.
2. Hearing Impairments: Partial or total loss of the ability to hear sounds can occur following disease or injury. Injury is often the result of exposure to very loud noise.
3. Tactile Impairments: The ability to feel things—touch—is tactile sensation. It is possible to lose all or part of the ability to feel things, to discriminate between different objects by touching them, or to differentiate between hot or cold.
4. Olfactory and Taste Impairments: The senses of smell and taste relate to our enjoyment of food as well as our ability to distinguish dangers, such as gas in the air.

Cognitive and Speech Disabilities

1. Cognitive Impairments: A person may have difficulty remembering things, making decisions, or understanding more complicated ideas or instructions.
2. Speech Impairments: There are many "categories" of speech impairments. A person may suffer partial or total loss of ability to communicate verbally.

Other Disabilities

1. Mental Illness: There are a large number of diagnosed mental disorders that affect a person's ability to function.
2. Life Support: Some people require "high-tech" life support systems to stay alive. Examples include respirators for breathing, dialysis machines for cleaning the blood, and IVs for nourishment. While these machines may be "life supporting," they may also be

"handicapping," and assistive technology may be recommended to reduce the handicap.

Multiple Disabilities

Many individuals have more than one disability. This presents unique challenges for the applications of assistive technology. Multiple disabilities may require either more or less complexity in the user interface. Often there is not a commercially available device, and the professional must work closely with the consumer in the development of a useful solution for that person.

Variables in the Human/Technology Interface

The successful use of assistive devices (technology/tools) by persons with disabilities (tool users) depends on many factors. The human/technology interface should be viewed as an interrelated system of factors. The main variables influencing the outcomes of the human/technology interface fall into four categories: (a) human performance, (b) assistive device capabilities, (c) functional tasks, and (d) task environments. The variables under these four categories are shown in Table 1.1.

Taken in order, an assessment of a person's abilities (human performance) starts with the person's self-assessment. What can he or she do? What does he or she like to do? Not like? Prefer? What are his or her expectations and goals concerning functional tasks and task environments?

Once the person and the professional develop a clear understanding of the person's performance abilities and goals, together they can better assess the utility of device capabilities, and apply those assistive devices to functional tasks within the appropriate task environments.

Human Performance

Human performance variables such as intellect and motivation, motor and communication abilities, and strength and endurance all influence the selection and successful use of an assistive device. The requirements for operating a device should be well matched to a person's abilities. People will not effectively use a device that is excessively challenging to control or operate, regardless of the device's potential capabilities. Conversely, people will outgrow a device with excessively simple controls and correspondingly limited functions. Both cases may lead to abandoning the device, which translates into lost personal and financial investments in technology. In the latter case, an individual's potential performance may not be reached if the capabilities of the device are too limited.

Human performance must be carefully assessed and then matched to appropriate devices. Successful task performance results from a combination of human and technology performance. A person must be able to use the assistive device. A keyboard with enlarged keys is not accessible if the person with a visual impairment also has quadriplegia. An assistive device providing an alternative method for keyboard control, such as a light-pointer or sip-and-puff switch, allows a person with such a disability to access the computer system.

Cost/performance trade-offs are necessary to attain the best human/technology interface. Some devices with complicated operating requirements offer more capabilities, room for learning, and skill acquisition, but they require more complex levels of human performance. Other devices build the operating complexity into the hardware and software, permitting the user to accomplish complex functions via simple controls. Maximizing the role of human performance minimizes the cost of acquiring technology performance; the more the person can do, the less the technology must do. The following attributes of intellect, motivation, abilities, and endurance will determine the trade-offs.

Human Intellect and Motivation

Level of intellectual function influences the types of assistive devices people can operate effectively. A person with a higher level of intellect can operate more sophisticated devices than a person with a lower level of intellect. Assistive devices may require mental skills of learning, retention, and memory with respect to the proper activation, control, and safe use of an assistive device. Mental stamina is important for learning and task performance. Complex instructions should be divided into training modules that the person can comfortably complete.

Personal motivation also plays an important role. A highly motivated person will devote more effort to learning. People with higher motivation levels can learn to operate devices with more sophisticated capabilities. They will also devote more time to acquiring greater skills in device use. High motivation should be matched to device capabilities with room to grow. The person's commitment to acquire, master, and apply an assistive device is considered the single most influential factor in the human/tool interface because inappropriate devices can be

Table 1.1. Variables in the Human/Technology Interface.

Variable Categories	Variables
Human Performance	Intellect and Motivation
	Motor and Sensory Abilities
	Strength and Endurance
Assistive Device Capabilities	Functions and Options
	Cost and Availability
	Maintenance and Repair
Functional Tasks	Task Type
	Task Variety
	Task Attributes (frequency, duration)
Task Environments	Home Environment
	School and Work
	Recreation
	Transportation
	Support Networks
	Community/Commercial

replaced, access can be improved, environmental factors can be mitigated, and designs can be altered. Modifications are part of the learning cycle inherent in assistive device use. However, the value of assistive devices as tools for extending human functions is limited by the attitudes of the user. The professional must work closely with consumers to help anticipate their reactions as device users.

Human Motor and Sensory Abilities

Physical—motor—and sensory abilities largely determine both the type of device a person needs and the type of device a person can operate effectively.

A person with full use of upper extremities and fine motor skills can use standard switch and control systems such as keyboards, toggle switches, and mouse controls. Persons with motor impairments may gain access to the same devices through alternative-input (switch and control) systems that are adapted for use by body parts under the person's voluntary control. Joysticks, pressure pads, single switches, and head-mounted controls are fairly common. Sophisticated controls activated by voice or visual contact are also available in the marketplace, for a higher price.

After a user provides input to an assistive device through a switch or control, the device generates some form of output—a message to the user such as a screen display or printed material. The output from a device may not be directly accessible to persons with sensory impairments in vision, hearing, or touch. The device may need to generate alternate output formats such as synthesized speech, enlarged print, refreshable braille, tactile Morse code, vibrations, or flashing lights. Depending on the device, these output features are available as standard features or add-on components.

Providing technology access to persons with multiple disabilities presents additional challenges, but these users' unique requirements for alternative input and output formats may be met through a combination of assistive devices.

Human Strength and Endurance

Physical strength and endurance affect the frequency, intensity, and duration of assessment and use of assistive devices. People who fatigue quickly will spend less time on a task. This may translate into extended elapsed time for assessment and training as well as added time to reinforce information presented at prior sessions. The extra time required does not reflect poorly on the device user. It is simply a factor to consider when planning acquisition, training, and use.

Physical strength is a factor in device selection because the activation, control, and use of some devices require physical effort. Some devices require physical strength to lift, move, or transport. A device constructed from lightweight materials may cost more than other options, but the lighter weight may make the difference between a usable and an abandoned device.

Assistive Device Capabilities

An assistive device must be capable of performing the necessary function to complete the desired task. The *function* of the device is of great importance to the user; the type of technology involved is less important. A keyguard for a computer keyboard will not help a person with low vision see characters on a keyboard and screen. An enlarged keyboard and screen magnifier are more appropriate assistive devices for this person.

Assistive devices have specific capabilities. Devices produced and marketed through commercial channels have clearly defined capabilities targeted at specific applications. For example, alternative keyboards may be large or small, but they are intended for use with specific computer hardware and software. Implementing commercially available assistive devices in the intended manner typically provides the end user with product warranties, support services, and an organized maintenance and repair program.

Some user needs are complex enough or sufficiently unique to render commercial devices inappropriate or inadequate. Making modifications to a commercial device extends its capabilities or tailors the device to the user's needs. An example is rewiring an alternative keyboard to accept commands from a single switch. Modifications may make the device more difficult to operate or less reliable. In addition, modifications usually void the manufacturer's warranties and make mechanical or electrical shops reluctant to maintain or repair the devices.

Some needs are so novel that commercial solutions are either nonexistent or prohibitively expensive. Fabricating a new device to meet a person's needs may deliver a combination of benefits and problems—the customized design is more useful to the person, but the device experiences more problems in operation because the modified design suffers from a lack of testing and development.

Beyond an assistive device's capability and accessibility is its appeal to the user and perceived acceptance by others. Appearance is less important than function, but not much less, from the user's perspective. A useful device that is unpleasant to the eye or ear, or creates an unnecessary obstruction for others, will end up in the closet or the trash. People want the acceptance of others. It is less expensive to consider design and aesthetics during the development stage; it may add little or no cost to the final product.

Device Functions and Options

Working together, the professional and consumer assess the intended and potential functions of an assistive device. A device designed to magnify printed text on a video screen is intended for use by persons with a visual impairment. The device's function is print magnification. What if the person has difficulty moving the text material? A manual system may not suit the particular needs of a person with limited arm motion. A system with two functions, magnifying print and moving the text material, is more appropriate. What if the person intends to pursue education or employment involving computers? A magnification system that can present output from a computer also satisfies this potential application.

Identifying all available options for the components of an assistive device is time consuming, but it provides the user and the professional with the broadest range of choices. Optional equipment may increase the device's utility. In fact, as in the example of a print magnifier with the moving text option, some users may only be able to operate the device if it has this option. A print magnifier may have an optional power-driven platform to move the printed material. A low-technology option is a platform mounted on rolling casters and guided by tracks or bumpers. The platform is moved by a hand, foot, or drive mechanism.

Device Cost and Availability

The full cost of an assistive device includes the cost of the initial assessment, the device, all options and peripheral components, documentation and training, planned maintenance, expected repairs, and warranties. More sophisticated or complex devices cost more to purchase and maintain, but they typically fall within two product lines offering predictable performance and modification options. In the above example, the commercial device may cost more or less than the fabricated device. While the vendor has the cost of research and development, product materials, assembly labor, and overhead, the vendor may achieve savings through mass production, marketing a proven design, and providing cost-effective support services. The fabricated device may have none of those features.

Device Maintenance and Repair

Maintenance and repair are issues of practical concern beyond the financial cost. People grow increasingly reliant on the functions provided by an assistive device as it becomes integrated into their personal, social, and work environments. A person who depends heavily on the functions of a device will suffer serious hardships by a device failure that eliminates access to the critical functions. The failure of an important assistive device is analogous to suffering a debilitating illness. The result for the person is becoming unable to function at the level required to sustain routine activity.

As an example, consider a person who does not drive a car. The person has established a set of methods and expectations for traveling that involves alternate systems like public transportation schedules and fees. Acquiring an automobile and learning how to drive drastically alter the person's methods and expectations. A car breakdown has a serious impact on ability to function. The person is dependent on the car and can no longer readily access the alternative transportation system's schedules and fees. Like a car, an assistive device also becomes integrated into multiple facets of daily life. Anticipating maintenance and repair needs, and developing a regular maintenance plan for the consumer to follow, are critical contributions to successful long-term device use.

The user's location also relates to maintenance and repair. People in urban areas have greater access to transportation networks and skilled labor pools than people in rural areas. Plans for support contingencies should consider time, cost, and access. It is important to inquire about vendor loan programs and identify possible substitutes.

Functional Tasks

People use devices to perform some desired task. Human performance and device capabilities combine to produce a function. For example, a person's residual vision and a print magnifier combine to produce the function of reading printed material. The functions produced relate to successfully performing particular tasks. In this example, the person may need to read printed materials to sustain tasks related to education (studying), employment (managing paper flow), or recreation (reading mystery novels).

Optimizing the human/technology interface requires a thorough assessment of the functional tasks to be performed by the person. This assessment must address functional tasks in terms of their context—their type, variety, and attributes.

Task Type

The type of functional task the assistive device must perform depends on the person's level of impairment and abilities. Functional task types are broad definitions of general system requirements. Examples of functional tasks are mobility, communication, computer access, and environmental control. A person with a physical disability of the lower extremities needs assistance with mobility tasks. A person with a physical disability involving lower and upper extremities needs assistance with mobility, computer access, and environmental control tasks.

The type of functional task the device must perform largely determines the type of technology involved (e.g., electrical versus mechanical) and the range of professional expertise required to develop and deliver a useful combination of assistive devices.

Task Variety

Task variety is the number of different functional tasks the assistive technology must perform. The task variety depends on both the person's level of impairment and the life roles he or she plans on fulfilling. A child may need a device to function in school tasks, play with friends, and do home chores. A worker may only need a device for work-related tasks. A computer system adapted to the needs of a person with low vision may only perform the task of enlarging characters on the video screen. If the person also has quadriplegia, the computer system would require more task variety: enlarging characters, activating power, and accepting input and control without a keyboard. It would also require a position enabling the person to access the computer and work materials.

Task variety may exceed the capabilities of any one assistive device. A combination of devices may be required to accommodate task variety. Task variety has implications for accessibility and accommodation in the task environment.

Task Attributes

The attributes of each task are quantifiable in terms of frequency of occurrence, task duration, and task intensity. The terms *frequency, intensity,* and *duration* are used to quantify such forms of human activity as studying, working, and exercising. Quantifying task attributes provides detailed specifications about performance requirements for an assistive device.

The frequency of occurrence represents how often the task is performed within a given time frame. Is the device needed to perform one task in the morning every day, in the afternoons each weekday, or is it used throughout the evenings and on weekends? A device in constant use requires greater durability than a device used only upon awakening or during dinner. Frequency of occurrence also suggests how critical the device may become for the user. Frequency attributes of day and time influence plans for providing routine maintenance and repair support as well as special considerations such as glare and heat from sunlight, or lighting during darkness. For example, a mobility device that will be used outside at night should include a reliable power source, lights, and reflective surfaces, as well as moisture and rust protection. In contrast, a device used only indoors or only in fair weather can reduce these additional requirements and associated costs.

Task duration is a measure of how long the task takes to complete—the elapsed time in which the user is operating the device. Task duration addresses the level of comfort during operation, sustained intellectual attention and muscular control required by operation, criteria for a power supply, concerns of heat and noise, and the user's sustained dexterity under fatigue. Prolonged task duration magnifies the potential effects of these variables on the user's performance.

Functional task intensity addresses the amount of effort the user must expend to successfully accomplish the task. Task intensity may be mental, physical, or both. It will vary between people and between tasks. For example, a task involving multiple sequential commands, such as a computer scanning program, requires intense mental concentration. People with certain physical disabilities must expend high levels of energy to maintain the fine motor control needed to operate a joystick.

Task Environments

The person and the assistive device interact within the surrounding environment. Task environments encompass all places where the functional tasks may be performed by the device user. Task environments are located within the person's home, workplace, school, recreation facilities, transportation systems, and community and social centers. Using the home as an example, the kitchen task environment encompasses the functional activities of cooking, eating, and cleaning. These tasks involve tools like the stove, refrigerator, dishwasher, sink, cupboards, and table. The bedroom task environment encompasses activities like sleeping, dressing, engaging in sex, and studying.

Even if an assistive device has appropriate capabilities and is functional for the person, the task environment may present barriers that negate the device's value. Using devices for persons with visual impairments as an example, inadequate room lighting can make the enlarged keys on a keyboard illegible, while glare from excessive light may wash out a magnified screen image. Task environments and functional tasks represent multiple variables, each with the potential to influence task performance with assistive devices. A powered wheelchair that works well within the school's task environments may not fit within the doorways and passages at home. Accommodating the assistive device in all relevant task environments is crucial to optimizing the human/technology interface. This, in turn, emphasizes the need to involve the consumer in all assessment and selection processes. The user typically knows best.

Home Environment

Assistive devices are used to perform the greatest variety of tasks in the home. Activities of daily living, school and office work, recreation and leisure, and social interaction all occur in the home. If devices designed for the classroom and workplace also fit in the home, the user can gain economies by using one device in multiple locations. Important features of the home environment include the following:

Space. The typical home has a finite amount of space available for the use of an assistive device. Device selection is influenced by the amount of floor space available compared to the amount required. Floor-standing devices need space for the base, and desktop devices need room on a desk-height surface and ceiling clearance. Securely anchoring some support or mobility devices to the wall, floor, or ceiling may require structural reinforcements.

Accessibility. Accessibility of the task environment concerns the person's ability to enter and function within the environment both alone and with the assistive device. Determining physical accessibility for a new device, such as passage between rooms or entering the home, may involve measuring objects and simulating movement. Devices requiring electric power need outlets and power that can be controlled by the device user. A device may require specific lighting levels, heating or cooling, or other special conditions. To be accessible, a task environment must meet these needs or be modified. Accessibility may also be achieved by considering alternate solutions such as different devices.

Accommodation. Accommodation addresses the fit between the task environment and the assistive device. How will the person use the assistive device to perform functional tasks within the home's limited space? How many tasks will the device perform, and where will task performance occur? Accommodation planning is minimal if a device is dedicated to one functional task in one location, such as completing homework in the person's bedroom. The number and type of accommodations that must be planned increase with the variety of activities that involve the assistive device. A speech synthesizer may perform multiple communication tasks—from telephone calls in the kitchen to family discussions in the living room.

Family needs. Considering family needs within the task environment is important to ensure the device is assimilated into the home routine. A device generating excessive light or noise may disrupt other members of the household and their activities, unless these extraneous impacts are mitigated. Poorly located power lines, control cords, or the device itself might create obstacles or hazards for family members. Mitigating impacts of assistive devices on family members may involve costs that should be considered in the cost–benefit evaluation of a device. With proper planning, most devices can be installed with minimal disruption to the family.

School and Work

Task environments at school and work involve considerations similar to those in the home, and others specific to the classroom or office.

Space. School desks and work offices have a finite amount of space for an assistive device, so floor space, work surfaces, and anchor positions are important. Unlike the home, where space may be dedicated to the user and the device, space at school and work may serve multiple uses and people in the course of a day. Assistive devices should not represent an insurmountable obstacle for others. Security is also an important issue for devices used in public or shared areas, requiring protocols for using and securing the assistive device.

Accessibility. Accessibility issues described in the home are multiplied in school and work settings. Accessibility issues involve school rooms and offices, cafeterias, elevators, restrooms, gymnasiums, and any other locations reached by the student or worker. As in the home, a portable device used in multiple sites must have the required power and lighting available.

Accommodation. Accommodating an assistive device within the school or workplace may require modifications to the tasks performed, to the task environment, or to the device. A person performs a wide range of functional tasks at school or work, each with particular accommodation issues. A thorough plan for accommodating all anticipated tasks will maximize the device's utility.

The plan should involve the expected progression of students graduating to the next level and workers being promoted to more responsibility or new job duties (e.g., local or distant travel). The task environment may change as the person gains proficiency with the device. Planning should consider an assistive device's utility in the context of the person's probable future progress.

Peers. Peers in the task environment are fellow students or coworkers. Mitigating any adverse effects of using assistive devices, such as noise or physical disruption, helps increase acceptance by peers. Peer acceptance is a vital source of encouragement and support for device use.

Recreation

An assistive device may be useful in leisure pursuits. For instance, a wheelchair that allows a person to sit or stand while in motion allows persons with paraplegia to participate in golf, archery, or darts. People who are blind play baseball using a ball that emits a beeping sound—they pitch to their own teammates. New wheelchair designs are even used, like mountain bicycles for downhill racing. Consumer agencies in rural areas, along with some companies, are developing new devices specifically to make outdoor recreation more accessible. The recreational task environment involves understanding the person's past and present interests, and determining how an assistive device might support continued recreational activity.

Transportation

The transportation task environment addresses the variables the person will encounter while moving between environments of home, school, work, and recreation. Transportation includes private automobiles, public buses, taxis, and van services. Each form of transportation presents opportunities and problems for the assistive device user. A device may not fit in a private passenger vehicle or a taxi. The public bus system may not be accessible or within reach. A person using public transportation may face obstacles in transporting a device used in several locations. Van services are another option that might accommodate devices.

Transportation options vary across locations. An urban setting usually has more transportation options (e.g., bus, taxi, light rail, subway) and different obstacles (e.g., light rail platforms, subway escalators) than a rural setting. Suburban locations lack the mass transportation and pedestrian networks found in cities, and they involve the longer distances and reduced services associated with rural areas.

Support Networks

Family, friends, and caregivers. Family members, friends, and caregivers are the most critical part of the support network. Assessing the utility of an assistive device should include identifying any people who are willing to help use and maintain the device. For example, a portable device for use in multiple locations may only be feasible if some third party is willing to transport and connect the device at each

site. People in the support network can also help in sustaining regular maintenance programs.

The assistive device may also be of value to people in the support network. The device may help the user perform tasks with more independence, or directly perform tasks previously completed by family members, friends, or caregivers. In these instances, the assistive device frees people to interact with the device user in other ways.

Community resources. Community resources include members of advocate organizations with related interests. Other persons with similar disabilities may provide support to the user, or the user may become a role model for others considering assistive devices. Community support provides instruction, encouragement, and access to information networks valuable to assistive device users. Service agencies can provide immediate technical support. Local professionals may have expertise relevant to device use.

In summary, the human/device interface involves numerous variables that may be either opportunities or obstacles for the device user. Identifying and accommodating all relevant variables exceeds the skill of any one professional or discipline. The following section describes different professions with expertise relevant to providing assistive devices. Depending on the variables involved in a particular human/device interface, professionals from these fields can provide valuable assistance as consultants or as part of a team.

Professions in Assistive Technology

The applied field of assistive technology is based on contributions from disciplines in the natural sciences, biosciences, medical sciences, and social sciences. Ten professions are especially involved in delivering technology-related services to persons with disabilities. Alphabetically, these are:

- Architecture
- Medicine
- Nursing
- Occupational therapy
- Physical therapy
- Rehabilitation counseling
- Rehabilitation engineering
- Social work
- Special education
- Speech-language pathology and audiology

A summary follows for each profession, describing its education requirements, certification standards, and potential role in the technology services team (Bureau of Labor Statistics, 1989). The summary of other professions includes law, computer science, industrial design, psychology, and sociology. These professions all have a place in improving the human/technology interface.

Architecture

Architects design structures to be safe, functional, useful, and aesthetically pleasing. All states require persons who call themselves architects or who contract for architectural services to be registered. Licensure in New York state requires at least a Bachelor of Architecture degree from a program accredited by the National Architectural Accrediting Board plus 3 years of qualified experience in an architect's office. Other states vary the length of the internship. A registered architect is legally responsible for all design work performed, and can be hired to advise an owner about the quality and workmanship of a specific contractor.

Architects receive training in design, mechanical drawing, construction, mathematics, and related aspects of engineering. The architect's knowledge of building codes and structural requirements, as well as a grasp of spatial relationships, are useful for planning and implementing modifications that increase accessibility. Examples include ramps, doors, work stations, and work surfaces. Expertise in human factors and ergonomics is important to ensure a comfortable fit between the person and the task environment for an assistive device.

Medicine

Physicians provide medical examinations, diagnose illness from symptoms and tests, and prescribe treatment for persons with illness, disease, or injury. Physicians are general practitioners or specialists. The Doctor of Medicine (MD) and Doctor of Osteopathy (DO) both apply treatments of drugs, surgery, and therapy, but osteopathic physicians pay additional attention to the musculoskeletal systems.

All states require both DOs and MDs to graduate from an accredited professional school of medicine, pass a licensing exam given by the National Board of Medical Examiners (MDs) or the National Board of Osteopathic Medical Examiners (DOs), and in most states complete 1 or 2 years of residency/internship, (i.e., supervised practice in an accredited graduate medical education program). Graduates of foreign medical schools must complete a 1-year residency program in a U.S. hospital, then pass the Federation Licensure Examination (FLEX).

Several specialty areas in the field of medicine are directly involved with assistive devices, including family practice (general care), geriatrics (aging), orthopedics (locomotive structures), and physiatry (physical interventions). Physicians bring knowledge of relevant medical interventions and their predicted consequences. This knowledge is crucial to planning long-term requirements for assistive devices. Physicians also write prescriptions that obtain assistive devices of medical necessity and help obtain third-party reimbursement for certain devices.

Nursing

Registered nurses are responsible for health promotion and disease prevention, health maintenance, and health restoration. In caring for people who are ill, nurses consider their patients' physical, functional, psychosocial, and economic needs. They are prepared to assess, plan nursing care, prescribe nursing therapy, and evaluate interventions as well as record the progress of symptoms. Their activities reinforce therapies administered by other disciplines to patients who are in the process of convalescence and rehabilitation.

Registered nurses qualify for a license by graduating from an approved school of nursing and passing a national examination given in each state. Education involves coursework in biological, physical, and behavioral sciences as well as supervised nursing practice in medical facilities. Entry-level nursing programs include 2-year associate degrees from community colleges, 2- or 3-year diploma programs in hospitals, and 4-year bachelor degree programs. Some states now require a bachelor's degree in nursing to qualify for licensure as a registered nurse.

Several nursing specialties may be involved with rehabilitation and assistive technology. Hospital-based nurses provide skilled care during acute rehabilitation. Home-based nurses work with persons in long-term convalescence and with older persons. Community health nurses work in schools, clinics, and retirement communities. Occupational health nurses provide services to persons in the workplace. Assistive technology is applicable in all of these settings. Registered nurses can assess a person's progress in the rehabilitation process to help anticipate functional needs that can be addressed with assistive technology.

Occupational Therapy

Occupational therapists work to maintain or restore functional skills for persons with physical, sensory, developmental, or mental disabilities. Restoration of functional skills may be accomplished through treatment aimed at diminishing the disability, through compensatory strategies taught by the therapist, or through the therapeutic application of assistive devices. The occupational therapist's rigorous training program includes physical, biological, medical, and behavioral sciences, along with occupational therapy's accepted theories and specific intervention strategies. School training is followed by a required 6-month supervised clinical internship. The title Registered Occupational Therapist (OTR) is awarded through a national certification examination given by the American Occupational Therapy Certification Board, following completion of an entry-level professional baccalaureate or master's degree. An associate's degree in occupational therapy can lead to certification as a Certified Occupational Therapy Assistant (COTA).

Occupational therapists conduct functional assessments, provide therapy, and identify useful interventions that meet client needs. They work closely with other professionals in the evaluation, development, and provision of adaptive devices.

Physical Therapy

Physical therapy is primarily concerned with restoring functions and preventing additional disability following the onset of a disease or injury. Physical therapists plan and implement treatments to reduce pain; to improve physical functions such as strength, range of motion, and mobility; and to train patients in the use of assistive devices such as wheelchairs and prosthetic devices. Practicing physical therapists must hold state licensure, which is obtained after graduating from a program accredited by the American Physical Therapy Association and passing a state examination.

The physical therapy curriculum includes courses in anatomy, physiology, neuroanatomy and neurophysiology, biomechanics, human growth and development, and physical therapy procedures. Treatment modalities include exercise, physical agents (e.g., heat, cold, electrical stimulation), and instruction in device use. The physical therapist can determine if a person is able to operate a specific device and if the device will provide the intended function (National Academy of Sciences, 1988).

Rehabilitation Counseling

The vocational rehabilitation counselor is the central service provider for eligible clients associated with public vocational rehabilitation programs. Rehabilitation counselors help persons with disabilities gain independence and become more productive through education or employment. Counselors evaluate a person's level of impairment in terms of the potential for employment or education. They arrange for any necessary medical care, rehabilitation, job training, and work placement programs. The rehabilitation counselor develops a broad picture of the person's needs and abilities, including discussions with family members, caregivers, physicians, psychologists, occupational therapists, and potential employers. The rehabilitation counselor are responsible for recommending a course of rehabilitation and training that leads to successful placement in school or employment.

Vocational and rehabilitation service agencies usually require a master's degree or a bachelor's degree and relevant experience. Half the states require counselors in private practice to have a state license. State vocational rehabilitation agencies require employees to pass a written examination and be evaluated by a board of examiners. Most employers look for certification. Certification requires counselors to meet the education and experience standards of the Commission on Rehabilitation Counselor Certification and pass a written examination to be called a Certified Rehabilitation Counselor (CRC).

Rehabilitation counselors understand the process of making transitions to home, education, and employment. They identify the critical factors in making successful transitions from rehabilitation to gainful activity, help to define the role of an assistive device in the process, and assist in developing training for using assistive devices.

Rehabilitation Engineering

Engineers apply the theories and principles of science and mathematics to solve practical technical problems. They design, develop, test, produce, operate, and maintain machinery, products, systems, and processes. A bachelor's degree from an accredited institution is sufficient to work as an engineer in the fields of mechanics, electronics, chemistry, and industrial or civil engineering. However, engineers working in fields that may affect life, health, or property, and those who offer their services to the public, must be registered. Registration requires a degree from an accredited school, 4 years of related work experience, and passing of a state examination. Each state has a Society of Professional Engineers that administers licensure or certification.

The application of engineering to the field of rehabilitation—rehabilitation engineering—is only now becoming a formal training program in select schools of engineering, almost always in cooperation with a school of medicine or rehabilitation sciences. The practice of rehabilitation engineering can be defined as "the application of science and technology to ameliorate the handicaps of individuals with disabilities" (Robinson, 1993). A typical rehabilitation engineer has an advanced degree in a traditional engineering discipline (e.g., mechanical, electrical, or biomedical), coupled with coursework in human factors and anatomy and physiology, and some experience in clinical service provision to persons with disabilities. A rehabilitation engineer can provide technical expertise to the rehabilitation team. Possible roles include combining different technologies into an integrated system, assessing the biomechanics and function of a person to determine optional device access or seated posture, designing or modifying electrical (assistive) or mechanical devices to meet a particular need, and evaluating devices and modifications (i.e., car or home modifications) for safety and usability.

Some people in the field of assistive technology lack formal training in engineering, but they are certified, licensed, or eligible to practice in a basic clinical discipline (e.g., PT, OT, SLP). If they have sufficient experience, they may apply to a professional credentialing board (e.g., RESNA) as an assistive technology practitioner. If a practitioner has no formal credentials, he or she can only assess the person's knowledge and skills based on previous work and personal referrals.

Social Work

Social workers provide direct counseling and referrals to other service providers for persons and families coping with medical, social, and financial problems. Employment as a social worker usually requires bachelor's degree training in the social sciences and a master's degree in social work (MSW). Forty-one states require licensure for the title Academy of Certified Social Workers (ACSW), or registration for clinical social workers. Health insurance providers may require licensure or registration to reimburse social workers for services rendered.

Social workers deal with all facets of service delivery systems. They have skills and experience in coordinating service provision and have a case-based orientation toward each client. Social workers have broad knowledge of community resources and methods for accessing public and private service provider systems in their region. Their knowledge of reimbursement mechanisms, particularly third-party payment systems (e.g., Medicare and Medicaid), can be critical for a person to acquire an assistive device, or obtain reimbursement for the device from a third-party payer, in a timely fashion.

Special Education

Educators convey knowledge about numbers, language, science, and social studies to children, youth, and adults. Educators must be certified by their state's board of education or a certification advisory committee. A bachelor's degree—or a master's degree in some states—and completion of an approved teacher education program are generally required. Thirty-five states also require competency testing in basic skills, teaching skills, and a specialty area for certification. Almost all states require additional education to renew a teacher's certificate; many require a master's degree.

Special educators develop school-based programs for students with disabilities that address short-term, immediate educational needs (e.g., information about language, social skills, and core subjects) in both self-contained and inclusive educational environments. They are also responsible for long-term transition planning needs (e.g., what a person will do after high school in terms of higher education, vocation, residential needs, and leisure/recreation activities), identified by age 16 within each student's Individual Transition Plan. Generally, special educators work with students ages 3 to 21 in preschool, elementary, and secondary education settings, but infants and older adults may also have special educators involved in treatment planning.

Today, special educators frequently provide consultative and resource room support to children with disabilities in regular education settings. They play an integral role on the assistive technology service team through their direct experiences with classrooms, modifying curricula to meet the unique needs and abilities of individual students.

The Individuals With Disabilities Education Act (IDEA) guarantees each student access to "a free and appropriate public education," which is defined for each student in his or her Individualized Education Program (IEP). The IEP is determined annually by the student's parents, teachers, and related service personnel according to an individualized assessment of the student's needs. In order to effectively ensure the use of assistive technology devices within the goals of the IEP and to meet the needs of traditional classroom procedures, the service team must receive input from the special education teachers. Educators can design and implement support capabilities based on faculty expertise and school-based resources. They must also look ahead to the long-term needs of their students, both inside and outside school. The guidance and active involvement of special educators will facilitate device use by children and students with disabilities.

Speech-Language Pathology and Audiology

Speech-language pathologists diagnose speech and language problems, provide treatment, and counsel family members. Audiologists identify, assess, and treat problems with hearing. A master's degree in speech-language pathology or audiology is the entry-level professional requirement in most states. Coursework includes anatomy and physiology, language acquisition, neuroscience, analysis and measurement of speech, language and auditory processes, psychosocial aspects of communication, and instrumentation.

After graduation, clinicians obtain a Certificate of Clinical Competence (CCC-SLP in speech-language pathology or CCC-AUD in audiology) that involves a 9-month internship and a national written examination. In addition to ASHA certification, 36 states require licensure for a person to work in schools, private practice, or clinical settings. Licensure involves an examination and 300 hours of supervised clinical experience beyond the master's degree.

Assistive devices used to supplant spoken or written communication are called *augmentative communication devices*. Augmentative communication devices based on microprocessors provide an increasingly diverse range of applications, such as synthesized speech and voice-recognition systems.

Other Professions

The number of professions involved with assistive technology continues to expand as technology applications expand. Psychologists and sociologists study individual and group behaviors connected with the use of devices to increase acceptance, reduce abandonment, and decrease residual stigmas about technology and disability. Industrial designers enhance the aesthetic appeal of assistive devices by altering their shape, color, sound, and image. Computer programmers and analysts develop new hardware and software applications tailored to the needs of particular disability groups. Attorneys devote time to interpreting disability-related legislation and consulting with advocates for persons with disabilities.

Some of the expertise and resources that the physical and applied sciences devoted to military applications are being redirected to meet human needs. Many technological advances achieved for military and aerospace purposes have direct relevance to the functional needs of persons with disabilities. Research and development in composite materials, superconductivity, human genome identification, and micro/nano engineering are generating new fields of expertise with unprecedented value for persons with disabilities. This work is introducing more disciplines to the field of assistive technology.

Transdisciplinary Teamwork

Requirements for Technology Expertise

Delivering assistive technology services requires a team approach. The collective expertise of rehabilitation professionals working in partnership with the consumer is crucial to proper assessment, appropriate interventions, and successful use. Including the consumers in the entire service delivery process—both the person with a disability and caregivers—is essential to ensuring a positive outcome.

Three major trends are shaping the requirements for broad expertise in the assistive technology team. The first trend is that the diverse populations using assistive devices require professionals who draw upon increasingly diverse service modalities. Health care professionals must focus more on disability than on illness, more on maximizing independence than on providing a "cure." Further, most new services involving assistive technology applications fall outside the medical system. Educational, vocational, and advocacy agencies are applying devices to enable persons with disabilities to realize their full potential.

The second trend is that information on new techniques and products is being disseminated at a rapid pace. Professionals must learn new techniques for functional assessment, therapeutic interventions, and team management skills. New applications of technology that reduce or mitigate the effects of impairments—especially microprocessor-based assistive devices—are reaching the marketplace at an accelerating rate. New products are available to off-set the impact of decreased strength and endurance, visual and hearing impairments, and speech disorders. While the technology exists in increasing amounts, its delivery to people with disabilities and their knowledge of the technology are somewhat limited. One major limiting factor is the lack of knowledge about the applications of this technology among professionals in the field.

The third trend is that changes in social attitudes, legislation, and health status are expanding opportunities for persons with disabilities in education, employment, and recreation. Federal legislation has language and emphases increasing the demand for assistive devices through protection, advocacy, and inclusion policies, and increasing supply by changing funding eligibility and requirements. For example:

- *Individuals With Disabilities Education Act of 1990* extends children's rights to a free and appropriate education to include assessment for provision of assistive devices and services.
- *Older Americans Act of 1991* includes language about the availability and use of assistive devices.
- *Rehabilitation Act of 1992* describes assistive devices and services as a means to sustain or regain employment. Given the potential of these devices, no person can be presumed to be incapable of gainful employment.
- *The Americans With Disabilities Act of 1990* defines equal access for persons with disabilities as a civil right. It also requires all places of employment, transportation, education, accommodations, services, and telecommunications to become accessible through reasonable accommodations.
- *Technology Related Assistance for Individuals With Disabilities Act of 1988* defines assistive devices and services, and establishes a program so every state can develop an information and referral network.

Each new opportunity involves unique functional tasks and task environments for assessment. Evolving societal trends present new challenges for applying assistive technology as society increasingly recognizes special populations of persons with disabilities, including those in racial, ethnic, and economic minorities; those in rural areas; and those with mental illness and developmental disabilities. The families and other caregivers of persons in these spe-cial populations also benefit from the application of assistive devices.

The professional literature recommends multi-disciplinary assessment teams for persons with disabilities (Brandenburg, 1987; Enders & Hall, 1990; Smith, 1991). Professionals in the applied sciences and health fields often approach assessments as a multidisciplinary team. Each member of the team brings a particular expertise that augments the expertise of other team members. Consider the client as a member of the team. The other team members work with the client to assess the client's level of impairment, the capabilities of the assistive device, and the work/home context in which the person uses the device. This approach encourages the interaction of knowledge from formal training and practice by relaxing professional boundaries. The assessment process has three components:

1. Client assessments.
2. Assessments of work and home environments.
3. Functional specifications for devices.

Client assessments. These assessments include the client's actual and perceived abilities regarding mobility, sensory, and cognitive limitations and needs, task performance capabilities, workstation design requirements, use of adaptive devices, and equipment to make devices accessible. After reviewing existing assessment records on the client's physical, sensory, functional, and motivational status, the team gathers additional data on task-related functions. Important considerations include: What sensory channels are readily used? Can assistive devices mitigate sensory deficits? What are personal capabilities in terms of stamina, speed, and accuracy in task performance? What gaps exist between personal capabilities and work performance or independent living functions?

Assessments of work and home environments. These assessments address the adaptability of the client's workstations and work tasks, requirements for independent living, and related aspects of the physical environment. The assessments also delineate environmental and social constraints on assistive devices. The social adaptability of assistive devices is an equally important consideration. Other aspects to think about include: What accommodations might be made in the home or workplace to accommodate the person? Is the person dependent on others for assistance with any particular task or function? What training has the person received in the use of devices, and what additional training is available? What environmental conditions in the home and workplace will affect the use of assistive devices (e.g., noise, light, and space)?

Functional specifications for devices. After the client and environment assessments are completed, the team—including the consumer—considers how an assistive device or a device modification can bridge existing gaps in function, (i.e., tasks that cannot be completed). For example, is the problem with task completion a problem in the person's input to the device, a problem in the device's output to the person, or both? Are the person's skills congruent with the task requirements? How does the device meet user access and control needs, seating and positioning requirements, and motor/perceptual limitations?

The appropriate use of adaptive technology often requires therapeutic interventions or consultations from specialists. For example, an employed person who suffers a hand injury might initially need an adaptive device for fine motor manipulation. Occupational therapy treatment modalities may improve residual hand function, allowing the person to use a less sophisticated (and less expensive) device. Further, the therapist can help configure work tasks to take full advantage of the person's abilities. The architectural and design specialist can provide a device design that is functional and aesthetically pleasing to the individual by considering both the configuration of equipment and the entire task environment. The rehabilitation engineer can lead the final design and production of the device, including calculating the necessary tolerances and fabricating the device from appropriate materials. The rehabilitation counselor directs the team effort to accomplish the gainful activity objectives of employment or education for the individual. The occupational therapist actually "delivers" the device to the person and provides training in its use. Remember, multidisciplinary teamwork is most effective when the person with the disability is directly involved in all stages of assessment, design, development, and placement.

The Team

Ten years ago it was generally recognized that the occupational therapist was the professional trained and experienced in assessing and "prescribing" assistive devices. With the increased power and complexity of devices available today, no one profession can—or should—claim assistive technology as its "territory." However, occupational therapy remains in a central role with assistive technology. In most cases, the occupational therapist can be the profes-

sional who takes responsibility for assembling the appropriate assistive technology team. The occupational therapist has the breadth of training and experience with assistive devices, the understanding of human capacity and disability, and the assessment and intervention expertise required to deliver assistive technology services. This book should help occupational therapists understand their role in delivering assistive technology services and, most important, their role in relation to other service providers. Figure 1.1 shows the relationship of the occupational therapist to the other potential team members.

In some cases the occupational therapist independently prescribes an assistive device. For example, the occupational therapist may prescribe "buttonless" clothes (i.e., Velcro® or no fasteners) or a button hook for a person with fine motor impairment who has difficulty with buttons. In other cases the occupational therapist works with other professionals, including the following:

- Architect—when there is a need for structural home modifications or building modifications in a client setting.
- Special educator—with preschool, primary, and secondary school students who have disabilities that affect learning.
- Physical therapist—when the person with a disability has a motor impairment that affects seating or mobility.
- Speech pathologist—with persons with communication disorders. For individuals with only a communication disorder, the occupational therapist may not participate in the assessment or intervention. However, many persons with communication impairments also have motor impairments that must be recognized and addressed with the occupational therapist's expertise.
- Social worker—when an individual requiring an assistive device needs assistance with funding options, or for an individual whose progress across "systems" (e.g., acute hospital to rehab facility to home to school) requires close coordination.
- Rehabilitation nurse—for individuals in health care facilities or home health care, with additional health care needs for assistive devices.
- Rehabilitation engineer—for persons with unique assistive device needs where there is no existing device or where an existing device must be modified.

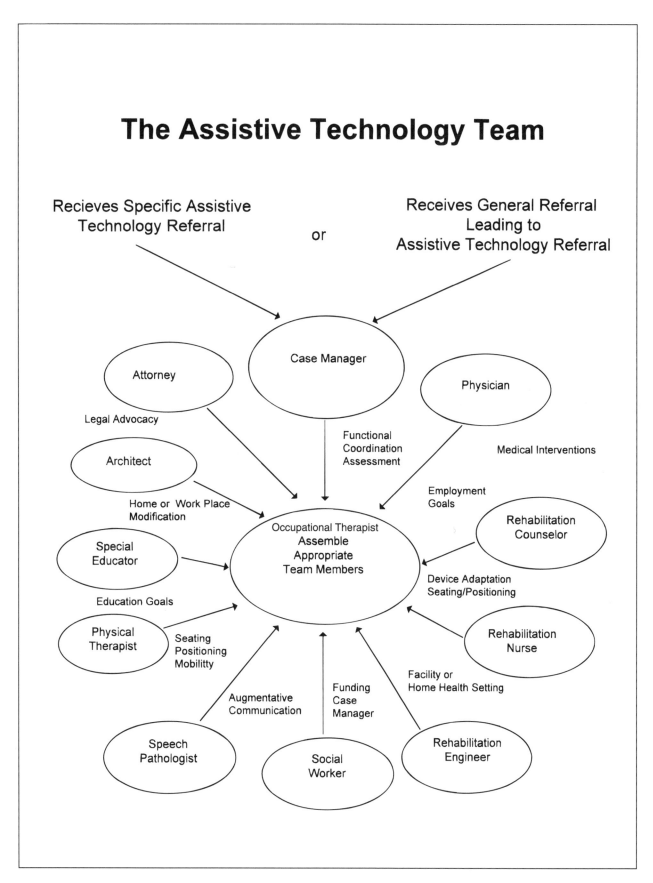

Figure 1.1. Interdisciplinary relationships in assistive technology services.

- Rehabilitation counselor—for persons requiring assistive devices or environmental adaptations who have an employment goal or who are already employed.
- Physician—for persons with medical needs that require oversight by a physician. Much assistive technology falls outside the medical model; in fact, devices can be purchased in neighborhood electronics stores. However, much assistive technology does require involvement of a physician to ensure its safe use.
- Attorney—for persons eligible for public funding of assistive devices who require legal advocacy to ensure the funding is made available.

The role of "coordinator" for the assistive technology team carries the responsibility of being knowledgeable in applying technology to the needs of persons with disabilities. This book provides a general overview of many applications. The practitioner needs additional training in a selected specialty area. Keeping up-to-date is critical to delivering state-of-the-art services. The last unit of this book offers advice on how to maintain one's skills.

In summarizing just what a practitioner should know, Smith (1991) lists four major areas:

1. A familiarity with existing assistive devices, including both low technology and high technology.
2. An understanding of the appropriate prescription of existing devices, and the use of specially fabricated or adapted devices.
3. An understanding of all aspects of the assistive technology service delivery process, including the required training with the device.
4. An understanding of when to recommend a device and when not to recommend a device. (p. 753)

The remainder of this book will address these questions. However, reading a book is not enough. Understanding the applications of assistive devices requires hands-on experience with the devices as well as experience with people using them.

Service Delivery Process

Delivering assistive technology devices and services to persons with disabilities has four general components:

1. the assistive technology marketplace,
2. the process of personal assessment and device selection,
3. the context of service delivery, and
4. information resources on assistive technology.

The assistive technology marketplace. The professional team needs an overall understanding of the range of assistive devices in the marketplace and their general areas of application to specific types of disabilities. Unit II: Assistive Technology Types reviews the different types of assistive technologies available for persons with physical, sensory, and cognitive/speech disabilities.

The context of service delivery. People of different ages and abilities use assistive devices in different contexts. Special considerations for the environments of pediatric, school-based, work-based, and geriatric and long-term-care populations are discussed in Unit III: Assistive Technology Applications.

The process of personal assessment and device selection. This is the process of determining the specific needs of the individual, identifying the capabilities of device options, and selecting the best combination within the environmental context. Unit IV: Assistive Technology Services describes the process of assessment, selection, implementation, and training, and provides information about funding and maintaining assistive devices.

Information resources on assistive technology. Given the pace of new innovations and the advancement of knowledge, professionals should consult available resources to confirm the basis for their decisions. Unit V: Assistive Technology Information describes the organizations, conferences, publications, and electronic resources active in the field of assistive devices for persons with disabilities.

Chapter 1 References

American Occupational Therapy Association Inc. (AOTA). (1994). *Policy manual of the American Occupational Therapy Association.* (Policy Number 5.3.1). Bethesda, MD: Author.

Brandenburg, S. (1987). *Overview: Evaluation/assessment defined in relation* to P.L. 94142 and P.L. 99–457. Madison, WI: Weisman Center.

Bureau of Labor Statistics. (1989). *Occupational outlook handbook,* 1989–90 Edition, Bulletin 2300. Washington, DC: U.S. Government Printing Office.

Enders, A., & Hall, M. (1990). *Assistive technology sourcebook.* Washington, DC: RESNA.

National Academy of Sciences, Institute of Medicine, Division of Health Care Services. (1988). *Allied health services: Avoiding crisis.* Washington, DC: National Academy Press.

National Institutes of Health. (1993). *Research plan for the National Center for Medical and Rehabilitation Research,* (NIH Publication No. 93.–3509). Washington, DC: U.S. Government Printing Office. Modified from work published in *Disability in America: Toward a national agenda for prevention,* 1991, Institute of Medicine, Washington, DC: National Academy Press.

Robinson, C.J. (1993). *The electrical engineering handbook,* Boca Raton, FL: CRC Press.

Smith, R. (1991). *Technological approaches to performance enhancement.* In C. Christiansen & C. Baum (Eds.), *Occupational therapy: Overcoming human performance deficits* (pp. 747–788). Thorofare, NJ: Slack.

Webster's New Twentieth Century Dictionary (Unabridged) (1977). Cleveland, OH: William Collins and World Publishing.

Chapter 1 Study Questions

1. What role do occupational therapists perform in providing assistive technology to persons with disabilities?

2. List the four categories of variables influencing the outcome of the human/technology interface, and identify one variable in each category.

3. Give two examples of how these variables in the human/technology interface interact to influence the outcome.

4. Describe five professions (besides occupational therapy) that are involved in assistive technology services.

5. How can these different professions work as a team to deliver assistive technology services? What are their respective and collective roles?

Unit II: Assistive Technology Types

Introduction to Unit II

Assistive devices are tools for persons with limitations in their functional abilities. Assistive devices are as varied in their design and purpose as are the types, severity, and mix of functional limitations. Equally varied are the interests and activities of persons with disabilities.

Unit II reviews assistive devices for different categories of functional needs. The devices shown represent entire groups of devices. Every device can be further modified or tailored to the individual. The categories are used as a convenience, and are not intended to categorize individuals or their needs. The content shows that even within categories, the devices vary in terms of their form and function.

Chapter 2 reviews devices for persons with physical disabilities. Physical disabilities are limitations in the use of arms, legs, hands, feet, and trunk. The devices assist in functional activities such as sitting, moving, reaching, carrying, lifting, transferring, and manipulating other objects in the environment. Most of the devices shown in this chapter perform a single, discrete function. Instrumental activities of daily living involve multiple, complex tasks. Thus, multiple devices might be used in combination to achieve the desired functional outcomes.

The section on computer access shows multiple alternatives, because accessing a computer is key to controlling and manipulating many other devices. The review of robotics indicates that future developments will combine multiple functions within a single device, or link multiple devices within a single environment.

Chapter 3 addresses devices for persons with sensory impairments. The senses of vision and hearing are critical to daily living. Assistive devices are available that address limitations in each. The other senses of touch, taste, and smell have not yet received much support from assistive devices. Vision and hearing permit a person to safely and effectively interact with the environment. Some devices help a person identify important signals such as pedestrian crosswalk light or ambulance sirens. Still other devices enable the user to send and receive information, such as personal correspondence, books and periodicals, and electronic media. Changes in mass market products, such as captioned television programs and decoders in every television, are gradually reducing the need for certain assistive devices.

Chapter 4 covers assistive technology for persons with speech and cognitive impairments. Augmentative communication devices provide the essential ability to interact with other people. Such devices enable the user to express thoughts to other people by generating speech. For people with cognitive impairments, devices help learn, retain, or use knowledge. Devices also assist care providers by monitoring a person's activity or location.

Unit II provides an overview of the devices and applications available. Chapter 12 describes resources for accessing much more information about assistive devices and about functional impairments and the resulting disabilities.

Chapter 2:
Assistive Technology for Persons With Physical Disabilities

I. Assistive Devices for Persons With Physical Disabilities
   A. Assistive Devices and Acceptance Issues

II. Assistive Devices for Upper-Extremity Gross Motor Deficits
   A. Environmental Control Devices
      1. Types of Environmental Control Devices
      2. Functions of Environmental Control Devices
      3. SmartHouse Technology
      4. Considerations for Rehabilitation Technologists
   B. Robotics
      1. Types of Robots
      2. Robotic Functions
         a. Daily Living Functions
         b. Education and Vocation Functions
         c. Robotic Applications in Development
         d. Considerations for Rehabilitation Technologists
   C. Physical Extension Devices
      1. Mouthsticks
      2. Headpointer Devices
      3. Considerations for Rehabilitation Technologists

III. Assistive Devices for Fine Motor Deficits
   A. Switches and Controls
   B. Computer Access
      1. The Mouse and Other Pointing Devices
      2. Keyboards
      3. Alternate Input Methods
      4. Assistive Software
      5. Integrated Systems
      6. Considerations for Rehabilitation Technologists
   C. Assessment for Adapted Computer Access

IV. Assistive Devices for Lower-Extremity Motor Deficits
    A. Wheelchairs
        1. Manual Wheelchairs
        2. Powered Wheelchairs
        3. Other Wheelchairs
        4. Considerations for Rehabilitation Technologists
    B. Seating and Positioning Devices
        1. Cushions
        2. Pelvic, Trunk, and Head Positioners
            a. Pelvis
            b. Trunk
            c. Head
        3. Custom vs. Modular Systems
    C. Functional Electrical Stimulation
        1. Considerations for Rehabilitation Technologists

V. Assistive Devices for Daily Living

2.

Assistive Technology for Persons With Physical Disabilities

Stephen Sprigle, PhD, and Joseph P. Lane, MBPA

Physical disabilities include paralysis, weakness, contractures, amputations, tremors, spasticity, and other limitations to coordinated musculoskeletal movement. Physical disabilities result from development, disease, or injury. Examples of disabilities due to development are incomplete growth or articulation of limbs, back or spine curvature, and incomplete neurologic networks. Diseases that damage muscles, bones, or neural pathways, such as motor neuron degeneration, rheumatoid arthritis, and osteomyelitis/bone disorders, may result in physical disabilities (LaPlante, 1988). Injuries may result from vehicular accidents, falls and diving, gunshot wounds, and burns. Injuries account for the majority of preventable disabilities in the population. Over half (52.1%) of the 14.8 million impairments caused by injuries result in limitations on physical activity. Over two thirds of the impairments caused by injuries are physical deformities or orthopedic impairments (Kraus & Stoddard, 1989).

Physical disabilities present dynamic, rather than static, conditions. The effects of some physical disabilities become more debilitating over time, while there is stasis or even improvement over time with others. As an example of the former, amyotrophic lateral sclerosis is a progressively degenerative motor neuron disease marked by increasing muscular weakness, spasticity, and hyperreflexia. The effects of other physical disabilities, particularly those caused by injury, can be mitigated through the body's regenerative processes and the interventions of rehabilitation professionals. Therapists train persons to restore impaired functions or to replace them with compensatory strategies.

For this chapter, we group disabilities into three major categories of function/dysfunction:

1. Upper-Extremity Gross Motor: Deficits in the large muscles of the back, shoulders, and arms; bone deterioration; or deficits in the nervous system that impair the arm functions of strength, coordination, or joint range of motion. Technologies for upper-extremity gross motor deficits encompass environmental control systems and robotics.

2. Upper-Extremity Fine Motor: Deficits in the small muscles, bones, and nerves of the wrist, hand, and fingers that impair the functions of precise movement and grasp. Technologies for fine motor deficits include switches, controls, and keyboards.

3. Lower-Extremity Motor: Deficits in the large muscles, bones, and nerves of the lower trunk, legs, and feet that impair the leg functions of strength, coordination, balance, or joint range of motion. Technologies for lower-extremity motor deficits span balance aids, wheelchairs, seating systems, and functional electrical stimulation.

These three major categories are not mutually exclusive. Persons with a lower-extremity disability use robotics and environmental controls, and persons with upper-body gross motor impairments use switches, controls, and adapted keyboards. Persons with physical disabilities often have deficits in more than one major category of function, so they may need more than one device or devices from more than one category.

Assistive Devices for Persons With Physical Disabilities

A national household survey conducted in 1969 determined that 6.2 million persons with physical disabilities in the United States required the use of 7.2 million assistive devices to maximize independence in self-care, work, and leisure activities (National Health Survey, 1969). A similar survey in 1977 found that 6.5 million people with physical disabilities required 8 million assistive devices (National Health Interview Statistics, 1977). The assistive devices included canes and walking sticks, special shoes, braces, walkers, wheelchairs, crutches, and prostheses.

We know that persons with physical disabilities have used assistive devices based on low technology for centuries. Wooden crutches, peg legs, and metal hand hooks became stereotypes for adventurous buccaneers who acquired physical impairments on the high seas and in the low ports. Device developments continued as new technologies emerged. In 1268 Roger Bacon described framed optical lenses for reading; Benjamin Franklin invented bifocal glasses in 1784; Thomas Edison's phonograph was used to create talking books for people who were blind in the 1870s (Crewe & Zola, 1983). As we move toward the 21st century, science and industry offer an array of high-technology devices that have immense potential for assisting persons with physical disabilities.

Assistive Devices and Acceptance Issues

There is a growing body of literature on applications of technology for individuals with disabilities. Much of the literature relates to low-technology assistive devices that have been available for many years. Issues of acceptance or use of assistive devices have also been studied with varied results. Results show low use of devices after only a few months: 50% nonuse in one study (Bray & Wright, 1980), 79% nonuse in another (Kaplan, 1966).

A recent survey of technology use found that 29% of devices had been abandoned (Phillips & Zhano, 1993). The authors identified four factors related to abandonment—lack of consideration of user opinion by the provider, easy device procurement, poor device performance, and change in user needs or priorities. Changes in training and funding policy were identified as ways to reduce abandonment. Devices have the highest abandonment rate during their first year of use, so equipment rental might be a better alternative to purchase. The importance of adequate training has also been well documented (LaRocca & Tirem, 1978). Training of both users of assistive technology and the professionals prescribing it would lead to better purchasing decisions.

Assistive Devices for Upper-Extremity Gross Motor Deficits

Environmental Control Devices

Applications of electronic technology provide persons with disabilities with the potential for increased control over their environments. Devices with the capacity to regulate aspects of a person's physical surroundings are called *environmental control devices*. Environmental control devices were first designed in the early 1960s for use by persons with high-level quadriplegia and poliomyelitis (Symington, Lywood, Lawson, & MacLean, 1986).

Today, many mainstream consumer environmental control devices are available. From the infamous Clapper to programmable remote controls, products are available to simplify our lives. However, not all of these products are appropriate for persons with upper-extremity deficits. Some have small control buttons, or are too bulky. Many devices are just too complex—they have too many buttons or excessively complex operations for ready programming or use.

Types of Environmental Control Devices

Environmental control systems have five parts (Haataja & Saarnio, 1990):

1. Switch Device—The input mechanism that enables the user to activate the environmental control system. Switches come in a variety of forms described later in this chapter.
2. Control Device—The mechanism that allows the operator to transmit instructions to perform a function. The ubiquitous remote control unit for the television is a limited-function environmental control device. More elaborate control devices—based on a microprocessor—operate numerous functions. Control devices rely on infrared light, sound waves, mechanical connections, or even voice commands.
3. Target Device—The appliance (television, microwave), furnishing (lamp, bed), or equipment (door locks, garage door) that functions in response to commands from the control

device. One control device may operate several target devices, as in a stereo component system. In an environmental control system, the multiple target devices may serve very different functions.

4. Connections—The electrical and mechanical components that connect the control and target devices, such as the wiring and sensor on a lamp or the mechanical arm on a garage door opener.

5. Feedback Device—A signal communicating to the user the status of actions taken. Feedback signals may be visual, auditory, or tactile.

Feedback is critical to the appropriate operation of environmental control systems, since it tells the user when to activate, alter, or deactivate the control system through the switch (Symington, Batelaan, O'Shea, & White, 1980).

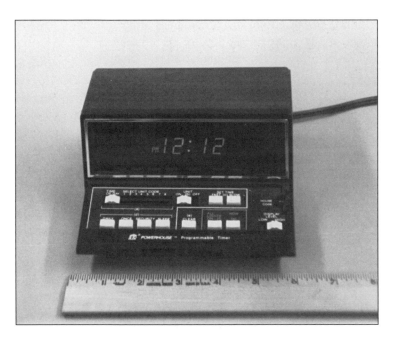

Figure 2.1. An example of a basic ECU is this programmable timer, which controls lights and appliances.

Figure 2.1 shows a basic environmental control unit (ECU), a programmable timer to control electrical appliances in the home.

Functions of Environmental Control Devices

A relatively early study of environmental control devices compared the features and utility of various units. The study conducted a 3-year evaluation of environmental control units for persons with high-level quadriplegia. It addressed device use in the laboratory, clinical bedside, and home, and it assessed reliability, suitability, and acceptance. The results demonstrated the feasibility of independent functioning with the assistance of environmental control devices (Sell-Heimer, Stratford, Zimmerman, Youdin, & Milner, 1979).

Another early study examined the impact of environmental control units on daily living (e.g., activity patterns, adjustment, and locus of control) of high-level spinal cord–injured patients. The authors found that the environmental control devices had the greatest impact on the area of activity patterns: "The users participated in more activities and spent considerably more time educating themselves than the nonusers" (Efthimiou, Gordon, Sell, & Stratford, 1981).

Another study of environmental control devices examined cost savings. Using a sample of 15 persons with severe physical disabilities living in institu-

tions, and providing them with a device that could perform five functions, the authors found that patients used the device an average of 10 times per day. It was estimated that this level of use saved 2 hours of nursing care per day. The cost of the equipment was estimated to be $1.35 per day. Thus, just from a cost-benefit analysis, environmental control units were found to be effective in this setting (Symington et al., 1986).

Many recent studies of environmental control units for persons with disabilities concentrate on the elderly. The elderly are a large and growing population with a high incidence of physical disabilities—many of which worsen over time. The incidence of acute illness decreases with age, while the probability of the development of a chronic condition increases (Maguire, 1985; Rice & Feldman, 1983). These chronic conditions experienced by the elderly often limit daily functioning, but environmental control units offer the potential for greater independence.

According to the U.S. Senate Special Committee on Aging (1982), more than 80% of the population over age 65 has at least one chronic physical impairment, the most frequent being arthritis. Arthritis or osteoarthritis of the hands may cause pain and limitations of function in one or more activities of daily living, especially those activities requiring fine movements of the hand such as management of switches or controls.

In a 2-year study of one environmental control system, the Possum PSU3, 60% of the 48 elderly subjects were using the equipment after 9 months (Bell, Whitfield, & Rollet, 1987). Examining the 40% of elderly subjects not using the equipment revealed the following: 7 persons (15%) still had the devices but were not using them; 7 subjects (15%) had asked to have the equipment removed; 5 subjects (10%) had died. Future studies must address the issue of abandonment for devices in general. The answers will lead to better device designs, more constructive prescription and use, and better follow-up.

A recent study considered the use of hand-held environmental control devices by patients in nursing homes. In this experimental study, it was found that persons who had environmental control devices used their radios and lights significantly more than the control group, who had to rely on staff or their own operation of traditional on/off switches to work their lights and radio (Mann, 1989). In a typical nursing home environment there is minimal positive environmental stimulation, and patients have little control over decisions and objects. This study demonstrated the value of an inexpensive intervention.

Commercial environmental control units range from single-device to whole-home configurations. Some are designed for the assistive technology market while others have appeared, in part, because of the advancements in computers or the miniaturization of electronics. Table 2.1 lists a sample of environmental control units representing more than 110 models available in the marketplace (CO-NET, 1993). The capabilities of units vary widely, with some requiring connection to a personal computer while others use plug-in modules.

The most commonly available environmental control technology has been developed by X-10 USA. X-10 technology allows a person to control lights and appliances from push-button consoles, programmable timers, remote controls, and personal computers. X-10 systems consist of a combination of transmitters and receiver modules. Lights or appliances are plugged into an existing outlet. Control signals are sent from the transmitter to the module through existing power lines in the home; therefore, no additional special wiring is needed.

Its simplicity and wide availability make X-10 the most common ECU. It is compatible with Radio Shack's ECUs, among others. However, as electronic development progresses, other standards may emerge.

SmartHouse Technology

The most comprehensive and complex scenario for environmental control systems is termed the SmartHouse (SmartHouse L.P., 1988). The SmartHouse is envisioned as a means of integrating all electrical, gas, water, heating and cooling, security, appliance, and media components into a single system. All the home's functions will be connected to a control unit in charge of distributing energy to and controlling all devices (appliances and media). The control unit represents the capability to use and monitor every household function from a single location. The SmartHouse project combines the research and development efforts of 40 major companies under the guidance of the National Association of Home Builders. This collaborative approach should deliver standards that ensure compatibility of all new household products. The implication for persons with physical disabilities is that the system's single control unit can be adapted for alternate access, increasing an individual's opportunities for independent living (Lesnoff-Caravaglia, 1988).

Considerations for Rehabilitation Technologists

A descriptive article (Dickey & Shealy, 1987) presents questions to consider with selection of an environmental control device:

- How difficult will the system be to operate?
- Does the product have a reputation for reliability and durability?
- Is it easy to install?
- Is it portable?
- Is the manufacturer likely to be around in 5 years to support or repair the system?
- What sources of feedback are available (e.g., auditory, visual)?
- What are the training requirements necessary to operate the system successfully?

Haataja and Saarnio (1990) add four more considerations for selecting a suitable environmental control device:

1. The user's level of impairment and residual functions.
2. The user's motivation for acquiring and using a device.
3. The specific appliances and utilities the user needs to control.
4. The environment in which the control will operate.

Each of these areas must be considered by the

Table 2.1. Environmental Control Units.

Name	Description	Manufacturer	Cost
Environmental Control	Computer interface providing up to 128 selective switch closures.	David Favin Little Solver, NJ	Free
X-10 Receiving Modules	Various models, control lamps, lights, stereos, fans, etc.	Radio Shack, Fort Worth, TX Home Automation Labs, Roswell, GA	$12.95–$15.95
X-10 Mini Console	Controls up to 8 light and appliance modules.	Radio Shack, Fort Worth, TX Home Automation Labs, Roswell, GA	$10.95
Timer Console	Timer can be programmed to control 8 modules—also permits manual control.	Radio Shack, Fort Worth, TX Home Automation Labs, Roswell, GA	$29.95
Wireless Controller and Base Transmitter	The remote control signals a base unit to control 8 light and appliance modules.	Radio Shack, Fort Worth, TX Home Automation Labs, Roswell, GA	$39.95
Power Minder	110 VAC power cord with automatic power interrupt via built-in timer switch.	TASH, Inc. Markham, Ontario	$100
Stove Minder	Interval timer with alarm and automatic power shut-off for electric ranges.	TASH, Inc. Ajax, Ontario	$125
Ultra 4 Remote System	Remote control of four remote appliance modules.	TASH, Inc. Ajax, Ontario	contact manufacturer
Training Aid 2	Two switches operate two appliances with internal timer controller.	Prentke Romich Co. Wooster, OH	$595
SMARTHOME 1	Sixteen radio and 16 power-line sensors for appliances and alarm system.	CyberLYNX Computer Products Boulder, CO	$600
KINCONTROL	Three to 10 outputs operated by single or dual switch scanning mode.	TASH, Inc. Markham, Ontario	$650–$800
EZRA	Single switch system selects commands from menus displayed on TV screen.	Long Beach, CA	$950–$1,775
DEUCE	Controls telephone and appliances through scanning or direct input.	DU-IT Control Systems Group Shreve, OH	$1,350–$1,800
CONTROL 1	Controls eight receptacles in base unit up to 256 receptacles through modules.	Prentke Romich Co. Wooster, OH	$1,700–$3,465

(Continued)

Table 2.1. Environmental Control Units (continued).

Name	Description	Manufacturer	Cost
MICRODEC II	Remote appliance control operated by two-switch scanning.	Medical Equipment Distributor Lubbock, TX	$1,886
HECS-1	Select electric functions from back-lit menu using a variety of switch options.	Prentke Romich Co. Wooster, OH	$2,900–$3,500
Butler-in-a-Box	Voice-activated with speech output for hands-free operation of appliances.	Mastervoice Los Alamitos, Ca	$2,995
Simplicity Series 5	Voice-input appliance control system.	Quartet Technology Tyngsboro, MA	$3,750
VOCAL 1	Voice-input system for controlling most electrical appliances and systems.	Power Translation Co.	$4,495
SenSei	Full-range computer-based control of home environment, telecommunications, and computer functions (Mac Classic 2).	Safko International, Inc.	$9,500

therapist when helping a person select an environmental control device.

Environmental control systems can operate specific appliances, primarily to turn them on or off, or manipulate controls like channel selectors or volume on home electronics. Persons with physical disabilities may have needs that cannot be met with an environmental control unit; for example, mechanical functions such as lifting, moving, and manipulating objects. Robotic devices serve these functions with increasing frequency.

Robotics

Robotic personal assistance devices are still in the early stages of development. The patchwork of various components in systems, the laboratory prototype testing, the great expense of many components, the large size of existing systems, and the limited functions they perform are all hallmarks of a technology in its infancy. However, single purpose robotic systems have been used by rehabilitation technologists for many years. Automated page turners and feeding devices are simple systems that illustrate the role of robotics in rehabilitation. Robots have the potential to reduce dependence on health care attendants, perform menial or labor-intensive chores, provide continuous monitoring of vital functions, and control environmental conditions. All of these areas offer benefits (e.g., reduced cost of human services, increased independence for the person), and new

problems (e.g., cost of robotics, maintenance and repair, reduced human interaction). Rehabilitation technologists are interested in the promise of robotics but cautious about the problems (Glass & Hall, 1987).

Types of Robots

The automation of industrial facilities precipitated the concept of using robotics as assistive devices. If robotic devices could substitute for human labor in the workplace, then other devices could augment or replace human functions for persons with physical disabilities. While much of the technology (hardware and software) is readily transferable, industrial robots perform automated and repetitive tasks and are often isolated from people. The special needs of persons with disabilities are less defined and controlled, and multipurpose robotics require high levels of safety, reliability, and accuracy. Still in its infancy as an area of investigation, the development of personal assistance robots includes research on needs assessment, perception, training, monitoring, and safety (Engelhardt, 1989). Personal assistance robots will basically integrate systems of electronic and mechanical components.

Current robotic systems can be roughly grouped according to function (vocational, personal) and mobility (independently mobile, desk or table mounted, wheelchair mounted). Each has benefits and drawbacks with respect to capabilities, complexity, and expense. All robotic systems generally have four components.

1. *Manipulator*—The robot's "arm," with a designed range of motion. Many personal assistance robots use modified versions of industrial manipulators, such as the Unimation PUMA-260, Rhino Robotics Rhino XR-3, and Universal Machine Intelligence Limited's RTX robotic arm. The Rhino XR-3 robotic arm, shown in Figure 2.2, is being used in experimental automated workstations.

   Simpler, easier tasks use smaller versions of robotic arms. The mechanism holding a book on an automated page turning device is a miniature robotic arm, as shown in Figure 2.3.

2. *Gripper*—The robot's "hand," capable of grasping objects of various sizes, weights, and materials. Grippers may be configured as pincers, implements, or even prosthetic hands, depending on the tasks required and aesthetics desired. Early models were preprogrammed to grasp only specific objects set in exact locations of the workspace. Newer versions of robotic grippers have multiple sensors or permit the user to relay information to enable handling of different objects (Amanat, Riviere, & Thakor, 1994; Seaman & Napper, 1988).

3. *Control*—The robot's "brain" that translates the user's commands into the robot's actions. Robot controls run the full range of direct and adaptive control devices such as head motion, eye movement, joystick, keyboard, sip-and-puff, and voice recognition (Cannon, 1990; Cheatham, Mulner, & Verberg, 1994; Dallaway, Mahoney, & Jackson, 1993; Regalbuto, Krouskop, & Cheatham, 1992).

   Many robotic systems are programmed to perform repetitive tasks in structured environments, such as moving a drinking cup from a resting point to a position in space where it tilts for drinking. The cup and the person must be in the preprogrammed space for the system to work. An increase in a robot's capabilities increases the complexity of control. The

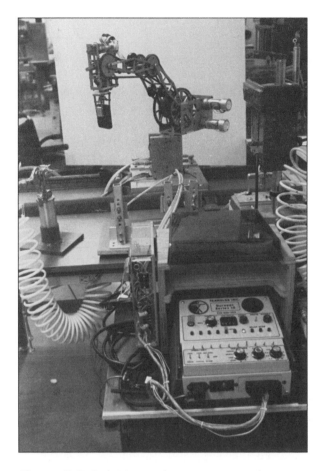

Figure 2.2. Robotic arm in prototype workstation. Photo courtesy of Scott Segner, Adelante Techworks, Albuquerque, NM.

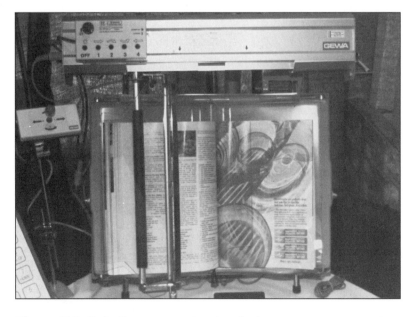

Figure 2.3. Robotic arm page-turning device.

user must be able to instruct the robot to perform unprogrammed tasks. The interface between the user and the robot is very important for complex control. In the past, users had to be well versed in computer languages and programming, but today's systems operate similarly to the menu-driven environments of Windows-based or Macintosh computers. Using the example from above, more advanced control would allow a person to receive a drink at the kitchen table, in a living room chair, or even in bed.

4. *Transport*—Rehabilitation robots are either stationary or mobile, depending on the functions performed. A stationary arm is mounted on a desktop or rail. A mobile robotic arm is mounted on a rail or on a wheeled base. Of course, a stationary robotic arm becomes mobile if it is mounted on a wheelchair. A wheelchair-mounted arm could enable a person with quadriplegia to shop in a grocery store unassisted because the arm could reach products. Or the arm could reach products and appliance controls in the home without requiring extensive adaptations to shelf heights and control panels. Independently mobile robots are typically the most complex because they must adapt to ever-changing environments. Vocational robots have been desk mounted and programmed to perform paper and book handling tasks within a workstation.

Robotic Functions

Studies have demonstrated the utility of robotic arm/workstations for persons with various physical disabilities including spinal cord injuries (Seamone & Schmeisser, 1985), multiple sclerosis (Hillman, 1987), and muscular dystrophy (Bach, Zeelenberg, & Winter, 1990). Robotic systems have numerous applications for persons with physical disabilities. In an excellent overview of the application of robotic devices to human service areas, Engelhardt (1989) divided tasks that robots could address into nine descriptive categories:

1. Transport–lift–transfer
2. Ambulation assistance
3. Daily living tasks
4. Housecleaning
5. Therapy delivery and therapist training
6. Personal surveillance and monitoring
7. Vital signs monitoring
8. Mental stimulation and cognitive rehabilitation
9. Other tasks

Daily Living Functions. Expanding the range of tasks performed by different robotic systems and increasing each robotic system's ability to perform multiple tasks enhance opportunities for personal independence. However robotic systems with multiple functions are expensive and complex, which has limited their use as assistive devices.

Robotic devices are already suitable for performing activities of daily living that are preprogrammable, because they involve a limited range of movements, are repetitive, and always occur in the same location. Robotic feeding devices have been available for several years. The system consists of a plate and an attached arm. A spoon is attached to the arm, which scoops food from the plate and positions it near the user's mouth. While simplistic, this device illustrates the utility of devices in other programmable activities such as washing the face, shaving, and drinking.

Bach et al. (1990) studied commercially available industrial robot manipulators with modified control panels to increase independence in daily living for persons with Duchenne muscular dystrophy. These persons, some with only residual finger movement and others with ventilator dependence, mastered the robotic tool and used it full time. The device reportedly saved about 3 hours of attendant care per patient per day.

Education and Vocation Functions. A 4-year project to design and implement a robotic-based assistive system for use in educational environments has summarized the critical hardware and software design issues. Although these issues were prepared as guidelines for robotics developers, they are equally appropriate for therapists involved in comparative evaluations of the utility of different robotic systems. For example, the robot's hardware must be adaptable and versatile, have reliable mechanical and electrical components, balance utility with safety, and consider aesthetics and cost-effectiveness for user acceptance. The robot's software must be easily understood while maintaining useful interaction speed; control features must be clear, accessible, and complete; and the defined robotic motions must accomplish the intended education tasks (Howell & Hay, 1989). The last issue is crucial. Regardless of how technically impressive the robotic device may appear, its ability to perform specific tasks for a certain client is its most important feature.

Several programs have incorporated robotic systems into classroom and educational settings. In Michigan, four mechanical systems were integrated into special education programs (Phelps &

Erlandson, 1994). These devices were simple robotic systems: a switch-activated packaging dispenser, an assembly trainer, a soap dispenser, and a turntable. Students with cognitive impairments demonstrated decreased reliance on staff and increased self-esteem after the systems were installed. Additionally, a commercially available robot has been used to increase the educational opportunities of children with severe physical disabilities (Beitler, Strange, & Howell, 1994). The UMI RTX robot was used to allow children to participate in finger painting. The ultimate goal is to integrate the robot into the curriculum. For example, a robot could be used to permit students with disabilities to perform their own experiments in science class.

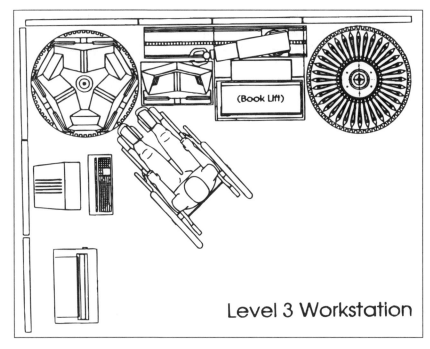

Figure 2.4. AbleOffice Level 3 Workstation. Developed at the Center for Rehabilitation Technology, College of Architecture, Georgia Institute of Technology, Atlanta, GA. Reprinted with permission.

Robotic devices are demonstrably adequate substitutes for human assistants in work settings. Although the robot may require longer elapsed time to perform a task, the robot is immediately available to the user. Some projects integrate the robotic system within a wholly redesigned workstation.

The AbleOffice is a modular office workstation system consisting of 14 interchangeable components allowing custom configuration. It was developed at the Center for Rehabilitation Technology, College of Architecture, Georgia Institute of Technology. The 14 components include a computer station, reference and file carousels, book lifts, and a robotic arm on a track. The AbleOffice system provides three levels of automation. Level 1 consists of manually powered components; Level 2 has powered components controlled by momentary switches or a computer; and Level 3 involves computer-controlled automated components with integrated robotic assistance. Figure 2.4 shows one possible configuration of components in a Level 3 automated workstation.

Two robot systems aimed at increasing vocational capabilities have also been developed and tested. The RAID workstation performs paper and book handling. A recent evaluation resulted in positive feedback but improvements in control and flexibility are needed to perform different (unprogrammed) tasks (Danielsson & Holmberg, 1994). Another vocational robot, the DeVar Manipulator, was found to reduce attendant time needed for the subject to perform his job (Hammel, Van der Loos, & Perkash, 1992). It combines book and paper handling with environmental control functions. The DeVar Manipulator costs between $50,000 and $100,000, but the study's authors argue that this cost could be recouped within 6 years if it reduces attendant time. The authors also state that the vocational robots are best suited for jobs that involve a majority of cognitive work.

Robotic Applications in Development. Many rehabilitation robotics programs are active in North America and Europe, each pursuing a unique approach to robotics development for specific applications in basic research or clinical settings. New applications for robotics often prompt modifications to existing products. For example, a commercially available industrial robotic arm was redesigned for use in a robotic workstation after pilot testing revealed performance limitations for the intended applications (Hillman, Pullin, Gammie, Stammers, & Orpwood, 1990).

The design of wheelchair-mounted arms has been advanced by the development of small manipulators. Evaluations of two wheelchair-mounted arms (ART and Mannus) identified some design and functional attributes necessary before those systems become practical (Moynahan, Stranger, Harwin, & Foulds, 1994). Issues such as adding weight and width to the wheelchair, arm and hand strength, control interface, and safety must be addressed before the systems become viable. However, subjects in both evaluations gave positive feedback and encouraged further development.

Independently mobile robots offer many potential uses, but are the most complex and expensive. Most are still in the development stage. A robot developed at Baylor and Rice is a modified HERO 2000, a commercially available educational tool (Regalbuto et al., 1992). The control system combines robot control with environmental and wheelchair control functions to increase its utility.

Another mobile robot, the MoVar, was designed to turn and move in any direction, track the location and state of motion of its own mobility platform and its manipulator, and avoid collisions with objects in the environment (Van der Loos, Michalowski, & Leifer, 1988). The prototype MoVar is shown in Figure 2.5.

Robotic devices are fairly new to the marketplace. Many are still in development or prototype stages, or they are built to order. A sample of robotic devices is provided in Table 2.2.

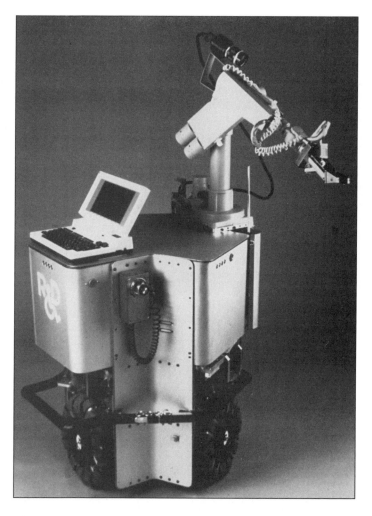

Figure 2.5. MoVar mobile robotic assistant. Photo courtesy of H.F. Machiel Van der Loos, Rehabilitation Research and Development Center, Veterans Administration Medical Center, Palo Alto, CA. Reprinted with permission.

Considerations for Rehabilitation Technologists. The successful use of robotic devices as assistive devices requires a careful match between the person and the device. Clinical testing of one robotic appliance showed users want full control over all capabilities of the robot. Providing users with broad control enhances acceptance of the device but requires more sophisticated software programming, backup operating systems, and fail-safe safety mechanisms (Cameron et al., 1990). This added complexity is needed to monitor user commands and device actions in order to avoid accidents, damage to the device, or injury to the person. Another study, which explored the willingness of children with disabilities to use a robotic arm as a tool, found that all children in the study with a cognitive age of 7 to 9 months or greater used the robotic arm, were not fearful of the arm, and were able to use a joystick

switch to control the arm's movement (Cook, Liu, & Hoseit, 1990).

One team of rehabilitation technologists has developed screening criteria for potential users of a voice-controlled robotic workstation (Bush & Peterson, 1989). Another team of rehabilitation technologists and rehabilitation engineers has developed assessment criteria for vocational workstations (Hammel & Van der Loos, 1990). These sets of criteria are grouped and summarized as:

1. User criteria: Voice level and stability for voice recognition; muscle control and positioning for system access; sensory and cognitive abilities for successful operation; stamina for length of use; psychosocial states (i.e. motivation); interpersonal and job skills necessary for employment.

Table 2.2. Robotic Devices.

Name	Description	Manufacturer	Cost
Automatic Page Turner	Book stand (horizontal or vertical) with mechanical arm moved by single switch.	Lakeland Products Burnsville, MN	$525
Automaddak Page Turner	H73200 reading stand has motorized arm, page clips, and various switches.	Maddak, Inc. Pequannock, NJ	$990
GEWA Page Turner	Automatic system accommodates most books, turns pages in either direction, has self-adjusting rubber roller, tilts in space.	GEWA Rehabteknik Zygo Industries, Inc. Portland, OR	$3,995–$4,200
Robotic Workstation Attendant	Robotic arm with "hand" options handles files/pages.	Regenesis Development Corp. N. Vancouver, BC	Contact manufacturer
Voice Command 1	Voice-activated workstation with an IBM PS/2 Model 30 computer, voice capability, robotic arm, and office equipment.	PRAB Command, Inc. Kalamazoo, MI	$34,995
AbleOffice	Modular workstation with controller and robotics arm for full automation needs.	CRT, Inc., Georgia Tech, Atlanta, GA	Contact manufacturer

2. Robotic workstation criteria: System accessibility from user's physical position; availability of alternate control devices; required equipment and appliances; safety parameters such as robotic features and user proximity; broad system capabilities; and aesthetics.

3. Environmental criteria: Space requirements to accommodate the user/wheelchair while permitting intended maneuverability for the robot; ambient factors such as light, temperature, and noise; availability of work materials; access to other work-related equipment such as telephone or computer; emergency aid plan; and the involvement of coworkers for peer acceptance.

Considering all the design, implementation, and training involved in such a complex technology, how useful is robotics? One group is developing protocols for client evaluation and productivity assessment, to quantify the level of function restored through the use of robotics. The evaluation instrument is incorporating measures for learning time, control accuracy, task difficulty, task repeatability, and the value of accrued experience for the user. Longitudinal studies using this instrument will establish baseline measures for comparing robotic systems (Horowitz, Webster, Hausdorff, Gordon, & Quintin, 1989). As with other assistive devices such as wheelchairs and seating cushions, quantifying evaluation criteria and performance outcomes will greatly help rehabilitation technologists make recommendations for robotic systems.

Physical Extension Devices

Persons with upper-body gross motor disabilities, including quadriplegia, poliomyelitis, spinal cord injuries, degenerative diseases, and cerebral palsy, may benefit from a device or implement that extends the body's reach. These persons may have substantial motor control only over their neck and head. Useful physical extension includes mouthsticks and headpointers.

Mouthsticks

The typical mouthstick device, shown in Figure 2.6, has two sections:

1. Extraoral section: The portion of the mouthstick extending outside the user's mouth. This section has three parts: (a) the *tip* of the mouthstick may press against, grasp, or pull against the object to be manipulated; (b) the *shaft* is the extending portion of the mouthstick, which may be fixed, telescoping, or folding; and (c) the *holder* attaches the mouthstick's shaft to the intraoral section (see Table 2.3).

2. Intraoral section: The mouthpiece portion of

Table 2.3. Extraoral Components for Mouthsticks.

Function	Mechanism	Method of Activation
Telescoping action	Extending wand	Tongue activates external battery power to extend shaft.
Telescoping action	Interlocking (docking) action	Pressure exerted through the mouthpiece and shaft with a friction grip snap locks shaft to tip portion.
Telescoping action	Ball-and-socket action	Protrusive-retrusive (anterior-posterior) jaw motion activates ball and socket, which extends shaft portion.
Prehensile function	Pincer	Bite closes pincer arms. Tongue protrusion closes pincer arms. Protrusive-retrusive jaw motion activates ball and socket.
Prehensile function	Suction	Slipping action creates vacuum to hold lightweight objects.

the mouthstick, which users grasp and hold with their teeth to manipulate the extraoral section. The mouthpiece section varies in design, size, material, and location within the mouth. The mouthpiece section is of particular concern to dentists as well as therapists because it is in direct contact with the user's teeth, tongue, and jaw muscles.

Early versions of mouthsticks lacked adequate design and fabrication. People stopped using them because of problems with dental malformation, tooth pain, and jaw muscle fatigue. Better mouthpiece design, stan-dard fabrication methods, and more appropriate materials reduced discomfort and thereby increased the utility of mouthsticks (Mulligan, 1983). Improvements in mouthpiece designs and materials continue. The dental profession and the rehabilitation field are applying new knowledge to the development of better mouthpieces (Hock, 1989), and pioneering the application of new materials for mouthpieces. For example, inexpensive thermoplastics or self-curing acrylics are useful materials because they are malleable and readily customize to fit the user (Budning & Hall, 1990).

Smith's (1989) thorough literature review of mouthstick design issues addresses current dental theories, potential problems with use, and dental standards for mouthpieces and mouthstick fabrication. It also organizes the extraoral components of mouthsticks, showing the sophisticated operation of these "sticks."

Commercially available mouthsticks come in a variety of shapes and materials to serve different functions. Table 2.4 shows the range of mouthsticks available (CO-NET, 1993).

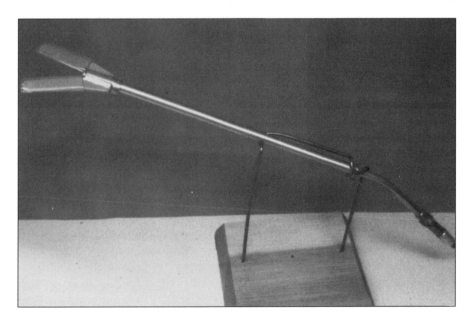

Figure 2.6. Mouthstick.

Table 2.4. Mouthsticks.

Name	Description	Manufacturer	Cost
H73217 Mouth Held Page Turners	Heart-shaped, flat, rubber-coated mouth-pieces, equipped with rubber tips to grip pages.	Maddak, Inc. Peuannock, NJ	$13.50–$15.90
Mouth Held Page Turner 88-1066	Heart-shaped, flat rubber mouthpiece, with serrated rubber tip for paper contact.	Cleo, Inc. Cleveland, OH	$13.89
Vaccum Wand	Suction mouthstick, aluminum shaft and plastic mouthpiece with two inter-changeable ends.	Woodrow Wilson Rehab Center Fisherville, VA	$20
Vacuum Wand BK6002	Mouthpiece with suction cup tips (two interchangeable), with aluminum shaft.	Fred Sammons, Inc. Brookfield, IL	$25.95–$29.95
Mouthstick, Page Turner Mouthstick, or Typing wand AD-8008	L-channel aluminum with Y-shaped pro-tective coated bite.	Adlib, Inc. Huntington Beach, CA	$28.95
Pincer Mouthstick AD-212	Tongue-activated plunger between Y-shaped bite plate opens and closes padded pincer at end.	Adlib, Inc. Huntington Beach, CA	$50
Mouthsticks	Wand, clamp-on, or vertical pincer mouthsticks with V-shaped mouthpiece for tongue movement.	Fred Sammons, Inc. Brookfield, IL	$25.95–$64.95
Arrow Mouthstick BK6004	Includes all materials except mouthpiece for making mouth sticks (shafts, tips, clamps).	Fred Sammons, Inc. Brookfield, IL	$89.50
Heyer-Abadie Modular Mouthstick	V-shaped mouthpiece gripped by molars, made to individual's bite pat-tern. Shafts of several lengths provided, with various optional tips available.	Extensions for Independence, San Diego, CA	$89–$415
Cloran Oral Telescoping Orthosis	Variable speed, battery-powered telescoping mouthstick with custom fitted mouth piece, six tips, accessory table, and mounting clamps.	Arthur J. Cloran East Liverpool, OH	$1,500

Headpointer Devices

A person with sufficient range of motion in the head and neck to use physical extension devices can avoid the intraoral complications of mouthsticks by using devices affixed to other parts of the head. There are several headpointing devices in the marketplace, each using different technologies.

Headsticks. Headsticks function and look like mouthsticks (see Figure 2.7). As with a mouthstick, the user controls the headstick by moving the neck and head. The user can activate the headstick's tip through the same methods used for the mouthstick—tongue, jaw, or sip-and-puff. The headstick can also be activated through other motions of the head or body. Unlike a mouthstick, the headstick fastens to the user with a headband or fits over the head like a cap.

Noncontact Headpointers. The headstick requires physical contact between the user and the assistive device, but there are three variations to the mechanical headstick, and the light, ultrasonic, and eyegaze pointer. These variations provide user con-

trol through means other than a
mechanical shaft—they are noncontact headpointers. Noncontact headpointers offer psychological advantages to the user because the user is
not physically connected to the
device, nor is there an obvious
implement protruding from the
user's head. The disadvantage is
that noncontact headpointers cannot
physically press or grasp objects.
Their use is confined to objects
designed to receive their signals.

Light Pointer. The light pointer
is a variation of the headstick that
uses a light beam to activate the
assistive device. The light beam is
either visible or infrared. The infrared light pointer
functions exactly like an infrared remote control
device.

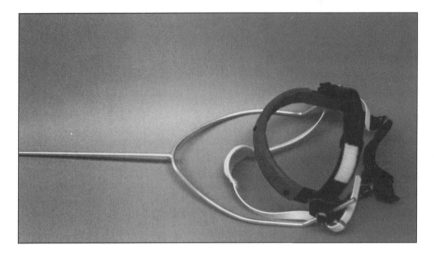

Figure 2.7. Headsticks.

Headpointing devices from commercial sources
differ according to function, technology, and price.
Table 2.5 gives examples of headpointing devices
available in the marketplace (CO-NET, 1993).

Considerations for Rehabilitation Technologists

Of the physical extension devices, the mouthstick has
received the most coverage in the press. However, the
professions of dentistry and occupational therapy
both urge caution in the design, fabrication, and use
of mouthsticks. An early article called for standards
based on 14 points, summarized below (Blaine &
Nelson, 1973):

• In order to allow normal vertical growth, the
  mouthpiece should not exert pressure on
  newly emerging teeth, but it should contact
  all fully emerged teeth in the posterior and
  anterior segments.

• To reduce fatigue, the two sets of opposing
  teeth should stabilize the device when the jaw
  is nearly closed in the resting position, and
  the device should be balanced laterally and
  vertically to rest lightly in the mouth without
  pressure.

• The device should distribute the biting force
  to all possible teeth to reduce injury to the
  structures supporting the teeth, and it should
  fit the existing pattern of teeth rather than
  attempt to correct irregularities.

• The device should be relatively inexpensive,
  sanitary, easily cleaned, and free of taste and

odor, while also being sturdy—virtually
unbreakable in routine use.

• The user should be able to access the mouthstick independently, have a clear line of
  vision with the device, and be able to communicate, swallow, and keep lips moist during use.

Despite the publication of such thorough standards, a recent survey reported "limited adherence to
the dental standards for mouth stick design" (Smith,
1989). The report shows limited collaboration
between rehabilitation technologists and dentists in
clinical settings, and practitioners from each profession have insufficient knowledge to substitute for the
other. For example, rehabilitation technologists lack
knowledge about key oral safety factors, while dentists lack the knowledge to train clients in the use of
mouthsticks and about their task environments.

More general recommendations for all types of
headpointers (headsticks and noncontact headpointers) also appear in the literature (Ludovici &
Brockman, 1989):

• Easy donning, adjustment, and removal permits the greatest independent use of the headpointer. Resting the headpointer in a sheath
  that the user can reach with head movements
  permits independent access.

• Headband size should be adjustable for
  secure fit. Headpointer effectiveness depends
  on pointing accuracy; a secure fit reduces
  shifting of the pointing device during use.

• Adjustable pointer length for headsticks
  enables the user to shift positions and reach
  objects located at different distances.

Table 2.5. Headpointing Devices.

Name	Description	Manufacturer	Cost
BK6001 Adjustable Head Pointer	Aluminum pointer on elastic headband projecting from above the forehead.	Fred Sammons, Inc.	$27.95–$31.25
Adjustable Head Pointer H71830	Attaches to head with adjustable plastic bands. Rod has adjustable length and angle.	Maddak, Inc.	$69
Clearview Head Pointer BK6000	Six-way adjustable pointer projects out at jaw level, leaving clear filed of vision for user.	Fred Sammons, Inc.	$95
Head Pointers AD-1, AD-2, and AD-3	Uses chin rather than forehead as reference, for standard model, tiny-tot and hook closure model.	Zygo Industries, Inc.	$170
Pointer Gripper	Switch-operated gripper at end, with activating switch according to user's capabilities.	Enabling Devices	$425
Light Pointer	Mounted on user's head and pointed at objects to project a spot of light to activate light switch.	Linda J. Burkhart	$28.95
Talking Beam	Cap-mounted light pointer, with bulb mounted on end of 10-inch flexible shaft.	Crestwood Company	$45.95
Viewpoint Optical Indicator 6 (V01-6)	Small light beam projector mounted on headband. Adjustable position and angle.	Prentke Romich Co.	$339
Light Pointer	Cylindrical device that can be attached to head or other body part. Projects a red light spot.	Adaptive Communication Systems, Inc.	$350
Light Beam Indicator, Model 2	Lightweight, flexible plastic headwand with Velcro® closure. Focused light beam is switch-adaptable.	Jims Instruments Mfg., Inc.	$370

- The device should be compact for storage and transport so it can be used in multiple locations.
- It must be possible to access switches and controls for mobility and computer use.

The therapist must remain mindful of the long-term impacts of device use. Expensive devices are usually expensive to maintain and repair. Systems with high complexity or relatively new technology may be a cost burden to the user. The purpose and context of device use are important indicators of cost and benefit.

Assistive Devices for Fine Motor Deficits

Switches and Controls

Switches and controls are the interface between the person and a device. Switches and controls send signals from the user to the connected device. These signals activate and direct the device's activity. Switches and controls either are separate components or are integrated into a device. Integrated switches and controls, such as the buttons on a television or

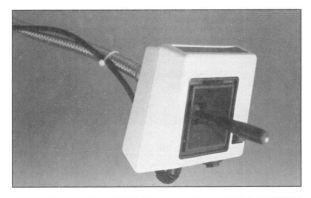

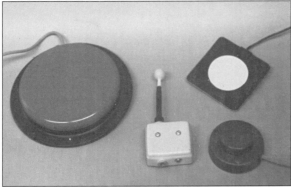

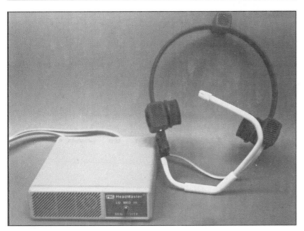

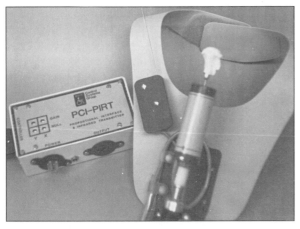

Figure 2.8. Several switches, each of which can be configured for multiple access points.

microwave, define device access. Only people capable of operating the integrated switch/control can access the device. Separate switch/control components enable a person to customize the method of device access to his or her preference and ability. The type of switches and their locations can be optimized for the user (see Figure 2.8 and Table 2.6).

Many alternative switches and controls are available to meet the varied needs of people. One resource catalog lists more than 100 different types of switches and controls (Brandenburg & Vanderheiden, 1987). This wide variety in switches and controls enables a person to gain device access through multiple approaches—access through any body part the person uses to make volitional movements. For example, switches in existing systems have been positioned to be activated by movement of the head (Hamann, 1990; Harwin & Jackson, 1990), tongue (Ortiz, Fortune, Brooks, & Chroust, 1990), mouth (Kozole, 1986), jaw (DiPietro, Warfield, & Bradshaw, 1986), eyelid (Grattan, Palmer, & Sorrell, 1986), chin (Everson & Goodwyn, 1987), and neck (Van Laere & Duyvejonck, 1986), along with more traditional points of switch/control positioning such as the arm, finger, hand, leg, and foot.

Switches are frequently used in combination with other devices. Low-technology aids that improve functional ability also increase a person's switch type and placement options. For example, slings or mobile arm supports increase shoulder and arm motion, while orthoses and splints increase wrist, hand, and finger stability. Pressure switches and rocking levers can be activated by shifting the weight of a body part. These switches offer the advantage of not requiring any fine motor manipulation (O'Leary, Saxena, Lindner, & Perkash, 1990).

The variety of mechanisms available for switches also exists for switch activation. Switch activation options include light reception, pressure from air, physical contact, magnetic fields, and sound waves. Physical contact switches include buttons, pads, levers, paddles, joysticks, plates, and flexible tubes. Switch activation and control involves a single switch or multiple switches. A keyboard represents a large array of switches, each linked to a specific function.

Switches can be latched or momentary. Latched switches, such as a light switch or the "power" button on a stereo, alternate between "on" and "off" positions. A momentary switch remains "on" only as long as it is engaged. A key on a keyboard is a

Table 2.6. Commercially Available Switches.

Name	Description	Manufacturer	Cost
Push Switch	Activated by direct pressure. They vary in size, shape, and amount of pressure required for activation. A push switch can be single- or multi-button, with a protruding or recessed pressure plate . It can be activated by any body part and designed for almost any pressure desired.	Pres Air Trol Corp. Luminaud Tash, Inc. AbleNet Don Johnston, Inc. Zygo Industries, Inc. DU-IT Control Systems	$10 $35 $40–$80 $42–$52 $50–$70 $80–$290 $45
Large Surface Switch	Enlarged surface area provides easier switch access for those with limited fine motor control.	AbleNet Don Johnston, Inc. BAH, Inc. Tash, Inc.	$42 $50 $75 $80–95
Lever Switch	Switch mounted at one end, with other end free to move between fixed or variable positions. Toggle switch activated by pushing into alternative position. Lever may be any length and shape.	Therapeutic Toys Don Johnston, Inc. SpellerTeller Communication Tash, Inc.	$24 $75 $60–$80 $100–$135
String or Pull Switch	Activated by pulling or releasing a string attached to the unit.	Enabling Devices AbleNet	$19–$42 $26
Rocking Switch	Located under a broader plate making it easier to activate. Any body part can activate switch with minimum pressure of 1 ounce.	Tash, Inc. Prentke Romich Co. Zygo Industries, Inc.	$35–$110 $80–$105 $60–$345
Treadle Switch (or Foot Switch)	Similar to the rocking lever except it is hinged on one end so it can only be depressed from a specific angle.	Radio Shack Tash, Inc. Therapeutic Toys Creative Switch Industries Linemaster Switch Corp. (light to heavy duty)	$4 $35 $25 $60 $25.20– $310.15
Thumb Switch	Small device that can be held in the hand and the button is depressed on the top by the thumb.	Enabling Devices Zygo Industries, Inc.	$21 $50
Pillow Switch (or pad switch)	Pressure-sensitive element wrapped in a soft or flexible covering. Sensitivity, size, and shape vary.	Enabling Devices Adaptive Aids Tash, Inc.	$22 $26 $75–$80
Ribbon Switch	Flexible switch activated by pressure of variable amounts anywhere along length of ribbon.	Dufco Electronics Tapeswitch Corp. of America	$45 N/A
Joystick Switch	4-position joystick; certain models have fifth switch.	Rehab Equipment Systems Enabling Devices Prentke Romich Co. Tash. Inc. Dufco Electronics	$40–$65 $50 $230 $230–275 $350–$625

(Continued)

Table 2.6. Commercially Available Switches (continued).

Name	Description	Manufacturer	Cost
Wobble Switch	Similar in construction to the joystick except movement does not correspond to movement of target. It is off when in the resting position and activated when pushed off-center in any direction.	Enabling Devices Prentke Romich, Co.	$41–$66 $115
Chin Switch	Similar to joystick but mounts on rigid bib that hangs around the user's neck. Switch moved by contact with chin or shoulder shrug.	SpellerTeller Communication Rehab Equipment Systems DU-IT Control Systems	$75 $229–$467 $480
Tongue Switch	Lever protrudes enough to permit activation by the user's tongue or face. Activation requires minimal amount of force and slight travel distance.	Enabling Devices Prentke Romich Co. DU-IT Control Systems	$26–$52 $125 $195
Leaf Switch	A flexible protrusion activated by a slight bending.	Enabling Devices Zygo Industries, Inc. Tash Inc.	$26 $43–$65 $100–$135
Pneumatic Switch	Activated by the pressure or vacuum created by the sipping or puffing of air through a tube.	Therapeutic Toys, Inc. Enabling Devices Zygo Industries, Inc. Tash, Inc. DU-IT Control Systems Prentke Romich Co.	$37 $37–$49 $90 $235 $240 $300
Pneumatic Bellows Switch	Similar to the pneumatic switch in that air pressure is used, but the force does not originate from the mouth. A bellows or bulb activates the switch.	Pres Air Trol Corp.	$12
Grasp Switches	Consists of a pressure transducer, a squeeze bulb, and a connecting tube. The squeeze ball is activated by squeezing or pressing on the bulb, creating an air force registered in the pressure transducer. Squeeze switch activates by bending.	Enabling Devices Adaptive Aids Tash, Inc. Maddak, Inc.	$21 $23–$35 $100 $100–$119
Air Cushion	Much like a rocking lever switch except that when the plate is depressed, an air current is transmitted instead of a switch being tripped.	Enabling Devices Prentke Romich Co.	$41 $125
Tilt Switch/Mercury Switch	Made from a glass tube containing mercury with electrodes attached to one end. The switch activates when tilted from its neutral position.	Enabling Devices Adaptive Aids Creative Switch Industries Tash, Inc. SpellerTeller Communication	$19 $23–$28 $28 $60 $60
Photocell Switch	Activated when an object or body part passes over a photocell.	SpellerTeller Communication	$200

(Continued)

Table 2.6. Commercially Available Switches (continued).

Name	Description	Manufacturer	Cost
Contact Switch	Closes a circuit by contact.	Enabling Devices Tash, Inc.	$43 $275
Blink Switch/Eyebrow	Sensor attaches to the eyelid and activates when the eye is closed for a certain amount of time. Sensor activated by movement of eyebrow or forehead.	Word +, Inc. SpellerTeller Communication	$35 $95
Sound Input Switch	Activated by user's vocalization (sound). Less sophisticated than voice recognition units.	SpellerTeller Communication Enabling Devices	$200 $76–85
Electromyograph (EMG)	Applied to the skin near muscle groups under volitional control. Muscle contractions operate switch.	Prentke Romich Co. Asaflex Manufacturing	$240 $595
Motion Switch	Activated by vibrations within range of the sensor or along radar or infrared beams.	Don Johnston, Inc. Prentke Romich Co.	$285 $229
Magnetic Switch	Activated by magnetic attraction when magnet is brought within range of sensor.	Luminaud	$35
Multiple Switches	Multiple switches (2–5) contained in one housing.	Tash, Inc. Prentke Romich Co.	$110–180 $360

momentary switch. Momentary switches can be interfaced to a switch latch or control unit to make electronic devices more accessible. Switch latch interfaces turn devices on when a momentary switch is depressed. Many have timers that allow the activation time to be varied so a single depression of a momentary switch will operate the device for a preset duration. Switch latch interfaces are usually limited to battery-operated devices. Devices that run off AC power can be plugged into a switch control unit and operated by an external switch in a manner similar to the switch latch interface.

Various switches are listed in Table 2.6. They are intended for use only as examples, because there are many hundreds of switches in the marketplace.

A single switch can control multiple functions by having alternate patterns of switch use represent different commands. The different patterns are then interpreted by electronics or software which execute the command. For example, some hair dryers use two switches to control four functions, high heat/high fan, high heat/low fan, low heat/high fan, low heat/low fan.

Computer Access

Computers have become more powerful, compact, and affordable, helping everyone with productivity and efficiency. Assistive computer technology can provide use of computers for persons with disabilities, granting independence and self-sufficiency. Although the use of computers holds much promise for all individuals, ways that computers are accessed may need to be modified for users with disabilities. Typical input methods include the standard keyboard and the mouse. The standard keyboard may present problems to some individuals due to the keys' layout and number, size, and labeling. Mouse use may be equally difficult for many as it requires coordinated, controlled movements. Fortunately, there are many devices that can be used in place of the standard input methods and they are often commercially available.

The Mouse and Other Pointing Devices

The majority of computers and software programs today require input from the mouse as well as the standard keyboard. The mouse is a small hardware pointing device used to control the movement of the pointer on the screen. It is used extensively in soft-

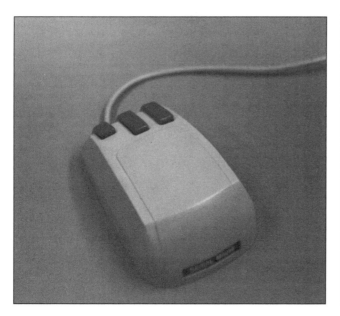
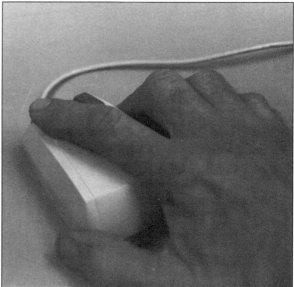

Figure 2.9. Mouse computer control device.

ware employing a graphical user interface (GUI) (see Figure 2.9). A roller ball on the underside of the mouse, when rolled against a flat table surface, controls the corresponding movement of the screen pointer. With the pointer on the desired position on the screen, a mouse button is activated to make a selection, open a file, or move to different parts of the program. Modifications to mouse movements can be adjusted through the computer's control panel options. Three mouse operations are common: clicking, double-clicking, and dragging. Other pointing devices can be used to imitate the mouse movements;

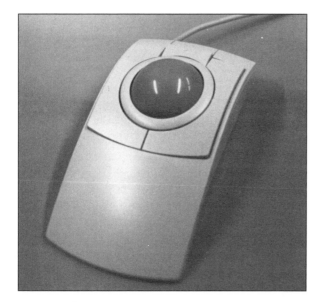

Figure 2.10. Trackball computer control device.

all control the directionality of the pointer on the screen and use various methods to "click."

A popular alternative to the mouse is the trackball, which functions like an upside-down mouse. Requiring less range of motion, it provides a more concrete experience as the user moves the ball itself in the desired pointer direction. Once the pointer is on the desired screen icon or menu bar item, the press of a button acts to select it. Trackballs come in a variety of shapes and sizes with differing features such as programmable mouse buttons. Most provide an area for resting the palm or heel of the hand. Other devices that resemble pens or crayons can operate on any surface to control the movement of the pointer (see Figure 2.10).

Touch screen technology is commonly used in community restaurants, grocery stores, and other businesses. Touch screens enable the user to make selections by directly pointing to an area on the monitor with a finger or stylus. For PC use, any software program designed to be used with a mouse will work with a touchscreen. Trackpads provide a surface where the pointer moves across the screen as a finger slides over the surface of the pad. The user points to a location on the pad and the pointer instantly appears in the same location on the screen.

Other devices that control the movement of the pointer include head pointing devices, which control the movement of the pointer-arrow with minimal head movement. Controllers interpret head movement through headsets (HeadMaster) and head dots

(Head Mouse). Joysticks also control the movement of the mouse. These can be controlled by hand, chin, or any other appropriate body part. When used in conjunction with an onscreen keyboard (see Table 2.7), independent typing ability is achieved.

Keyboards

Operating the standard QWERTY keyboard with function keys or key combinations for computer commands requires fine motor control, some gross motor range of motion, eye-hand coordination, and extensive practice or training in touch typing. Persons with physical or cognitive impairments can choose from a variety of keyboard alternatives that better address their individual needs (see Table 2.7). Adapted keyboards vary according to the accommodation required. Assistive software can also be used to further refine the adapted keyboard or mouse input.

Ergonomic Keyboards. A variety of keyboards are available that are designed to ensure safe and comfortable computer use by preventing repetitive muscular or skeletal strain injuries. Many offer flexible positioning options changeable throughout the day (see Figure 2.11), while others use "wells" for support (see Figure 2.12), or are fashioned for chording (e.g., BAT) or minimal finger/hand movements (e.g., DataHand).

Enlarged Keyboards. The enlarged keyboard is simply a larger version of the standard keyboard, in whole or in part. With enlarged key areas, the user finds it easier to strike the desired key. They can be quite effective with children and persons with cognitive and/or physical impairments because the larger key surface can be labeled with icons or symbols representing key functions (e.g., a symbol of a printer). An enlarged keyboard is shown in Figure 2.12.

Reduced Keyboards. Reduced keyboards are the opposite of enlarged keyboards, with smaller, more closely arranged key areas. They are useful for persons with an extremely limited range of motion but with some fine motor control. A stylus is often used to activate keys on reduced keyboards. Figure 2.13 shows the Magic Wand Keyboard.

Customizable Keyboards. Customizable keyboards can be fully reconfigured to provide larger and fewer keys for the user to select from, or to accept all key input from one side of the keyboard or another. These keyboards have extensive applications for persons unable to freely access more

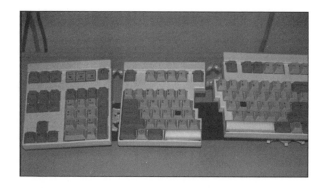

Figure 2.11. Adjustable ergonomic keyboard.

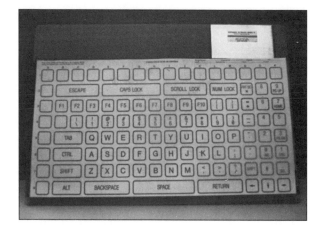

Figure 2.12. Ergonomic keyboard.

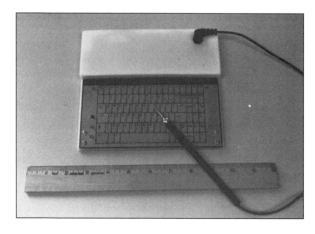

Figure 2.13. Reduced keyboard with striking pen.

typical input methods. Keys can be grouped together to act as a single key, and a string of characters or computer commands can be customized under a single key. Overlays are created that indicate the keys to be used and can be labeled with letters,

Table 2.7. Alternative Keyboards.

Name	Description	Manufacturer	Cost
PC King Keyboard	Expanded keyboard with separated and enlarged keys that are slightly recessed. Direct plug in.	Tash, Inc.	$1,000
King Keyboard	Similar to PC King. Requires keyboard emulator.	Tash, Inc.	$750
PC Mini Keyboard Mac Mini Keyboard	Small membrane keyboard with closely spaced keys. Direct plug in.	Tash, Inc.	$750
Mini Keyboard	Similar to PC Mini Keyboard but requires keyboard emulator.	Tash, Inc.	$375
Magic Wand Keyboard	Miniature keyboard operated by hand-held wand or mouthstick. Direct plug in for IBM or Macintosh.	In Touch Systems	$1,295
Datalux	Small-footprint keyboard and receiver for remote control of IBM computers. 100 keys.	Datalux, Inc.	$125
Dvorak Keyboard Converter	Alternate keyboard layouts with key configuration that increases efficiency of one-handed typing.	Microsoft Corp.	N/A
Kinesis Ergonomic	Ergonomically designed keyboard.	Kinesis Corp.	$690
IBM Ergonomic	Adjustable keyboard with ergonomic design.	IBM Corp.	$175
Microsoft Natural Keyboard	Adjustable keyboard with ergonomic design.	Microsoft Corp.	$110
Comfort	Adjustable keyboard with ergonomic design.	Health Care Keyboard	$700
Apple Adjustable	Adjustable keyboard with ergonomic design.	Apple Computer, Inc.	$219
BAT	Two cord-based keypads with ergonomic design.	Infogrip, Inc.	$495
IntelliKeys	Customizable overlay keyboard.	IntelliTools, Inc.	$395
Concept Keyboard	Customizable overlay keyboard.	Hach Associates	$495
Key Largo	Customizable overlay keyboard.	Don Johnston, Inc.	$320–$780

words, photos, or symbols (see Figure 2.14). Customized keyboards usually require the use of specialized software or a computer interface or both.

Any of the keyboards described above can be further modified to provide increased access to individuals. Keyguards, such as the one shown in Figure 2.15, are useful for persons with insufficient motor control to strike the intended key. Keyguards are plastic or metal overlays with finger-sized holes that correspond to the keys on a particular keyboard. Users can slide their hands over the surface without accidentally activating the keys. Some keyguards have a latch device to hold certain keys down while another is pressed (i.e., for shift, alt, control, etc.). Other keyboard modifications include the use of highlighters such as stickers or keycaps to stress the keys to be used. Conversely, the use of cardboard masks helps eliminate distracting unneeded keys.

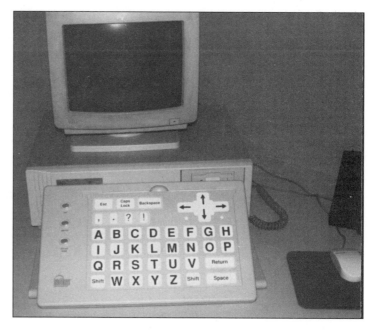

Figure 2.14. Customizable keyboard.

Alternate Input Methods

For users who are unable to access the computer via keyboards or pointing devices, other methods must be identified. Several methods require hardware for a computer interface to "translate" the nontraditional input into information the computer can understand, as well as specialized software to customize and drive the input method. This combination of hardware and software interfacing creates a highly customizable input system. Such interface systems are available for both Macintosh and IBM/compatible computers. Through these interface systems, single and multiple switch scanners, Morse code, and communication devices with ASCII output can be used for computer input.

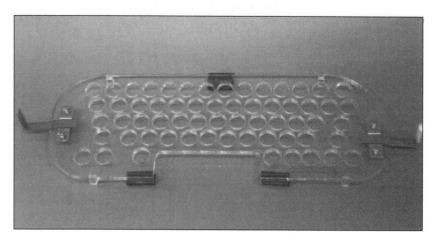

Figure 2.15. Keyboard keyguard.

Another input method increasing in use is speech dictation. These systems allow the user to dictate text into the computer by voice. Systems include dictionaries (up to 120,000 words) that "learn" the user's voice. Without having to use the keyboard, the user can dictate a fully corrected document at up to 70 words per minute. Voice also controls computer commands such as save, cut, paste,

and print. These systems also provide a method to create custom text macros that can enter large blocks of text with a single command, resulting in greater efficiency.

Assistive Software

Assistive software programs are available that further adjust the input method for increased independence and efficiency. These programs are often integrated with other software programs to make them easier to use. One example, onscreen keyboards, project the image of the keyboard on the monitor, focusing all motor, cognitive, and visual abilities to the same focal point. Any pointing device can be used to access the onscreen keyboards. Utility software programs, which affect all applications in a computer, are used to adjust the key repeat and response rates or to replace the need to "click" by simply dwelling on the selected onscreen key area.

Other assistive software programs intended for speed enhancement include word prediction, abbreviation expansion, and macro programs. *Word prediction* software programs are designed to reduce the number of keystrokes a person must make by predicting what will be selected next. These programs provide a more efficient method of written communication. A window appears on the screen with word choices available; these choices are stored in a dictionary that is modified to meet the user's needs. *Abbreviation expansion* software provides a way for the user to insert frequently used words or phrases by simply typing initials or another abbreviated form of the desired text. *Macro* programs allow the user to assign a wide range of computer activities such as entering text, opening files, or clicking buttons to single keystrokes.

Other software features and programs are available to assist the user. These include talking word processors, spell checkers, thesaurus, and dictionaries.

Integrated Systems

Integrated systems are available that allow persons with physical disabilities to control computer functions, their environment (e.g., lights, infrared devices, and intercoms), telephone communication, and frequently, powered mobility through a single central controller. Several systems exist and may be accessed by voice, a pointing system, keyboard, or single or multiple switch access. These include, but are not limited to:

- Sensei System—Safko International, Inc.
- Doors/PROXI—Madenta Communications, Inc.
- Universal Control System/Tongue Touch Keypad—newAbilities.
- LIAISON—DU-IT Control Systems.

There are many other computer software programs and alternate input systems with special features that provide easier access to persons with disabilities. Ongoing contact with national resources will help to maintain current information. Three major computer resources for persons with disabilities:

- **IBM**
  IBM Independence Series Center

(Information on VoiceType, AccessDOS, THINKable, Phone Communicator, SpeechViewer, Screen Reader/DOS and Screen Reader/2)
(800) 426-4832
- **Macintosh**
  Apple Worldwide Disability Solutions
  (408) 974-7910
- **Aisle 17: Product bundles**
  (includes peripherals and software)
  (800) 600-7808

Considerations for Rehabilitation Technologists

Alternative access devices such as switches, controls, and keyboards hold great promise for increasing personal independence through access to all types of assistive devices. Selecting or designing the proper access device is limited only by imagination, time, and resources. Even persons with severe physical disabilities can access high technology with the proper device. For example, a person with quadriplegia and spastic athetoid cerebral palsy can control an electronic communication device and an electric wheelchair through a single appropriate control interface (Pickering, Hauber-Wheeler, & Bristow, 1989)

The person's ability and preference determine the type of switch or control selected. One study suggested the following three-step process to assess the client and select a switch/control interface. The proper seating of the client and positioning of the device are imperative and assumed before initiating step one (Cook, Leins, & Hussey, 1988).

1. Identify an anatomical site under the client's voluntary control.
2. Identify and assemble the array of switch/control options that work with the identified anatomical site.
3. Conduct comparative evaluations of the switch/control options through actual use with the identified anatomical site.

The selected device must then be positioned in a manner that makes the best use of the person's ability. Improper positioning or inappropriate movement patterns often stimulate reflex patterns that interfere with controlled movement (Schuldt, 1990). Proper positioning maximizes control, minimizes involuntary movement and resulting fatigue to the user, reduces the likelihood of damaging the device through improper use, and successfully integrates the switch or control into the person's functional environment.

Selecting an appropriate keyboard requires similar considerations. Remember that technology can turn a 100-button keyboard into a single adapted switch directed by a person's eyeblink. Keyboards operate computer systems with immense potential, so it is also important to consider the user's future abilities in system selection. Is cursor speed variable? Can the user combine commands and alter icons to take advantage of learning? Will the system accommodate other keyboard configurations as the user's functions increase or decrease? Careful analysis results in an access method the user will not quickly outgrow.

Assessment for Adapted Computer Access

Computers have become a pervasive part of our lives and culture, and persons with physical disabilities must have the opportunity to participate fully in those educational, vocational, and leisure roles that require use of computer-based applications. Rehabilitation technologists play a crucial role in provision of assessment and training services necessary for someone with a physical disability to gain access to, and become proficient in the use of, a personal computer and its attendant application software.

Occupational therapists, rehabilitation engineers, adaptive computing specialists, physical therapists, special educators, and vocational rehabilitation counselors can make equally significant contributions toward a successful assessment and training outcome. Regardless of team composition, the following questions should be addressed in order to establish the initial goals for the assessment:

- What are the individual's immediate and long-term goals? Consider his or her educational, vocational and leisure roles when discussing this question.
- How would use of a computer help the individual achieve those goals? It is important to bear in mind that the computer is not an end unto itself, but rather a tool that can help people achieve a variety of goals.
- What is the anticipated context in which the individual would be using the computer?
- What is the availability of software training and technical support within the anticipated environment of computer use? The levels of support will vary widely among educational and vocational settings, yet ongoing training and technical assistance are among the most crucial factors influencing the long-term success of the computer as a productive tool for the individual.

There is not standardized protocol for assessment of computer access; however, it is generally agreed that the following performance areas and functional roles should be evaluated for the individual with a physical disability:

Physical Performance
- Gross range of motion
- Manual dexterity and fine motor resolution
- Sitting tolerance
- Working endurance
- Mobility

Cognitive Areas
- Existing computer knowledge
- Preferred learning style(s)
- Attention to detail
- Ability to follow multistep instructions
- Ability to work with visually presented information

Other
- Residential environment and familial role
- Medical history and anticipated changes in medical condition
- Personal care issues
- Current therapies being received and anticipated functional changes that will result
- Vocational and educational history
- Leisure activities

Basically, assessment of physical access to the computer involves evaluation of keyboards and keyboard-replacement devices as described earlier in this chapter. The goal, of course, is to identify an access method that will provide the individual with the most efficient and reliable method of inputting information into the computer. As described earlier in the chapter, access methods to be considered include:

- Direct access to the standard keyboard using fingers, headstick, or mouthstick.
- Use of a standard keyboard with an assistive device, such as a keyguard, or with a software enhancement program, such as those that include "sticky key," "delayed acceptance," "debounce," and "key-repeat defeat" features.
- Mouse, trackball, and other pointing device options.
- Rate enhancement software that includes macro, word prediction, and/or abbreviation expansion capabilities.
- Speech recognition software.

- Optical pointing systems used in conjunction with onscreen.
- Switch-controlled input, including Morse code and scanning software.

Finally, it is important to consider the necessity and desirability of integrating use of the computer with existing assistive technology, including augmentative communication, mobility, and environmental control devices.

Assistive Devices for Lower-Extremity Motor Deficits

Canes, crutches, and walkers are simple ambulation aids useful for persons with sufficient muscle tone, body strength, and coordination to hold themselves upright and provide controlled propulsion independently.

Conventional orthotic braces provide relatively stable support, and criteria for prescription are fairly well established. Mechanical orthoses provide support at various combinations of joints (foot, ankle, knee, and hip) depending on the level of impairment. Orthotic braces lock joints in place, so ambulation requires relatively high levels of energy output. Newer materials, such as carbon fiber epoxy resins, are improving the value of orthotics by reducing their weight while increasing their strength and flexibility.

Walkers are the most stable aid and therefore users require the most stability during ambulation. Walkers are designed to support the entire body weight, if needed. Many people limit their use of walkers to indoors and might utilize a wheelchair for outdoors or long distances. Walker users tend to ambulate less frequently and over shorter distances than users of the other aids. However, newer wheeled walker designs are more conducive to outdoor and long-range use.

The two basic types of crutches are the axillary and forearm. Axillary crutches are typically used by short-term crutch users. One or two axillary crutches can be used for assistance. Forearm crutches offer more stability than axillary crutches due to their ability to better distribute load through the forearm cuff. For this and other reasons, they tend to be used by long-term crutch users.

Cane users probably represent the largest population of ambulation aid users. Cane users need the least amount of support, and therefore most people use a single cane for assistance. Canes come in a variety of designs and are made primarily of wood and aluminum.

Some balance aids attach to the wheelchair and move the person from sitting to a standing posture either through mechanical means or through functional electrical stimulation (FNS) (Jaeger, Yarkony, & Roth, 1989). The role of FNS as an assistive device is described later in this chapter. More intricate balance aids involve orthotics. Sophisticated orthotic devices can even provide balance for persons participating in strenuous physical activities (Gawreluk, Raue, & Rugheimer, 1990).

Wheelchairs

Of all assistive devices, only balance aids such as canes and crutches predate the use of wheelchairs. Wheelchairs of the past century came in one size and functioned more like hospital gurneys—a means for attendants to transport patients from one location to another. Advances in materials and design led to lighter, collapsible wheelchairs in the 1930s. Casualties from World War II provided the impetus for the development of the modern hospital wheelchair (Grunewald, 1986). The past 20 years have seen continued advances in materials and design. Special wheelchair models are now available for use by small children, marathon racing, and strolling on the beach, for example.

Wheelchairs can be roughly classified into two categories: manual and powered. Manual wheelchairs come in two basic designs, depending on whether the user is self-propelling or being propelled by another. Self-propelled manual wheelchairs usually have a pair of large wheels that can be pushed by the user. Powered wheelchairs can be roughly divided into three designs: conventional, power based, and three-wheeled scooter models.

The present variety of chair makes, models, and features cannot be captured in a single chapter section. Several sources provide very thorough reviews of the available technology, as well as assessment, selection, and technical considerations:

1. The book *Rehabilitation Engineering* (Smith & Leslie, 1990) is the first to focus on assistive technology from medical considerations, through personal evaluations and device assessments, to particular areas of technology application. One chapter provides a concise summary of relevant issues in 60 pages (Hobson, 1990).
2. The publication *Choosing a Wheelchair System,* prepared by the Department of Veterans Affairs (1990) contains articles on clinical perspectives, technical considerations, and future developments for wheelchair selection.

3. ABLEDATA, an assistive technology database, offers information about wheelchair models, including an abstract of features.

Choosing the proper wheelchair for a particular person involves several factors. Functional ability helps determine if a powered or manual wheelchair is more appropriate, but other user and environmental factors also influence the decision.

Manual Wheelchairs

Self-propelled manual wheelchairs fall into two general categories:

1. Conventional manual wheelchairs are most commonly used in institutions (hospitals, clinics) and depots (airports) and are still popular among individuals because of their low cost. The conventional wheelchair is fairly heavy (35 to 50 pounds) with a chrome-plated steel frame. It has large rear drive wheels, front swivel castors, armrests, push handles, and footrests (see Figure 2.16). The seat and backrest are vinyl upholstery, which simplifies folding for storage or transport.

2. Lightweight or sports wheelchairs are increasingly favored for everyday use (see Figure 2.17). The lightweight is about half the weight of a conventional design (around 25 pounds) and is therefore more maneuverable and easier to propel and lift for transport. Weight reduction is achieved by using lighter frame materials such as aluminum or composites. The frame and upholstery come in dozens of colors, which adds to the appeal of these chairs. These chairs evolved from the desire of wheelchair athletes to maximize performance. Besides being lighter, these chairs offer a variety of features typically not found in conventional designs such as a rigid frame, adjustable rear axle location, absence of armrests and push handles, different foot plate designs, and optional sizes and types of rear wheels or front casters.

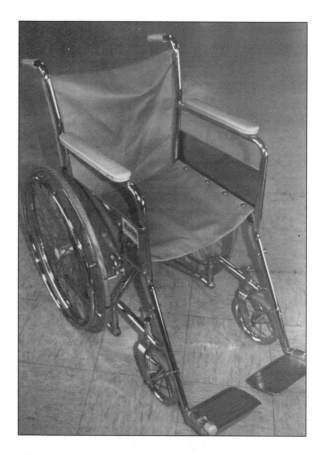

Figure 2.16. Conventional wheelchair.

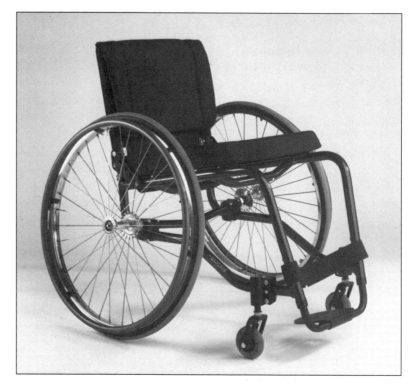

Figure 2.17. Lightweight wheelchair design. Picture provided by Quickie Designs, Inc.

Powered Wheelchairs

Powered or motorized wheelchairs use motors, batteries, a drive train, a controller, and an interface to control mobility. Powered chairs are typically used by people who need the added assistance for independent mobility. They can be classified into three general categories: conventional, power based, or three-wheeled scooters. The three designs reflect different capabilities that should be matched to the user's needs and desires. For example, a three-wheeled scooter disassembles to permit loading into a car's trunk.

Choosing the proper powered wheelchair is similar to choosing a manual wheelchair. In addition to the user's functional abilities, issues such as the means of transport, environmental terrain, and accessibility of home/work/school greatly affect the selection. Powered wheelchairs, as seen in Figure 2.18, are usually operated by a joystick that controls both speed and direction. However, many other interfaces are available to permit persons with severe physical disabilities or special needs to control a powered chair. Interface devices are as varied as the controls for other devices reviewed earlier in the chapter. Other alternative inputs include sip-and-puff (breath) control and voice-activation.

Figure 2.19 illustrates alternate wheelchair control systems and sites. The bold letters (A-I) indicate points of potential control. The bold arrows indicate potential directions of movement for control. The entire key is given in the caption underneath the figure.

Other Wheelchairs

Wheelchairs traditionally provide mobility. In recent years, several special-purpose and unconventional designs have become available. Stand-up wheelchairs, which allow users to approach a standing posture, are available in both powered and manual versions. Manual wheelchairs propelled by cranks or levers provide alternative control for everyday use or for exercising. Designs for use on snow, sand, and mountain trails, and designs that also float, are available to permit users to participate in these recreational pursuits.

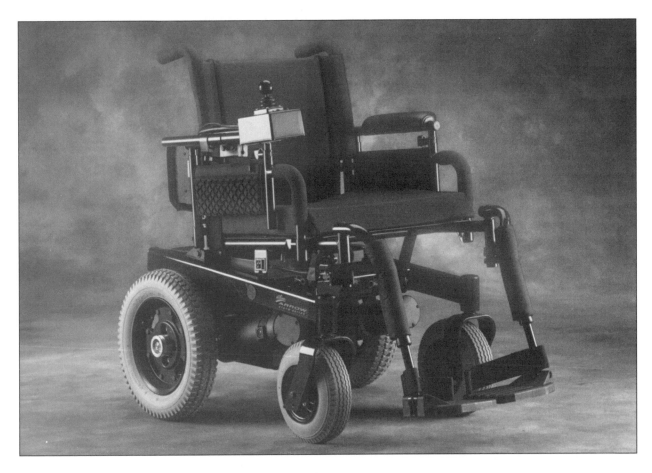

Figure 2.18. Powered wheelchair. Photo courtesy of Invacare.

Considerations for Rehabilitation Technologists

Selecting an appropriate wheelchair requires consultation with a team of experts who must, in turn, have access to information on a range of wheelchairs. One publication spends more than 100 pages simply outlining the considerations involved in wheelchair selection (Department of Veterans Affairs, 1990). The following section provides excerpts of these considerations. The general goals involved in recommending a wheelchair are as follows (Behrman, 1990):

I. Medical Goals

1. Compensate for a lost or absent function.
2. Prevent the occurrence of additional problems.
3. Optimize functional abilities through proper seated posture.
4. Accommodate or correct orthopedic impairments.

II. Personal Goals

1. Maximize access to school, work, and recreational opportunities.
2. Maximize access to communication options.
3. Optimize personal independence in mobility and transfers.

Powered wheelchairs are typically used by persons with severe physical disabilities—persons who lack the strength or coordination to propel themselves. Of course, mobility requirements vary between persons depending on their level of activity, the environments in which they function, and the tasks they expect to perform. Selecting the appropriate powered wheelchair system requires consideration of many of the same factors involved in selecting a manual wheelchair. In addition, the factors of motor power and driving speed, control type, control placement, and functions required of the powered wheelchair must be considered. Whenever deciding on complex and expensive equipment, a user trial should be arranged.

A recent report examined the actual

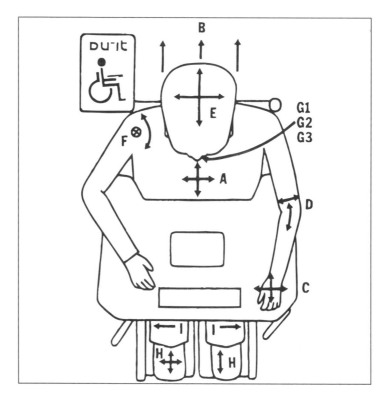

Figure 2.19. Wheelchair control diagram. Controls or switches can operate powered wheelchairs and ancillary assistive devices from virtually any location on the human body. Using multiple control activation points increases switch options and command complexity. Common control points are identified by letter as shown below:

A. Chin control—A joystick or pressure switch mounted on a collar or bar.

B. Headrest control—Pressing the head against the switch activates the forward or reverse power; rocking the head from side to side turns the wheelchair.

C. Hand control—Hand and finger motion or grasp activates numerous controls. The multidirectional joystick is widely used.

D. Arm/elbow control—Flexing and shifting the elbow, or sliding the arm.

E. Head control—Like the headrest control, activated through head movements.

F. Shoulder control—Horizontal and vertical movements.

G. Face control—Eyelids, cheeks, mouth, or chin movement activates switches. Mouth activation includes tongue or teeth pressure, breathing (sip and puff), or speech (voice).

H. Foot control—Moving the foot or shifting foot pressure.

I. Knee control—Horizontal movement of right and left knees.

Note: Diagram reprinted courtesy of David M. Bayer, President, DU-IT Control Systems Group, Shreve, OH.

mobility habits and requirements of persons with physical disabilities, and developed a five-point strategy to address mobility needs (York, 1989):

1. List all the environments in which the person will function now and in the future, including home, community, work, school, and transportation.
2. For each environment, identify the constraints and opportunities present for mobility such as distance, speed, other traffic, physical barriers (curbs), and terrain.
3. Consider all the mobility options available to the person in each environment.
4. Provide the person with access to, and training in, all the feasible mobility methods.
5. Evaluate the person's ability for each mobility option; then modify the mobility methods, environmental conditions, and mobility devices to optimize function.

Seating and Positioning Devices

Wheelchairs were designed as a combination seating and mobility device. However, the upholstery seat and back of most wheelchairs do not offer appropriate support for wheelchair users. However, many devices are available to provide a safe and functional seating system.

Seating systems perform two similar yet distinct functions: support and positioning.

1. Support: Seating devices support a person's body weight. The seat, backrest, armrests, and footrests combine to support the body. These supports should distribute body weight away from bony prominences to increase comfort and decrease the risk of pressure ulcers.
2. Positioning: Positioning devices orient a person's body in a useful posture. For example, proper positioning may alleviate excessive load-bearing of asymmetrical posture, or it may increase access to a computer by positioning the trunk in a functional posture.

Many seating and positioning devices perform both support and positioning functions and are chosen to meet the goals and needs of a particular person. The objectives of seating systems can be divided into three categories (Hobson, 1990):

1. *Seating for Postural Control and Deformity Management.* This is determined by the needs of children and youths with cerebral palsy or traumatic brain injury. The presence of varied levels of involuntary muscle activity and skeletal deformity requires diverse seating accommodations.

2. *Seating for Pressure and Postural Management.* This responds to the needs of persons with spinal cord injuries who are at risk of developing pressure ulcers in tissues surrounding the bony protuberances of the pelvic region. Dissipation of body heat to reduce moisture, and maintaining proper posture, are related concerns.

3. *Comfort and Postural Accommodation.* This objective concerns both geriatric and multiply disabled populations. Older persons are seated for prolonged periods, and they may require assistance sitting or rising to a standing position. Degenerative conditions caused by aging or disabilities require consideration of postural issues as well.

Proper seating and position has many benefits, including decreased abnormal tone or reflexes, increased stability, decreased risk of pressure ulcers, and increased range of motion (Bergen, Presperin, Tallman 1990). Proper seating maximizes function, and therefore it allows an individual to make the best use of assistive devices.

Determining the best seating system for someone can be a difficult process, depending on the person's needs and physical situation. Many different cushions and supports are available, and choosing the best system can be confusing. Regardless of the person, a functional assessment should be done before trying out different supports (Bergen, Presperin, & Tallman 1990; Taylor 1987).

A functional assessment involves a neuromotor summary of tone and reflexes, especially their effects when the person is in a seated position. An orthopedic summary identifies the available range of motion of the extremities and spine and determines which limitations can be corrected through proper positioning and which must be accommodated by the seating/positioning system.

After the assessment, determination of the proper components of the seating system may begin. Depending on the person's needs, the appropriate intervention might involve simply a cushion or a complex, customized system. Proper positioning starts with proper pelvic support, and then includes the trunk, head, and extremities. The seating/positioning system should accommodate current and expected daily living activities, educational and vocational goals, and the person's psychological and social orientations. Lastly, the seating/positioning system must be functional and practical to benefit the client.

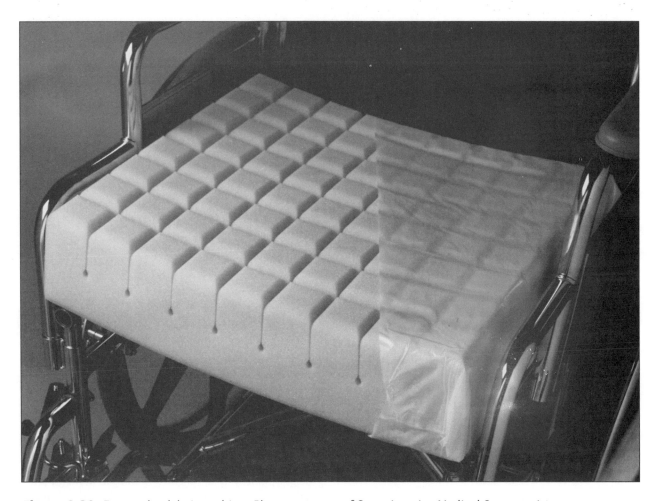

Figure 2.20. Foam wheelchair cushion. Photo courtesy of Span-America Medical Systems, Inc.

The use of simulation often ensures a successful seating outcome. Simulation involves trying different supports and postures until the most appropriate system is identified. A clinician can use the client's current wheelchair to simulate or might have access to a simulator. A seating simulator is a device that can be configured for different people and can interface with many types of seating or positioning equipment. A simulator can generally change size (seat width, back height, etc.) and position (seat tilt, back recline) to accommodate the needs of many clients.

Cushions

Just about every wheelchair user should use a cushion to properly support the buttocks. Many wheelchair cushions are commercially available and exhibit a wide range of features and costs. The most important fact about cushions is: No one cushion is best for everyone.

Many factors determine whether a particular cushion is appropriate for an individual. Ferguson-Pell (1990) listed factors that affect comfort, function,

and clinical safety. These factors include pressure distribution on the buttocks, moisture and heat accommodation, cushion stability, cushion weight, cushion thickness, maintenance, durability, and cost. These factors illustrate the importance of knowing the client and knowing the characteristics of the cushion.

Cushions can be divided into four general categories: foam, gel, air, and a combination of materials. Each of these materials is designed to cushion and support the body. However, the characteristics of the materials and the cushion's overall design affect the clinical factors listed above.

Foam cushions are common and generally inexpensive. Foam offers a stable and cushioned surface and is lightweight. However, foam has a relatively short lifespan and can increase skin temperature as it insulates against heat exchange. Foam comes in various density and stiffness ratings which determine the "hardness" or "softness" of a cushion. Combination foam cushions use foam with different properties to highlight the benefits of each and form a better cushion. A segmented foam cushion is shown in Figure 2.20.

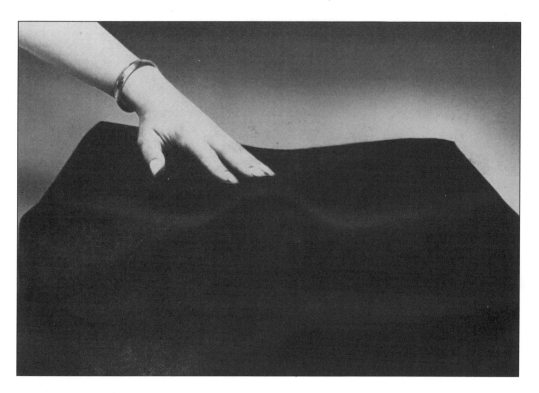

Figure 2.21. Gel wheelchair cushion. Photo courtesy of Southwest Technologies, Inc.

Gel cushions are heavier than foam cushions, often exceeding 7 lbs. Gel does not compress and is typically not as stable as foam because the buttocks do not sink in the gel. However, gel provides a good weight-bearing surface and does not raise skin temperature. Some cushions combine gel with foam to increase stability. A gel cushion is shown in Figure 2.21.

Air cushions are also fairly common and differ greatly in design and cost. All have an impermeable cover that encases the air and is a waterproof. Air is a good cushioning material, but these cushions distribute body weight well only when inflated properly. The foam air cushion requires periodic maintenance to ensure proper inflation. These cushions can be fairly light, and some designs allow moisture and heat to dissipate away from the buttocks. An example of an air cushion is shown in Figure 2.22 See Table 2.8 for a partial list of manufacturers and products.

Pelvic, Trunk, and Head Positioners

A person with orthopedic deformities, poor sitting stability, or pathological tonal influences might require external support to achieve and maintain functional posture.

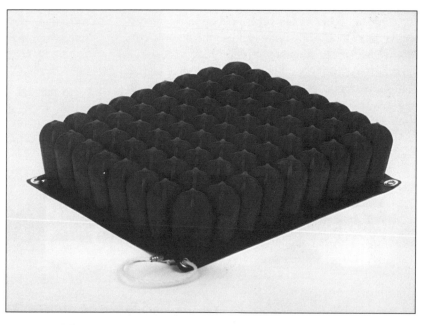

Figure 2.22. Air wheelchair cushion. Photo courtesy of ROHO Incorporated.

By their nature, external supports, as seen in Figure 2.23, restrict movement while providing support. For this reason, they must be used judiciously or functional motion will be compromised. A clinician could easily provide complete pelvic, trunk, and head supports for every client. Each client might have very good posture but will have problems accessing his or her individual environments. Postural support should be used to enhance function by providing body stability and alignment. As mentioned previously, the pelvic support is typically addressed first, followed by the trunk, head, and extremities.

Pelvis. Wheelchair cushions are integral to pelvic stability, and the previous discussion addressed stability in terms of material characteristics. The cushion can incorporate other features to increase pelvic support. Lateral pelvic supports can be used to prevent the pelvis from moving laterally. A cushion with one side carved lower than the other can accommodate pelvic deformity and offer improved support.

A lap belt is often used to help keep the pelvis in the seat, especially for individuals with extensor tone. Lap belts should act on the bony part of the pelvis to be effective and pull rearward and downward before attaching to the wheelchair. A lap belt that rides up to the abdomen will allow the pelvis to slide underneath and will also encourage slouched posture.

Trunk. Many wheelchair users require external trunk support to maintain a functional posture. Scoliosis, trunk muscle imbalance, and trunk muscle paralysis are reasons why support might be necessary. Maintaining an erect trunk posture is important to keep the head erect. A client who uses an arm to continually prop up the trunk can no longer use that arm for other purposes. Trunk supports include back supports, lateral supports, and anterior supports.

The sling upholstery of a wheelchair generally does not offer adequate back support, especially after the upholstery stretches with use. Several back inserts are available to provide appropriate support for wheelchair users.

Lateral supports attach to the wheelchair frame or seating system and are positioned to support the trunk in erect posture. Some supports are fixed while

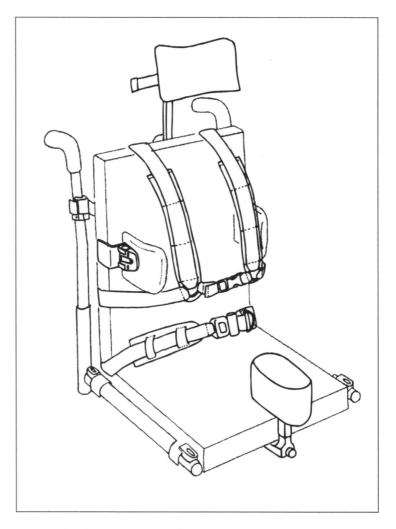

Figure 2.23. Head, trunk, lateral, and hip pads. Diagram courtesy of Adaptive Engineering Lab, Inc., copyright © 1994.

others swing away to facilitate transfers and positioning. Generally, lateral supports are used in pairs. They should be positioned to support the trunk while not interfering with the upper extremities.

Anterior trunk supports (or butterfly supports) are used to prevent an individual from falling forward. These supports include a chest pad or chest straps and are secured to the backrest and seat. They obviously need to be removed for transfers.

Head. Proper head positioning is crucial for feeding, swallowing, vision, and proper vestibular input. Some people with disabilities are unable to hold or move their heads without external support. Headrests can be used to support the occiput, or prevent lateral neck flexion or neck rotation.

Custom vs. Modular Systems

Some wheelchair users will require several supports to maintain a functional posture. When entire sys-

Table 2.8. Partial List of Cushions and Manufacturers.

Manufacturer	Description	Models and Cost
Dynamic Systems, Inc. Leicester, NC 704-683-3523	Visco-elastic foam in a variety of thicknesses, sizes, and stiffnesses. Foam-in-Place (FIP) kits for custom molded systems.	Sunmate Foam $7–$56 per sheet FIP Kits $56
Roho Inc. P.O. Box 658 Belleville, IL 62222 800-851-3449	Air and air/foam cushions in a variety of styles and sizes.	$370–$425 Hi-Profile, Low-profile, Enhancer, Quattro, Nexxus
Jay Medical P.O. Box 18656 Boulder, CO 80308-8656 800- 225-2610	Foam/gel cushions with a contoured foam base topped by a flowable gel.	$325–$450 Jay 2, JayCare, Jay Medical, Jay Active
Alimed, Inc. Dedham, MA 02026-9135 800-225-2610	Foam & foam/gel cushions in a variety of sizes, styles, and stiffnesses.	T-Foam $40–$60 T-Gel $88–$120 Latex Foam $28–$34
PinDot Products 2840 Maria Avenue Northbrook, IL 60062 800-451-3553	Custom-molded seat and back cushions and mounting hardware.	Contour-U $750 & up Silhouette $500 & up Performance $375 & up
Pryamid Rehabilitation P.O. Box 242153 Memphis, TN 38129-2153	Custom-molded seat and back kits with mounting hardware.	Bead seat $450 & up
Southwest Technologies 2018 Baltimore Kansas City, MO 64108 800-247-9951	Gel & foam/gel cushions in a variety of styles.	Elasto-gel $65–$200
SpanAmerica Medical Systems, Inc. P.O. Box 5231 Greenville, SC 29606 800-888-6752	Segmented foam and foam/gel cushions.	Geomatt $35 Geomatt PRT $40 Gec-T $50
Special Health Systems 90 Englehard Drive Aurora, Ontario L46-3U2 800-263-2223	Contoured foam cushions in various styles. Molded backrest and modular seating supports.	Ulti-mate Cushion $270–$300 Ulti-mate Back $435–$475
Action Products, Inc. 22 N. Mulberry Street Hagerstown, MD 21740 800-228-7763	Gel cushions in different sizes and thicknesses.	Action Flotation Pad $100–$125

tems are needed, the clinician, client, and family might decide between custom contoured and modular seating systems.

Custom-contoured or custom-modeled seating systems are fabricated from measurements of the client. Several custom systems are commercially available, such as PinDot's Contour-U, Dynamic Systems' Foam-in-Place, and Pyramid's Bead Seat. Custom systems are typically more labor intensive and require additional expertise or training. The size and shape of custom systems are not adjustable but fit closely around the client, even those with fixed deformities. They can offer a high amount of support and can withstand the strength of clients with the highest tone. A Contour-U system is shown in Figure 2.24.

Modular systems are fabricated from separate seating supports. Supports from different manufacturers can be mixed and matched to provide the appropriate positioning. Modular systems are more adjustable than custom molded systems and individual components can be easily replaced. Adjustability has its drawbacks and benefits. Adjustable seating systems can change as the user's needs change, but they can also become misaligned and provide poor support. Adjustability is one of many trade-offs warranting discussion when choosing a seating system.

Functional Electrical Stimulation

Functional Electrical Stimulation (FES), also known as Functional Neuromuscular Stimulation and Functional Neuromuscular Electrical Stimulation, refers to the application of electrical current to tissue to generate a response. FES has been used for many generations, but has recently become practical and effective in a variety of uses.

FES is often used for its therapeutic benefits, some of which are quite common, such as stimulation of cardiac muscle using pacemakers. Other applications include pain modulation, bladder management, electro-ejaculation, and wound healing. Another area of FES has been defined as the production of muscle contractions for joint stability and/or limb movement to augment muscle performance, modulate spasticity, or substitute for an orthosis.

Production of active movement with FES such as standing, walking, and grasping has received much attention, but its use is still primarily limited to research environments. The limitations of FES systems are a testimony to the complexity of volitional movement. FES systems simply cannot replace the motor and sensory pathways of the human body. Standing has both

therapeutic (Leo, 1990; Schafer, Jaros, Johnson & Boonzaier, 1989) and functional benefits and relatively simple FES systems have been used to allow subjects with SCI to stand. Improvement and restoration of walking in poststroke and SCI subjects has been intensively studied over the past decade and has received much attention. Gait restoration or improvement systems can be only FES or a hybrid system that combines FES with orthotics (see Figure 2.25). Upper-extremity FES research has been focused on two objectives: reduction of resting tone to permit colitional movement, and stimulation of muscles in an appropriate sequence to perform a function (Schafer, Jaros, Johnson, & Boonzaier).

Systems used to enhance motor performance vary widely in complexity depending on their purpose, but all possess some similar components and concepts (see Figure 2.26). Systems can use closed-loop or open-loop control. Closed-loop systems better reflect human motion but are more complex as they incorporate both "motor" and "sensory" pathways. Sensors monitor limb position, force, or acceleration, and the control system uses this input to regulate the stimulating current. FES systems stimulate muscle via surface, percutaneous, or implanted electrodes. Surface electrodes are the easiest to apply but are not able to stimulate deep muscles or provide precise, repeatable action. Percutaneous electrodes are fine wires with

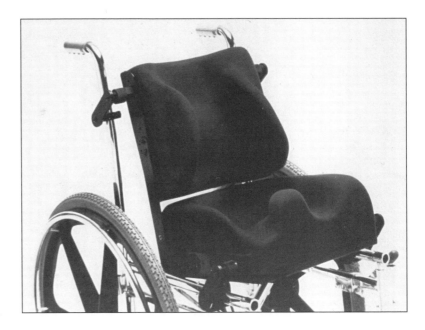

Figure 2.24. Custom-molded seating system.

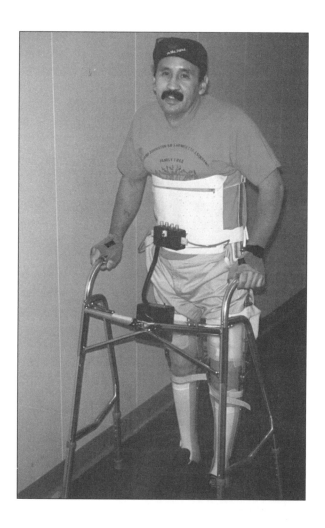

Figure 2.25. FES reciprocal gait orthoses—a hybrid system. Photo courtesy of Bioengineering Laboratory, Department of Ortho-paedic Surgery, Louisiana State University (LSU) Medical Center, New Orleans, LA.

tips that are embedded into muscular tissue. They provide a more consistent response and can remain in place for several months. Implanted electrodes are permanently positioned, and therefore provide a very consistent response. Implantation requires surgery, and these electrodes are still being developed. Therefore, most FES systems are based on surface or percutaneous electrodes.

Considerations for Rehabilitation Technologists

FES is important to the field of occupational therapy because restoring motor functions leads to restored task performance. Simple FES movements combine to complete entire tasks of eating, hygiene, work, and recreation. One study measured success in FES use by the completion of daily living tasks involving the manipulation of a book, telephone, computer disk, pen, toothbrush, drinking glass, finger food, and an eating utensil (Peckham, Keith, & Grago, 1988). Studies also applied FES to recreational exercise and physical fitness, and noted physiological improve-

Figure 2.26. FES system components (surface electrodes). Photo courtesy of Michael W. Keith, MD, and P. Hunter Peckham, PhD., Rehabilitation Engineering Center, Case Western Reserve University, Cleveland, OH.

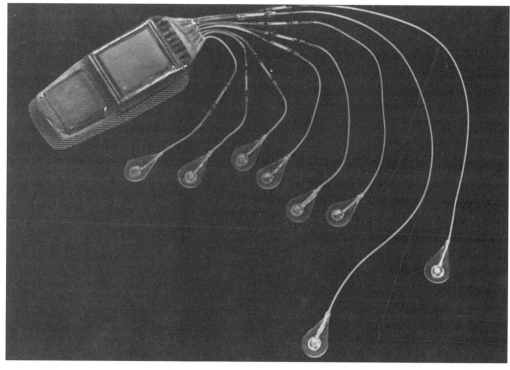

ments over time (Faghri, Glaser, Figoni, Miles, & Gupta, 1989; Mathews et al., 1989). Most FES work is occurring under controlled conditions in laboratories. However, FES systems with a variety of purposes are available commercially. These include systems that prevent foot drop, drive bicycle ergonmeters, assist with bladder control, correct scoliosis, and assist with pressure ulcer healing.

As with computers and mobility systems, new assessment methods are under development. Noninvasive stimulation of the neural pathways between the brain and muscles assesses the likelihood of motor recovery after injury and identifies candidates for early application of FES systems. The assessment involves magnetically induced central motor evoked potentials (CMEPs) and somatosensory evoked potentials (SSEPs) (Campbell, Monlux, Waters, Postigo, Haun, & Meadows, 1989).

Assistive Devices for Daily Living

The physical activity required to perform household tasks ranges from simple to complex. Assistive devices for the home follow the same distribution. Household devices range from simple low-technology gadgets (rubber jar openers) to complex systems (environmental control units) (see Figure 2.27). Several resource books described in Chapter 9 provide exhaustive descriptions of simple household assistive devices.

The Source Book for the Disabled (Hale, 1979) is somewhat dated, but includes descriptions of devices for eating, grooming, toileting, dressing, sex, child care, and recreation. *Coping with Daily Life: Handbook of Technical Aids* (1988) describes devices for the home and provides instructions for making these devices or similar ones that may not be available in the marketplace. *The First Whole Rehab Catalog* (Abrams & Abrams, 1990) contains device descriptions, vendor addresses, pictures, and prices

In addition to devices in the marketplace that meet basic needs, current developments are generating devices that expand the range of potential activities for persons with physical disabilities. A new modular wheelchair tray is designed to accommodate other assistive devices. The tray can be customized to fit the person and any seating insert, and it accommodates communication devices and wheelchair controls (Parnes, Naumann, & Ryan, 1989).

New devices for grooming are reaching the marketplace. For example, a makeup application board

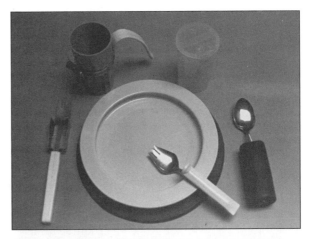

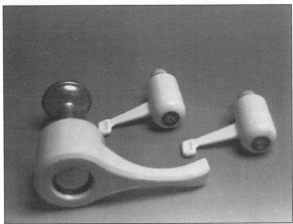

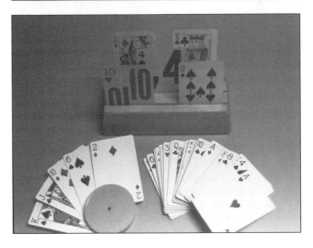

Figure 2.27. Assistive devices for daily living.

(Hage, 1988) and a positionable hairdryer (Feldmeier & Poole, 1987) both enable persons with upper-extremity impairments to perform complex motor tasks independently. Prior to the advent of these devices, people had to either refrain from wearing makeup and hairstyles or receive assistance from others. Although makeup and hairstyling are not necessary activities of daily living, these devices provide persons with access to socially desirable grooming options.

Incontinence remains a serious problem despite the variety of technology applied to other functions. One option is an electronic early warning device that alerts the person to an impending involuntary bladder evacuation and can prevent the occurrence. The device is also useful in biofeedback treatment programs (O'Donnell, 1988).

Rehabilitation technologists should have a general understanding of the range of available assistive devices and know where to go for additional information as the need arises. Reviewing vendor catalogs is another informative approach for identifying low-technology devices for activities of daily living. Several companies sell directly to users. Therapists should provide their patients with vendor information and encourage them to explore assistive technology options on their own.

Chapter 2 References

Abrams, J., & Abrams, M.A. (1990). *The first whole rehab catalog.* Crozet, VA: Betterway.

Amanat, I.Z., Riviere, C.N., & Thakor, N.V. (1994). Vibrotactile feedback for dextrous teleoperation. *Proceedings of RESNA 1994.* Nashville, TN.

Bach, J.R., Zeelenberg, A.P., & Winter, C. (1990). Wheelchair-mounted robot manipulators: Long-term use by patient with Duchenne muscular dystrophy. *American Journal of Physical Medicine & Rehabilitation, 69*(2), 55–59.

Behrman, A.L., (1990). Clinical perspectives on wheelchair selection. In choosing a wheelchair system. *Journal of Rehabilitation Research and Development: Clinical Supplement #2.* Baltimore, MD: V.A. Prosthetics R&D Center.

Beitler, M., Stange, C., & Howell, R., (1994). The design of an integrated interface to an educational robotic system. *Proceedings of RESNA 1994.* Nashville, TN.

Bell, F., Whitfield, E., & Rollet, P. (1987). Investigation of possum in Scotland. *Rehabilitation Medicine, 8*(3), 105–112.

Bergen, A., Presperin, J. & Tallman, T. (1990). *Positioning for function. Wheelchairs and other assistive technologies.* Valhalla Rehabilitation: Valhalla, NY.

Blaine, H.L., & Nelson, E.P. (1973). A mouthstick for quadriplegic patients. *Journal of Prosthetic Dentistry, 29,* 317–322.

Brandenburg, S.A., & Vanderheiden, G.C. (Eds.). (1987). *Resource book 2: Switches and environmental controls.* Boston, MA: College Hill Press.

Bray, J., & Wright S. (Eds.). (1980). *The use of technology in the care of the elderly and the disabled: Tools for living.* London: Frances Piner, for the Commission of European Communities.

Budning, B.C., & Hall, M. (1990). A practical mouthstick for early intervention with quadriparetic patients. *Journal of the Canadian Dental Association, 56,* 243–244.

Bush, M.A., & Peterson, C. (1989). User selection criteria for a voice-activated robotic work cell. *Proceedings of the 12th Annual RESNA Conference.* New Orleans, LA, 381–382.

Cameron, W., Birch, G., Fengler, M., Young, J., Carpenter, A., McIntyre, C., & McKay, K. (1990). Capitalizing on robot technology: MAD, MOM, DAD, and Next. *Proceedings of the 13th Annual RESNA Conference.* Washington, DC, 331–332.

Campbell, J., Monlux, J.,Waters, R.L., Postigo, P., Haun, C., & Meadows, P. (1989). Assessment of motor and sensory pathways: Enhancement of selection criteria for functional electrical stimulation. *Proceedings of the 12th Annual RESNA Conference.* New Orleans, LA, 397–398.

Cannon, D. J. (1990). The human-machine interface: A workspace-mouse concept. *Proceedings of the 13th Annual RESNA Conference.* Washington, DC, 131–132.

Cheatham, A., Mulner, M., & Verberg, G. (1994). Eye movement control of the MANUS Manipulator. *Proceedings of RESNA 1994.* Nashville, TN.

CO-NET (Cooperative Assistive Technology Database Dissemination Network). (1993). *Hyper-ABLEDATA Database, CO-NET CD-ROM Version* (6th ed.). Madison, WI: Trace Research and Development Center.

Cook, A.M., Leins, J.D., & Hussey, S.M. (1988). *Computer-assisted motor assessment of persons with disabilities to determine ability to use assistive devices.* ISA, Paper #88-0219, 125–131.

Cook, A.M., Liu, K.M., & Hoseit, P. (1990). Robotic arm use by very young motorically-disabled children. *Assistive Technology, 2*(2), 51–57.

Coping with daily life: Handbook of technical aids. (1988). Quebec, Canada: Les Editions Papyrus.

Crewe, N.M., & Zola, I.K. (1983). *Independent living for physically disabled people.* San Francisco, Jossey-Bass.

Dallaway, J.L., Mahoney, R.M., & Jackson, R.D. (1993). CURL—A robot control environment for Microsoft environment for Microsoft Windows. *Proceedings of RESNA 1993.* Las Vegas.

Danielsson, G., & Holmberg, L. (1994). Evaluation of the RAID workstation. *Proceedings of RESNA.* Nashville, TN.

Department of Veterans Affairs. (1990). Choosing a wheelchair system. *Journal of Rehabilitation Research and Development: Clinical Supplement #2.*

Dickey, R., & Shealy, S. (1987). Using technology to control the environment. *American Journal of Occupational Therapy, 41,* 717–721.

DiPietro, G.J., Warfield, D.K., & Bradshaw, A.J. (1986). A jaw-operated proximity switch for a paraplegic patient. *Journal of Prosthetic Dentistry, 56,* 711–715.

Efthimiou, M.A., Gordon W.A., Sell G.H., & Stratford C. (1981). Electronic assistive devices: Their impact on the quality of life of high-level quadriplegic persons. *Archives of Physical Medicine and Rehabilitation, 68,* 331–336.

Engelhardt, K.G. (1989). Health and human service robotics: Multidimensional perspectives. *International Journal of Technology and Aging, 2*(1), 6–41.

Everson, J.M., & Goodwyn, R. (1987). A comparison of the use of adaptive microswitches by students with cerebral palsy. *American Journal of Occupational Therapy, 41,* 739–744.

Faghri, P., Glaser, R.M., Figoni, S., Miles, D., & Gupta, S. (1989). Muscular effects of two FNS exercise modes for the spinal-cord-injured. *Proceedings of the 12th Annual RESNA Conference.* New Orleans, LA, 395–396.

Feldmeier, D., & Poole, J. (1987). The position-adjustable hair dryer. *American Journal of Occupational Therapy, 41,* 246–247.

Ferguson-Pell, M. (1990, March). Seat cushion selection. *Journal of Rehabilitation Research and Development,* Clinical Supplement No. 2: Choosing a wheelchair system, 49–73.

Gawreluk, C., Raue, V., & Rugheimer, P. (1990). Trunk support for a horseback rider with cerebral palsy. *Proceedings of the 13th Annual RESNA Conference.* Washington DC, 435–436.

Glass. K., & Hall, K. (1987). Rehabilitation technologists' views about the use of robotic aids for people with disabilities. *American Journal of Occupational Therapy, 41,* 745–747.

Grattan, K.T.V., Palmer, A.W., & Sorrell, S.R. (1986). Communication by eye closure: A microcomputer-based system for the disabled. *IEEE Transactions on Biomedical Engineering, 33,* 977–982.

Grunewald, J. (1986). Wheelchair selection from a nursing perspective. *Rehabilitation Nursing, 11*(5), 31–32.

Haataja, S., & Saarnio, I. (1990). An evaluation procedure for environmental control systems. *Proceedings of the 13th Annual RESNA Conference, Washington, DC,* 25–26.

Hage, G. (1988). Makeup board for women with quadriplegia. *American Journal of Occupational Therapy, 42,* 253–255.

Hale, G. (1979). *The source book for the disabled.* Philadelphia: Saunders.

Hamann, G. (1990). Two switchless selection techniques using a headpointing device for graphical users inerfaces. *Proceedings of the 13th Annual RESNA Conference.* Washington, DC, 439.

Hammel, J. M., & Van der Loos, M. (1990). A vocational assessment model for use of robotics technology. *Proceedings of the 13th Annual RESNA Conference.* Washington. DC, 327–328.

Hammel, J. M., Van der Loos, M., & Perkash, I. (1992). *Evaluation of a vocational robot with a quadriplegic employee, 73,* 683–693.

Harwin, W. S., & Jackson, R. D. (1990). Analysis of intentional head gestures to assist computer access by physically disabled people. *Journal of Biomedical Engineering, 12*(3), 193–198.

Hillman, M.R. (1987). A feasibility study of a robot manipulator for the disabled. *Journal of Medical Engineering & Technology, 11*(4), 160–165.

Hillman, M.R., Pullin, G.M., Gammie, A.R., Stammers, C.W., & Orpwood, R.D. (1990). Development of a robot arm and workstation for the disabled. *Journal of Biomedical Engineering, 12*(3) 199–204.

Hobson, D. A. (1990). Seating and mobility for the severely disabled. In R.V. Smith & J.H. Leslie (Eds.), *Rehabilitation engineering.* Boca Raton, FL: CRC Press, 193–252.

Hock, D. A. (1989). The use of the maxillary interocclusal splint as a mouthpiece for the mouthstick prosthesis. *Journal of Prosthetic Dentistry, 62*(1), 56–57

Horowitz, D.M., Webster, H., Hausdorff, J.M., Gordon, H., & Quintin, E. (1989). Clinical evaluation and human performance studies on prescribing robotic manipulators for severely disabled individuals. *Rehabilitation R&D Progress Reports, 26,* 160.

Howell, R., & Hay, K. (1989). Hardware and software considerations in the design of a prototype educational robotic manipulator. *Proceedings of the 12th Annual RESNA Conference.* New Orleans, LA, 113–114.

Jaeger, R.J., Yarkony, G.M., & Roth, E.J. (1989). Rehabilitation technology for standing and walking after spinal cord injury. *American Journal of Physical Medicine & Rehabilitation, 68*(3), 128–133.

Kaplan, L.I. (1966). A reappraisal of braces and other mechanical aids in patients with spinal cord dysfunction: Results of a follow-up study. *Archives of Physical Medicine and Rehabilitation, 47,* 393–405.

Kozole, K. (1986). A generalized wheelchair control system. In E. Trefler, K. Kozole, & E. Snell (Eds.), *Selected readings on powered mobility,* (pp. 47a–47n). Washington, DC: RESNA.

Kraus, L.E., & Stoddard, S. (1989). *Chartbook on disability in the United States: An InfoUse report.* Washington, DC: National Institute on Disability and Rehabilitation Research.

LaPlante, M.P. (1988). *Data on disability from the national health interview survey, 1983–1985: An Info Use report.* Washington, DC: National Institute on Disability and Rehabilitation Research.

LaRocca, J., & Tirem, J.S. (1978). *The application of technological developments to physically disabled people.* Washington, DC: The Urban Institute.

Leo, K., (1990). The effects of passive standing. *Paraplegia News, 39,* 45–47.

Lesnoff-Caravaglia, G. (Ed.). (1988). SmartHouse technology. *International Journal of Technology and Aging 1*(1).

Ludovici, A., & Brockman, R. (1989). An improved design for an adaptive headpointer. *Proceedings of the 12th Annual RESNA Conference.* New Orleans, LA, 418–419.

Maguire, G.H. (1985). *Care of the elderly: A health team approach.* Boston: Little, Brown.

Mann, W.C. (1989). Use of environmental control devices by nursing home patients. *Journal of Rehabilitation, Research, and Development,* Annual Supplement. *Rehabilitation R&D Progress Reports, 26.*

Mathews, T.M., Glaser, R.M., Figoni, S.F., Rodgers, M.M., Suryaprasad, A.G., Gupta, S.C., Enzenwa, B.N., Faghri, P.D., & Hooker, S.P. (1989). Evaluation of FES techniques for exercise. *Rehabilitation R&D Reports, 26,* 198–199.

Moynahan, A.J., Stranger, C.A. Harwin, W.S., & Foulds, R.A., (1994). The assistive research and technology wheelchair-mounted robotic arm: Prototype review. *Proceedings of RESNA 1994.* Nashville, TN.

Mulligan, R. (1983). A physiologic bitestick appliance for quadriplegics. *Special Care in Dentistry, 3*(1), 24–29.

National Health Interview Statistics (1977). *Vital and health statistics, series 10, number 135* (DHHS Publication No. FHS 81-1563). Washington, DC: U.S. Government Printing Office.

National Health Survey (1969). *Vital and health statistics, series 10, number 78* (DHEW Pub. No. HSM 731504), Washington, DC: U.S. Government Printing Office.

O'Donnell, P.D., (1988). Electromyographic incontinence alert device. *Rehabilitation R&D Progress Reports,* 293.

O'Leary, S., Saxena, K., Lindner S.H., & Perkash, I. (1990). Computer access for patients with spinal cord injury during rehabilitation. *Proceedings of the Fifth Annual Conference on Technology and Persons with Disabilities.* Los Angeles, CA, 501–510.

Ortiz, J.E., Fortune, D., Brooks, D.J., & Chroust, M.E. (1990). Communications and control for the severely disabled: The SmartLink system and the TongueTouch keypad. *Proceedings of the 13th Annual RESNA Conference, Washington, DC,* 93–94.

Parnes, P., Naumann, S., & Ryan, S. (1989). A modular wheelchair tray for the severely physically disabled. *Rehabilitation R&D Progress Reports, 26,* 131.

Peckham, H.P., Keith, M.W., & Grago, P.E. (1988). Upper limb applications: FNS for upper extremity control. *Rehabilitation R&D Progress Reports,* 184–185.

Pickering, C.L., Hauber-Wheeler, B., & Bristow, D.C. (1989). Facilitating independence. *Proceedings of the 12th Annual RESNA Conference.* New Orleans, LA, 432–433.

Phelps, J., & Erlandson, R. (1994). *Impact of Mechatronic Systems as Vocational Evaluators.* RESNA.

Phillips, B., & Zhano, H. (1993). Predictors of technology abandonment, *Assistive Technology 1993, 5,* 36–45.

Puckett, A.D., Sauer, B.W., Zardiackas, L.D., & Entrekin, D.S. (1989). Development of a custom-fit mouthstick appliance. *Journal of Rehabilitation Research and Development, 26*(4), 17–22.

Regalbuto, M.A., Krouskop, T.A., & Cheatham, J.A. (1992). Toward a practical mobile robotic aid system for people with severe physical disabilities. *Journal of Rehabilitation Research Development, 29*(1), 19–26.

Rice, D., & Feldman, J. (1983). Living longer in the United States: Demographic changes and health needs of the elderly. *Milbank Memorial Fund Quarterly Health and Society, 61,* 362–396.

Schafer, C., Jaros, G., Johnson, D., & Boonzaier, D. (1989). Effects of FNS on quadriceps: Muscle strength, bulk and fatigue in six spinal-cord-injured subjects. *Proceedings of the 12th Annual RESNA Conference.* New Orleans, LA, 393–394.

Schauer, J.M ., Vanderheiden, G.C., & Kelso, D.P. (1989). Keyboard emulating interface (KEI) standard. *Rehabilitation R&D Progress Reports,* 176–177.

Schuldt, M.E. (1990). Helping the physically handicapped access computers and utilize switches. *Proceedings of the Fifth Annual Conference on Technology and Persons with Disabilities.* Los Angeles. CA, 611–621.

Seaman, R.L., & Napper, S.A. (1988). Gripper automation and voice control of rehabilitation robots. *Rehabilitation R&D Reports, 25,* 144–145.

Seamone, W., & Schmeisser, G. (1985). Early clinical evaluation of a robot arm/worktable system for spinal-cord-injured persons. *Journal of Rehabilitation Research and Development, 22*(1), 38–57.

Sell-Heimer, G., Stratford, C.D., Zimmerman, M.E., Youdin, M., & Milner, D. (1979). Environmental and typewriter control systems for high-level quadriplegic patients: Evaluation and prescription. *Archives of Physical Medicine and Rehabilitation, 62.*

SmartHouse L.P. (1988). *Technical overview of the SMARTHOUSE system.* Upper Marlboro, MD: Advanced Design.

Smith, R. (1989). Mouth stick design for the client with spinal cord injury. *American Journal of Occupational Therapy, 43,* 251–255.

Smith, R.V., & Leslie, J.H. (Eds.). (1990). *Rehabilitation engineering.* Boca Raton, FL: CRC Press.

Symington, D.C., Batelaan, J., O'Shea, B.J., & White, D.A. (1980). *Independence through environmental control systems.* Toronto, Ontario: Canadian Rehabilitation Council for the Disabled.

Symington, D.C., Lywood, D.W., Lawson, J.S., & MacLean, N. (1986). Environmental control systems in chronic care hospitals and nursing homes. *Archives of Physical Medicine and Rehabilitation, 67,* 322–325.

Taylor, S.J. (1987). Evaluating the client with physical disabilities for wheelchair seating. *American Journal of Occupational Therapy, 41,* 711–728.

U.S. Senate Special Committee on Aging. (1982). *Developments in aging: 1981, Vol. 1.* Washington, DC: U.S. Government Printing Office.

Van Laere, M., & Duyvejonck, R. (1986). Environmental control and social integration of a high-lesion tetraplegic patient: Case report. *Paraplegia, 24,* 322–325.

Van der Loos, H.F.M., Michalowski, S.J., & Leifer, L.J. (1988). Development of an omnidirectional mobile vocational assistant robot. *Proceedings of the International Conference of the Association for the Advancement of Rehabilitation Technology (ICAART).* Montreal, 468–469.

York, J. (1989). Mobility methods selected for use in home and community environments. *Physical Therapy, 69,* 736–747.

Chapter 2 Study Questions

1. Name several examples of ECU technology used in homes. How might these benefit persons with disabilities?

2. What design differences would you expect to find between a robotic arm used to brush teeth and one used to cook a meal?

3. What is GUI-based software? Describe the alternatives used to operate this software.

4. Define "latched" and "momentary" switches. Provide two examples of each.

5. Identify three features that are often found in lightweight wheelchairs, but not found in conventional wheelchairs. Describe how these features could benefit a wheelchair user.

6. List wheelchair cushion types and identify one good and one poor characteristic for each type.

Chapter 3:
Assistive Technology for Persons With Sensory Impairments

I. Hearing Impairments
    A. Who Provides Services?
    B. Environmental Adaptations
        1. The Environment
        2. The Person
    C. Assistive Devices
        1. Hearing Aids
        2. Alerting Devices
        3. Assistive Listening Devices
        4. Telecommunication Devices
    D. Cochlear Implants
    E. Future Prospects

II. Visual Impairments
    A. Overview
    B. Who Provides Services?
        1. Adaptations for Persons With Vision Loss
        2. Individual Interactions
    C. Low-Technology Assistive Devices
    D. High-Technology Assistive Devices
        1. Stand-Alone Print Enlargement Systems (SPES)
        2. Character Enlargement Systems for Computers
        3. Braille Output Devices
        4. Voice Output Systems
        5. Audio Tactile Devices
        6. Scanning Systems
        7. Notetaking Devices and Laptop Computers

III. Tactile Impairments
    A. Overview
    B. Applications of Technology Using Tactile Sensation

3.

Assistive Technology for Persons With Sensory Impairments

Kathleen A. Beaver, BS, and William C. Mann, PhD, OTR

Hearing Impairments

Hearing impairments represent one of the most common chronic conditions. Prevalence is listed at 80 persons with a hearing impairment per 1,000 persons, and the percentage of persons affected increases with age. Almost one out of three persons over age 64 has a hearing impairment, and 42% of those over 85 have at least some hearing loss (Hotchkiss, 1989). Although there are many devices available for persons with hearing impairments, many elders accept hearing loss as a normal process of aging and do not seek assistance. Hearing loss can severely affect communication, and decreased communication can result in isolation and depression (Glass, 1986). Hearing loss can also affect health and safety in other ways, such as not being able to hear fire alarms or not being able to hear instructions for taking medications.

If a person has a hearing impairment, medical consultation should be sought first, because surgical procedures for some types of hearing loss may be an appropriate solution. When surgery is not appropriate, there is a wide variety of assistive devices. Early detection and intervention is an important factor in the successful prescription for assistive technology.

Hearing loss can be the result of exposure to loud noise over an extended time, hypertension, side effects of drugs, or stroke. There are three major types of hearing loss: conductive, sensorineural, and central. Mixed hearing loss is a combination of conductive and sensorineural impairments. Refer to Figure 3.1 while reading about each condition.

Conductive hearing loss occurs when sound waves are prevented from reaching the inner ear; it is similar to the sound reduction experienced by using ear plugs. Hearing aids are very effective in improving learning for those with conductive hearing loss.

Sensorineural hearing loss occurs with damage to the cochlea and surrounding hair cells. It is these cells that send electrical signals to the brain. A lay term for this condition is *nerve deafness.* A medical term for one type of sensorineural hearing loss is *presbycusis.* It is the most common form of hearing loss among older persons. In the early stage, and while the person is still young, presbycusis causes loss of ability to hear high-pitched sounds. As a person ages, middle and lower pitch sounds become more difficult to hear. Presbycusis typically affects both ears.

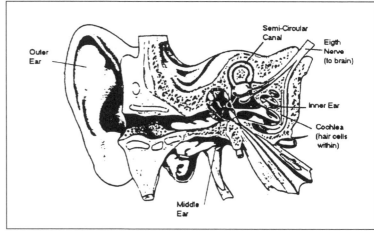

Figure 3.1. The ear.

Tinnitus is another sensorineural disorder. A person with tinnitus experiences a ringing or buzzing sensation. This ringing occurs without any external sound. A person with tinnitus typically has presbycusis as well. More than 90% of persons over age 64 experience tinnitus (Public Health Service, 1988). There is no cure for tinnitus, but "maskers" are sometimes used to provide a more acceptable sound than that produced by the tinnitus. Hearing aids may be used to offset the effect of the hearing loss that often accompanies tinnitus. Surgery is sometimes employed to reduce tinnitus, as are drugs, relaxation techniques, and biofeedback.

Central hearing loss is a result of damage to the nerves leading to the brain, or to the brain itself, which can be caused by stroke, traumatic brain injury, or vascular problems. Central hearing loss affects speech discrimination, and does not affect the volume of sound.

Who Provides Services?

Physicians (MD degree) who specialize in diseases of the ear are otologists, while physicians who specialize in treating the ear, nose, and throat are otolaryngologists. Audiologists (master's or doctoral degree in audiology) assess functional hearing, prescribe hearing aids and other devices, train patients to use prescribed devices, and train patients in auditory and visual communication. Hearing aid dispensers sell hearing aids but do not have formal training or certification for diagnosing and treating hearing loss. A number of other health professionals work with people with hearing loss, and occupational therapists often recommend assistive devices other than hearing aids.

Environmental Adaptations

While surgery, hearing aids, and other assistive devices are all very important in reducing the functional limitations of a hearing loss, environmental adaptations should also be considered. When working with individuals with hearing loss, think about both the environment and the person, as summarized in the numbered points below.

The Environment

1. Acoustics should be considered in the construction and renovation of any building or facility that will be used by persons with hearing impairments. In existing structures, the addition of carpets and drapes can absorb background noise.

2. Where groups of individuals will be meeting, personal sound amplification systems and/or assistive listening device (ALD) systems should be available for use by anyone with a hearing impairment.
3. Placement of furniture in a room should take into account the need for persons with hearing impairments to see others clearly when conversing.

In addition to these environmental considerations, there are several individual considerations to take into account when speaking with a person with a hearing impairment, as listed below.

The Person

1. Before initiating conversation, let the person know you are about to speak.
2. Look directly at the person you are speaking with, being certain that your lips and gestures can be seen.
3. Eliminate noises in the background, such as radios, stereos, and televisions.
4. Do not shout, but speaking somewhat louder than normal can facilitate hearing.
5. If it seems that the person you are talking with does not understand what you are saying, be patient, and rephrase what you have said.
6. It is often helpful to ask if you have been understood.

Assistive Devices

Hearing Aids

The most common assistive device is the hearing aid. While occupational therapists do not prescribe hearing aids, they often encounter individuals who use them. Those persons who use hearing aids and who also have vision or fine motor impairments may have difficulty replacing batteries, adjusting controls, and positioning the hearing aid. The therapist may work with the goal of independence in the use of the hearing aid. The therapist may also call on family members or others to provide assistance on a regularly scheduled basis, or the therapist, perhaps with a rehabilitation engineer, might work on finding "tools" that the person could use to work the controls or to assist in battery replacement. Typically, such tools would provide a larger implement for manipulating the device.

Alerting Devices

Among the most important types of devices for persons who are hearing impaired are those that alert them for some purpose. Those of us who have no serious hearing impairments take clock radios, doorbells, fire alarms, ringing telephones, and oven timers for granted. We use auditory signals to tell us important information about our environment. For persons with hearing impairments, failure to hear these auditory signals is not simply an inconvenience; it can be dangerous.

Today there are many applications of technology that help persons with hearing impairments receive signals from their environment. There are devices that can pick up the sound of specific appliances—telephones, doorbells, and others—and turn the sounds into tactile or visual signals, or even different sound signals that can be perceived. Vibration (tactile), light (visual), and sound are discussed below.

Vibration. For vibration to work as an alerting device, it must be in direct contact with the person. Vibration is a more private method than amplified sound or lights; a person can be "alerted" with vibration, and no one else in the area may be aware of the signal. This may or may not be a desirable feature, depending on the application. Some individuals are uncomfortable having a vibrator in constant contact with their body.

There are four types of vibrators that are used for alerting devices: (a) metal tube, (b) heavy-duty box, (c) extra-heavy-duty bedboard motor, and (d) wearable (Jensema, 1990). The first three types of vibrators are used to awaken people in bed. The fourth type, a wearable vibrator, is used by people as they move within their home or other building, or even outside.

The metal tube vibrator shown in Figure 3.2 is the most common. This vibrator can be sewn into a pillow, or bought already sewn into a pillow, and used for waking a person up. Unfortunately, vibrators use motors to create the vibration, and it is possible for a motor to overheat, especially if there is no automatic shut off. This is an important safety feature therapists should consider when purchasing a vibrator. The vibrator should have a shutoff so that there is essentially no risk of overheating.

Box-type vibrators work on a principle similar to the metal tube, but they contain larger and heavier parts. These may work better for heavy sleepers, but again, the danger of overheating must be considered.

The extra-heavy-duty bedboard motor is mounted directly on the frame of the bed. There is less chance of fire with these vibrators, because they are

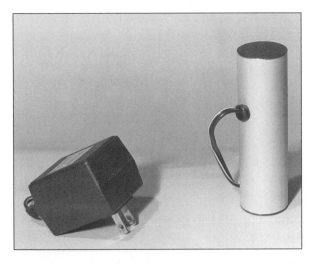

Figure 3.2. Metal tube vibrator.

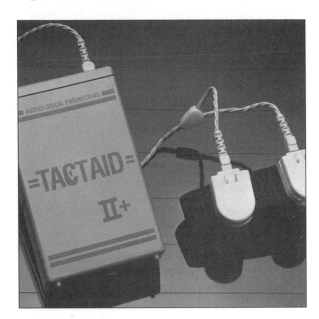

Figure 3.3. Wearable vibrator.

not in direct contact with the pillow or blankets. The permanence of the mounting is also an attractive feature; the user does not have to worry about tripping over electrical cords at night.

Wearable vibrators are attached to a belt, strapped against the body, or carried in a pocket. One type of wearable vibrator receives signals from special remote base units that pick up sounds of doorbells, telephones, and even the cry of a baby. Another type of wearable vibrator is self-contained, acting both to pick up the sound and to convert it into a vibration, but it is significantly more expensive. An example of a wearable vibrator is shown in Figure 3.3.

Table 3.1. Sample Alerting Products by Type of Display.

Device Description	Model No.	Manufacturer	Dealer	Cost
Sound				
Remote horn alert	SA-RH100	Sonic Alert	HARC	$55
Bell, indoor—extra loud	TEC 43015	TEC	Maxi-Aids	$15
Super Phone-Ringer	HAC-SR100	Ameriphone	HARC	$35
Vibration				
Quiet Awake—Silent Alarm Clock	QW-88	National Flashing Signal Systems	HARC	$50
Quest Alerting Systems	QS-Basic Sys	Quest Alerting Systems	HARC	$450
Shake-up Smoke Detector with Vibrator	CFU-5001-1	Global Assistive Devices	Maxi-Aids	$200
Light				
Micro-Strobe	MX-480	Tomar	HARC	$65
Alertmaster	15-AM-3000	Ameriphone	Maxi-Aids	$170
Sonic Alert—Personal Alert System for Deaf	M-731 Master Unit	Sonic Alert	HARC	$370 + Receivers

Light. Light is a lower-cost alternative to vibration, and it is also somewhat more flexible. Lights used as signals can vary from a very small LED up to a very powerful strobe. Some disadvantages of using light are that it may not be visible in a very brightly lit area, some lights are not as portable as vibration units, and a bright flashing light may distract or disturb to people.

One example of a special alerting device using light is a product that has a rotating light resembling the light on a police car. This sells for as little as $25.

Sound. Many persons with hearing impairments only have limited hearing. Increasing the volume of a sound may be sufficient to produce a recognizable alerting signal. The disadvantage of using loud sounds is the effect they have on others in the area who do not have a hearing impairment.

There are devices that will receive one type of sound and use the signal to set off a loud horn or buzzer. A comparison of products that use sound, vibration, and light is presented in Table 3.1.

Assistive Listening Devices

Assistive listening devices may be used when hearing aids are not sufficient to amplify sound, most often sounds produced by speech. An ALD consists of a microphone that captures the sound, an amplifier, and a headset for the person with the hearing loss (see Figure 3.4). There are three major types of ALD systems: FM, infrared, and hard-wired. Theaters and churches have begun to install FM and infrared systems. The hard-wired system is more often used in a home. While hearing aids are used to amplify all sounds, assistive listening devices are used to amplify sound while eliminating background noise. In the case of amplifying a speaker's voice, the assistive listening device has the effect of bringing the mouth of the speaker close to the ears of the listener with a hearing impairment. These devices are very portable, and prices range from $25 to $150. While the most expensive assistive listening devices have been shown to have more power and less noise, the $25 units may be more

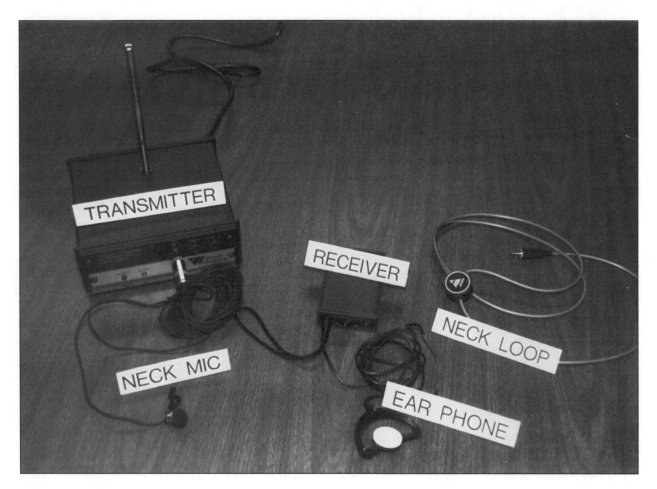

Figure 3.4. The components of an ALD system.

practical when background noise is not an important consideration.

Assistive listening devices are not a "miracle cure" for a person with a hearing impairment. They do increase understanding through amplification of sound without the background noise that a hearing aid would pick up in a large room. However, persons using assistive listening devices must also work at developing other skills to enhance understanding of communications. These other skills include taking advantage of the body language clues of the speaker and filling in gaps that might occur in the sounds heard. For persons who have had hearing impairments since they were very young, these skills are developed early in life. Someone who develops a hearing impairment in the later years of life may find it more difficult to develop these other skills and may withdraw from social interaction. Therapists should be alert for signs of withdrawal if a person has a hearing impairment.

Microphones. A microphone should be as near the source of the sound as possible to ensure an undistorted representation at the listener end, and to cut down on background noise. With one type of assistive listening device system, the microphone is directly wired to the amplifier. Microphones come in different sizes, and many very small microphones are now available that produce clear results. The advantage of a small microphone is that a person speaking can wear the microphone on a collar or clip it to a jacket or shirt pocket.

Systems. There are three methods available that eliminate the need to directly wire a microphone to the receiver/amplifier. The first is called an *audio induction loop*. This system uses electromagnetic induction to broadcast the microphone signal; the signal, in turn, is picked up by a telecoil within the hearing aid or other receiver. For relatively small installations, the audio loop system is least expensive. The disadvantage is that the signal is not of consistently high quality, because it

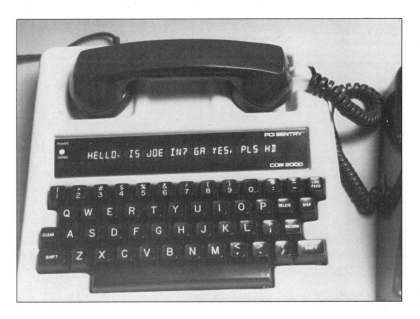

Figure 3.5. Text telephone (TTY).

depends on the location of the listener's telecoil relative to the audio loop.

A second method is *FM radio transmission*. The signal is broadcast from a transmitter, within or close to the microphone, and picked up by a small, pocket-size FM receiver/amplifier used by the listener. The advantages of the FM radio transmission system are that the FM signal passes through structures such as walls without weakening the signal, and it provides a consistent signal of good quality over a large area. The major disadvantage is the need to be sure there is no other similar FM radio signal being broadcast in the area.

An *infrared system* broadcasts a signal using infrared light, sent from the microphone-transmitter to an infrared receiver/amplifier. The major advantage of using an infrared system is that a single receiver can be used in a variety of settings, as the setup does not require tuning to a specific frequency. Physical barriers that block direct view of the infrared light beam will interfere with the reception of the infrared signal.

Receivers. There are many possibilities for the device at the listener's end. An earphone can be placed over the ear, or an ear bud can be placed into the outer ear canal. When earphones are placed over a hearing aid, feedback—a squeal—can result. Some hearing aids have a built-in telecoil, which can be switched on or off (referred to as the "T" switch). If there is an audio induction loop in the room, or if the person wears an induction loop around his or her

neck, the hearing aid with a telecoil can be used as the receiver for the assistive listening device. However, most hearing aids do not include a telecoil. In the past, the size of the coil and associated electronic parts required that a telecoil could only be incorporated into an over-the-ear type of hearing aid, rather than an in-the-ear type of hearing aid. However, new advances have now made it possible to place the telecoil within an in-the-ear hearing aid.

Assistive listening devices present a very useful technology for persons with limited hearing. Unfortunately, these systems are not very common. One reason is that few health care professionals are aware of assistive listening devices and therefore do not recommend them.

Telecommunication Devices

Telecommunication devices (TDDs), also referred to as text telephones (TTYs), are used to send printed messages through telephone lines. A TTY is simply a special telephone system. It consists of a small computer with a screen, keyboard, and modem. To communicate, there must be a TTY at each end of the telephone line. At one end the sender types a message into the telephone system. At the other end the message is visible as a line of text on a special telephone equipped with an LCD readout display. Ordinary telephone lines are used to transmit the signal, although special devices are needed at both ends. Figure 3.5 shows a picture of a TTY.

Coupled with a relay system, a TTY becomes a very powerful tool for persons with hearing impairments. Relay systems include a hearing operator who uses a TTY. A person with a hearing impairment can contact the relay system, send the message by TTY to the hearing operator, and have the hearing operator speak with the person whom the hearing-impaired person wishes to contact. Likewise, a hearing person who does not have a TTY can contact the relay system, and the relay operator can use the TTY to contact the person with a hearing impairment.

Telecommunication relay services are available nationwide. Under the Americans With Disabilities Act, relay services are required to operate 24 hours a day, 7 days a week. Operators are trained to ensure accuracy of conversations and are not permitted to limit the length of calls or disclose to others the contents of relayed conversations. The rates for relay calls do not exceed the rates charged for equivalent voice communications, based on such factors as duration of the call, time of day, and distance. There are now systems available that can be added to a computer to use TTY technology. A person with such a system could contact someone else with a more traditional TTY phone system, and the person with the traditional TTY phone system could communicate with the person with the computer system.

For individuals who have a hearing impairment but are not deaf, other assistive telecommunication devices are available. Most phone stores now carry telephone amplifiers and volume controls that either are built in or can be added to an existing phone. There are also hearing aid systems that permit a hearing aid to link directly with a phone.

Cochlear Implants

A new surgical procedure has been developed for profoundly deaf persons. Electrodes are implanted that bypass damaged hair cells that surround the cochlea, or inner ear. At present, the cochlear implant enables persons to hear sounds but not to discriminate speech. Most elders do not have the type of profound hearing loss that would require a cochlear implant.

The ear is a sense organ that captures and translates vibration in the air into signals that are transmitted to the brain. Within the cochlea, the organ of Corti has about 30,000 sensory receptor cells, called hair cells. When vibrations hit the small bones of the ear, this stimulates "waves" in the fluid of the cochlea. The waves are picked up by the hair cells and converted into electrical signals transmitted to the auditory nerve, which sends the signals to the brain. Severe hearing loss occurs when the hair cells do not function.

Cochlear implants were developed in the 1960s, and there are now more than 3,000 people using these devices. A cochlear implant has electrodes that bypass the hair cells and directly stimulate the auditory nerve. The UCSF/Storz cochlear implant is one of several now available. This implant has the following parts: an intra cochlear electrode, a surgical connector, a four-channel receiver, and an external speech processor. The patient information book describing the implant adds the following details:

Sixteen wire leads coming from the electrode in the cochlea are connected to the receiver capsule that is placed on the mastoid bone. The implanted receiver is capable of carrying four independent signal channels simultaneously. The signals are transmitted across the skin as radio waves and processed by the receiver to drive the electrode with a safety-limited signal. To accomplish this transmission there are four antennae implanted under the skin and a matching set placed externally behind the ear. The transmitters are located in the external antennae which sit on the side of the head with magnets. The transmitter is then connected to the speech processor, which hangs on a belt. The processor has a battery pack which lasts eight to ten hours. (Cochlear Implant Project: Patient Information Booklet)

Typically, a person with a cochlear implant will have several batteries and a battery recharger.

The cochlear implant has received much attention and has been hailed by some as "the cure" for deafness. It is indeed a remarkable application of technology, but it is not appropriate for all people, and it is not a miracle cure. The following statement was written by a woman shortly after receiving a cochlear implant. She had progressively lost her hearing over a period of 30 years. It expresses both the miraculous aspects of this technology and its limitations:

Exploration. I am trying to identify the sounds I hear. Some are obvious; tap water—the sound stops when I turn the tap off. I didn't know microwave ovens have a signal; I thought my computer board was silent. When I woke up this morning and put on the device, at first I couldn't identify a high whistling sound; then I realized it was the sound of my own breathing. Raindrops on the umbrella when I walked to work. I was surprised to realize that sound doesn't have direction. It's curious that I didn't think of that before. When I fantasized how it would be, the sound (mostly from people's voices) would come from wherever the person was. I'm getting a lot of sound, but voices are not readily identifiable as voices (except laughter— that characteristic rhythm is easy to understand). There is little (unless I am looking at the person) that distinguishes a voice from the background noise...sort of a low rumble and an occasional whistle. Hey! The turn indicator on the car makes a sound too—and when I pushed the button for the elevator, there was a "ping" when the red light went on and the elevator doors opened. The phone bell is loud, but the voice on the phone is not understandable, and I feel a little silly holding the receiver to my waist (the microphone is on the processor) instead of my ear. (Elliott, 1990)

We will see advances in surgical procedures that incorporate devices. Presently in the clinical trial stage, multi-channel cochlear implants consist of multiple electrodes inserted into the cochlea. The advantage over the first generation of single-channel cochlear implants is perception of distinct pitches or tones—which may lead to speech recognition.

Table 3.2. Definitions of Low Vision and Blindness.

Category of Vision Impairment	Best Possible Correction in Least–Impaired Eye
Moderate low vision	20/70 to 20/160
Legal blindness	20/200 or less in least impaired eye, or a visual field of 20° less diameter in less impaired
Total blindness	No usable vision

Future Prospects

A promising new technology is voice recognition systems for computers. This technology converts a person's speech into text output on a computer screen. At present the technology is still evolving. Because these systems offer great potential for the business community, there is much development work underway. With this large market, the systems will become more powerful and prices will fall. In the future, perhaps people with hearing impairment will be able to "read" what another person is speaking.

Visual Impairments

Overview

For noninstitutionalized persons, the prevalence of severe visual impairment is 6.5 persons per 1,000. There are significant differences in incidence according to family income (26.1 per 1,000 for the lowest income group versus 2.1 per 1,000 for the highest income group). For institutionalized persons, as many as 42% have at least some difficulty with vision, even with glasses, and 14% have severe visual impairment (Kirchner, 1988). Vision loss is greater among older persons than younger persons. More than 20% of noninstitutionalized persons over age 64

have difficulty reading due to a visual impairment. Five percent of persons over age 64 cannot see letters or words (Bureau of the Census, 1986). Most older persons with visual impairments have some functional vision. This residual vision is called *low vision.* Table 3.2 lists definitions for low vision and blindness.

The two major types of visual impairments are (a) central vision loss, and (b) peripheral field loss. Central vision provides the detail that is required for reading and recognizing people. Peripheral vision is not as clear as central vision, but enables a person to see a wider area. Loss of peripheral vision is sometimes referred to as *tunnel vision.*

Four major causes of vision loss are glaucoma, macular degeneration, a cataract, and diabetic retinopathy. Vision loss may also occur with stroke, retinal detachment, trauma, and tumors. Refer to Figure 3.6 while reading about each of these conditions in the following paragraphs.

Glaucoma (see Figure 3.7) is caused by pressure inside the eye that builds up as a result of a fluid that, under normal pressure, nourishes the eye and provides just enough pressure to maintain the eye's shape. There are no symptoms in the very early stages of glaucoma, which can occur as early as age 35. As the disease progresses, there is loss of periph-

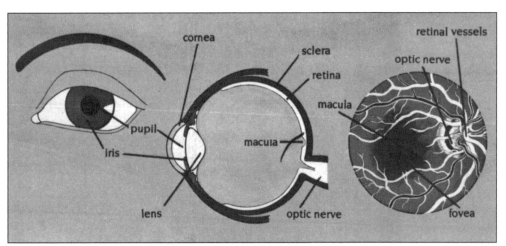

Figure 3.6. The eye. From *A Photographic Essay on Partial Sight.* Poster prepared by Eleanor Faye and Clare Hood (1989). New York: The Lighthouse. Used with permission.

eral field vision and blurred vision. Medication can be prescribed to reduce the intraocular pressure that causes glaucoma, but if glaucoma is not detected early, permanent loss of at least some vision can result.

A *cataract* (see Figure 3.8) is a clouding of the lens inside the eye. With a cataract on one or both eyes, a person will experience blurred vision, reduced ability to perceive color and contrast, and difficulty with driving at night and reading. Cataracts are typically removed surgically, and the lens of the eye is replaced by wearing thick glasses, contact lenses, or an intraocular lens that is surgically implanted.

Macular degeneration (see Figure 3.9) relates to a number of diseases of the macula—the back part of the eye that acts like the eye's camera and is responsible for detailed vision. Age-related macular degeneration occurs most frequently after age 50 and is the leading cause of vision loss among Americans over age 64. Macular degeneration causes loss of central vision, and symptoms include loss of clarity in the central visual field and distortion of straight lines. A new medical intervention uses laser treatment, which temporarily halts or retards the loss of vision.

Diabetic retinopathy (see Figure 3.10) occurs when retinal blood vessels "leak," which is associated with advanced or long-term diabetes. While not every person with diabetes will develop diabetic retinopathy, the chances of it occurring increase over time. In diabetic retinopathy, reading vision is impaired and variable. Print may be blurred or distorted. A cataract may also be present, in which case print is hazy as well as distorted.

Who Provides Services?

Eyeglasses are so common we do not think of them as an assistive device. Yet they are as much an assistive device as a button hook or an adapted computer. The authors of this book would not be able to drive to work, and would have great difficulty with reading and writing, without eyeglasses. The United States has one of the most advanced and organized systems of training professionals and providing services related to eyeglasses and contact lenses. These service providers include the following:

- An ophthalmologist is a physician (MD) who specializes in eye diseases.
- An optometrist (OD) is trained to assess vision loss and prescribe corrective lenses.
- An optician makes and dispenses corrective lenses.

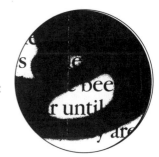

Figure 3.7. Glaucoma. From *A Photographic Essay on Partial Sight.* Poster prepared by Eleanor Faye and Clare Hood (1989). New York: The Lighthouse. Used with permission.

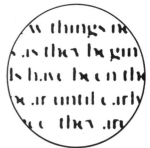

Figure 3.8. A cataract. From *A Photographic Essay on Partial Sight.* Poster prepared by Eleanor Faye and Clare Hood (1989). New York: The Lighthouse. Used with permission.

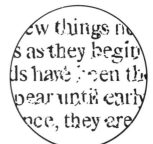

Figure 3.9. Macular degeneration. From *A Photographic Essay on Partial Sight.* Poster prepared by Eleanor Faye and Clare Hood (1989). New York: The Lighthouse. Used with permission.

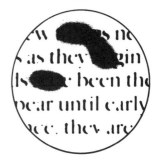

Figure 3.10. Diabetic retinopathy. From *A Photographic Essay on Partial Sight.* Poster prepared by Eleanor Faye and Clare Hood (1989). New York: The Lighthouse. Used with permission.

- Ophthalmologists, optometrists, and certain other professionals trained to work with persons with vision loss are referred to as *low-vision specialists.*

Orientation and mobility instructors are trained to work with persons with visual impairments on orientation to the home, orientation to areas outside the home, and travel skills. Rehabilitation teachers and occupational therapists provide rehabilitation and assistive devices for persons with visual impairments.

Some basic guidelines for assisting persons with visual impairments are provided in the numbered items listed below.

Adaptations for Persons With Vision Loss

1. Provide enlarged images.
2. Move objects closer to person, or move the person closer to objects.
3. Increase the amount of light.
4. Reduce or eliminate glare.
5. Provide contrast: light on dark, and reverse.

Individual Interactions

1. Let the person know you are talking with him or her.
2. Do not raise your volume of speaking unless you know that the person also has a hearing impairment.
3. When guiding a person with severe vision loss, allow the person to hold your arm and follow a few steps behind.
4. When leaving or entering a room, explain that you are doing so.
5. Don't wait to be asked to provide assistance. Ask the person with visual impairment if assistance is needed.

Low-Technology Assistive Devices

There are many very simple devices that can help people with low vision: pens that write in bold lines, paper lined for bold print, magnifying glasses, and so forth. Banks can print checks and deposit slips in large print, and writing guides are available that fit over a check and indicate where to write. Large-print reading materials are available for purchase in bookstores or for public use in libraries. Telephones with large-print buttons or dials are available from a number of sources. Self-threading needles and large-print versions of popular games provide opportunities for leisure activities. There are clocks and watches, thermometers, and blood sugar monitors with large print or voice output. The final chapter of this book lists sources for such products.

High-Technology Assistive Devices

In the last decade several new products have been introduced that offer very useful features for persons with visual impairments. These microprocessor-

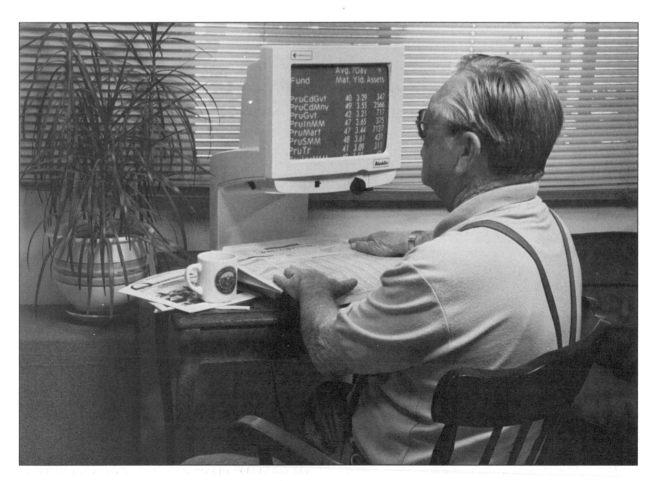

Figure 3.11. Aladdin CCTV. Photo courtesy of TeleSensory Corp.

Table 3.3. Character Enlargement Systems.

Product	Computer Platform	Company	Cost
CloseView	Macintosh	Included as part of the system software	Free
inFocus	IBM compatible DOS & Windows	AI Squared 802-362-3612	$149
inLarge	Macintosh	Berkeley Systems, Inc. 510-540-5535	$195
LP DOS Deluxe	IBM compatible DOS & Windows	Optelec US, Inc. 508-392-0707	$595
Lunar 2	IBM compatible DOS	EVAS 800-872-3827	$495
Lunar for Windows	IBM compatible DOS & Windows	EVAS 800-872-3827	$595
Screen Magnifier/2	IBM compatible DOS & Windows	IBM Direct Response Marketing 800-426-7630	$495
Magnum Deluxe	IBM compatible DOS & Windows	Artic Technologies 810-588-7370	$495
Magic Deluxe	IBM compatible DOS & Windows	Microsystems Software 508-626	$295
Vista	IBM compatible DOS & Windows	Telesensory Corp. 800-227-8418	$2,495
Zoomtext Plus	IBM compatible DOS & Windows	AI Squared 802-362-3612	$595

based products have become increasingly affordable as advances are made in the power of computers used in the mainstream economy. Enlarging the characters displayed on the screen, eliminating glare, adjusting contrast levels, and selecting foreground and background colors can make it possible for individuals with low vision to accomplish computer tasks. Large print labels on the keyboard make symbols easier to see, and therefore provide faster access to the keyboard. For individuals who are totally blind, speech or braille output devices provide access to the computer.

Stand-Alone Print Enlargement Systems (SPES)

Stand-alone print enlargement systems are sometimes referred to as closed-circuit television systems or CCTVs (see Figure 3.11). These are devices that electronically enlarge print and handwritten and graphic material onto a monitor screen. The compo-

nents include a camera with zoom lens and light source, a monitor, and a flat, moveable table. Material is placed face up on the table, which can be moved both horizontally and vertically. The area under the camera is displayed on the monitor in enlarged print. Models are available with 14", 17", and 19" monitors. Prices range from approximately $1,795 to $3,500 for a full-color display unit.

Character Enlargement Systems for Computers

Enlarging the size of the characters on a computer screen can be accomplished in a number of ways including using a magnification lens, selecting a large font size when available, using a large monitor, and using a character-enlargement program (see Figure 3.12). Character enlargement programs give the user many options. These include selecting magnification size (up to 16X), adjusting magnification

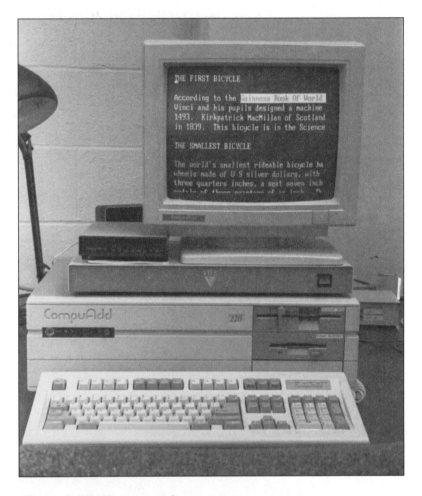

Figure 3.12. Character enlargement on a computer.

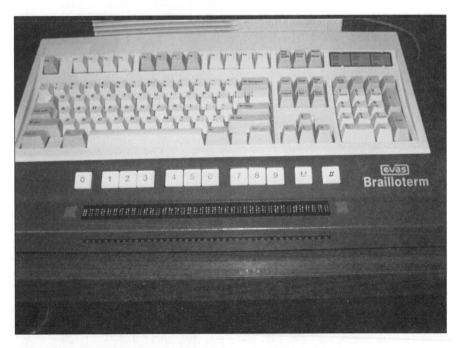

Figure 3.13. The Brailloterm "refreshable" Braille display system.

view (full screen, partial screen, single line), and selecting foreground and background colors for text and menu items. One disadvantage of a character-enlargement program is that only a small portion of the whole screen can be viewed at one time. The user must use keyboard commands or a mouse to move from top to bottom and left to right, in order to access all the information displayed on the current screen. Table 3.3 lists information on some of the major character enlargement systems.

Braille Output Devices

A number of devices produce braille. We are most accustomed to braille on a piece of paper. Many braille embossers are available that produce braille output when using a computer. Some are capable of printing sideways. This capability facilitates the printing of tables and statistical information in column format. The Duxbury Braille Translation Software is a program used to format information from a word processor into grade II braille for output to a braille embosser. This software costs $495 (available from Duxbury Systems, Inc.). A device called the Brailloterm (available from EVAS) offers a "refreshable" braille display (see Figure 3.13). Used with an IBM-compatible computer, characters displayed in a 40- or 80-character-long window on the computer screen are also displayed in braille. As the window on the screen moves, braille cells change.

Voice Output Systems

A number of systems are available that add a "voice" to the computer. For people who are blind, this provides a way of checking material they have typed. With material already in computer files, a person with a visual impair-

Table 3.4. Comparison of Voice Output Systems.

Product	Computer Platform	Company	Cost
ASAP	IBM compatible DOS	Microtalk Software 903-832-3471	$525
Business Vision	IBM compatible DOS	Artic Technologies 810-588-7370	$850 includes synthesizer
CompuSight Screen Reader	IBM compatible DOS	EVAS 800-872-3827	$395
Jaws	IBM compatible DOS	Henter-Joyce, Inc. 800-336-5658	$495
IBM Screen Reader	Versions available for DOS & OS/2	IBM Direct Response Marketing 800-426-7630	$648–$843
Master Touch	IBM compatible DOS	Humanware, Inc. 800-722-3393	$495
Omnichron Flipper	IBM compatible DOS	EVAS 800-872-3827	$495
outSpoken	Macintosh	Berkely Systems, Inc. 510-540-5535	$495
Protalk for Windows	IBM compatible Windows	EVAS 800-872-3827	$895
Screen Power	IBM compatible DOS	Telesensory Corp. 1-800-227-8418	$495
Soft Vert	IBM compatible DOS	Telesensory Corp. 1-800-227-8418	$495
Vert Pro	IBM compatible DOS	Telesensory Corp. 800-227-8418	$1,695 includes synthesizer
Vocal Eyes	IBM compatible DOS	G.W. Micro 219-483-3625	$450
Window Bridge	IBM compatible Windows	Syntha Voice Computers 905-662-0565	$595
WinVision	IBM compatible Windows	Artic Technologies 810-588-7370	$479

ment can have the computer "read" the contents of a file in spoken words. Hardware called a *speech synthesizer* may come as part of the computer system, as it does with a Macintosh computer; it may be sold separately; or it may come with software that provides the user interface. Table 3.4 lists information on some of the most popular voice output systems.

Audio Tactile Devices

The Nomad (see Figure 3.14) is a touch-sensitive pad with a built-in synthesizer that sends a signal to a computer, providing voice output. If you place a raised-line drawing on the Nomad, provide information to the computer about the drawing, and then touch a spot on the drawing, the computer will

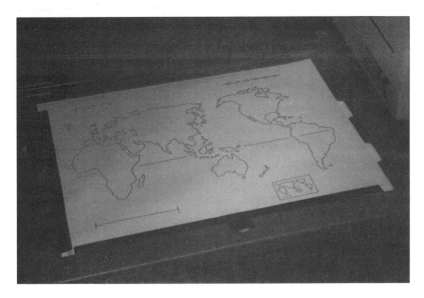

Figure 3.14. The Nomad can be programmed to "speak" when touched.

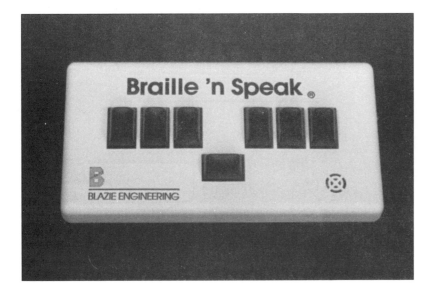

Figure 3.15. Braille portable notetaking device.

china marker. Once imaged, the tactile paper is inserted into the image enhancer, which creates a raised-line drawing. This device costs $895 and is available from Repro-Tronics, Inc. (800-948-8453).

Scanning Systems

A scanning system could be compared to a photocopy machine; some printed material is fed into the device, and it comes out in another form. With a photocopy machine you receive a second (or multiple) copies of the original printed material. With a scanner, you receive a second copy, but this second copy is digitized and may be stored as a computer file. The computer file can be used to produce (a) voice output, (b) print copy, (c) braille copy, or (d) braille on a refreshable braille display. The Open Book Unbound from Arkenstone includes a Hewlett Packard ScanJet IIIP scanner, optical character recognition software for IBM compatible computers with 8 megabytes of memory, and a software interface designed to work well with voice output systems. It costs approximately $1,600.

The Reading Edge, manufactured by Xerox Imaging Systems, combines a scanner, intelligent character recognition, and high-quality speech synthesis into a fully integrated, stand-alone reading machine for individuals who are blind or visually impaired. This devices weights 25 pounds and costs approximately $5,200.

"speak" a word or phrase related to the spot that is touched. For example, placing a raised-line map of the world on the Nomad would enable a person who is blind to explore the map and learn the shapes of the continents, and the relative locations of cities, rivers, and so on. The Nomad costs $1,495 (available from American Printing House for the Blind).

There are devices that produce raised-line drawings. The Tactile Image Enhancer is one such device. An image is placed on a piece of tactile paper using a copy machine or a laser printer, or drawn with a

Notetaking Devices and Laptop Computers

Portable devices are available to assist persons with visual impairments in taking notes. The Braille 'n Speak (see Figure 3.15) is a lightweight, portable electronic braille notetaking device with speech output. Internal memory in this device stores up to 800 pages of braille ($1,299, available from Blazie Engineering, 410-893-9333). A similar device, called the Braille Lite, includes the same features but incorporates an 18-cell refreshable braille display and costs $3,395. A third notetaking device marketed by

Table 3.5. Testing for Tactile Sensation.

Light touch	Touch person's fingertip with cotton or lightly with your finger.
Moving touch	Stroke person's finger with your finger.
Constant touch	Test with an instrument that applies a known pressure level to person's skin.
Two-point discrimination	Provide two simultaneous points of pressure.
Sterognosis	Test to see if person can identify objects in hand without seeing them.
Tactile localization	Test to determine if person can identify precisely where touch is applied.
Vibration	Touch person with a vibrating fork.

Blazie Engineering is the Type 'n Speak. Like the Braille 'n Speak and Braille Lite, it has a built-in talking word processor, spell checker, and scientific calculator. However, it uses a standard typewriter keyboard rather than the seven braille keys used by the Braille 'n Speak and Braille Lite for input. All these devices weigh less than 2 pounds and hold a battery charge for up to 15 hours.

Tactile Impairments

Overview

The skin holds receptors for the peripheral nervous system that provide very important information about the environment. While located throughout the body, they are most densely concentrated in the hand. With damage to the central or peripheral nervous system, loss of sensation can occur. This may lead to a need for an assistive device. The therapist must consider not only limitations of these senses, but also the presence of other impairments such as hearing or vision, because these senses have potential as a means of communication and interaction with the environment.

Pain is a protective sensation that alerts us to harmful elements in our environment. When we experience pain, we quickly seek a way to avoid or reduce it. When the sense of pain is absent, a person is more vulnerable to injury. Often the absence of pain occurs with other nervous system limitations, including those that affect cognition, making the potential for disaster even greater. Unfortunately, little attention has been directed at developing devices that address limitations of pain. Instead, therapists work with patients on developing habits to ensure safety.

Temperature sensation provides us with a means of knowing whether water, pots, and dishes are hot or cold. Like pain, temperature sensation is very important in avoiding injury, especially from burns. One common household device for people who have lost temperature sensation is a thermometer. Before bathing or drinking coffee, the temperature of the liquid should be taken. Therapists also help persons who have lost temperature sensation to establish safety practices, such as always using potholders when working with items on the stove.

Touch, or tactile sensation, is perhaps the most complex of the protective sensations. In determining impairments of touch, the therapist performs a number of short tests. Trombly (1989) provides an excellent description of these tests. Table 3.5 provides an overview of the types of pressure testing that therapists employ.

Applications of Technology Using Tactile Sensation

Applications of technology that call upon tactile sensation have focused more on the deaf population than on any other disability group. The primary mechanism for "alerting" the tactile system is vibration. Earlier in this chapter we discussed alerting devices that use sound and light or vibration.

Several studies have examined the use of vibration for communication with persons who are deaf. A relatively early study tested the efficacy of a vibrotactile aid, the SRA-10, over a 9-month period with four profoundly deaf preschool children; it determined that use of vibrotactile stimulation did enhance communication (Friel-Patti & Roeser, 1983). Two more recent studies found similar positive results of applying vibration for additional input for persons with residual hearing and with lip-reading. One study determined that "the electrotactile aid may be useful for patients with little residual hearing and for the severely to profoundly hearing-impaired, who could benefit from the high-frequency information presented through the tactile modality, but unavailable through hearing aids" (Cowan, Alcantara, Blaney, Whitford, & Clark, 1989, p. 2593). The other study determined increased recognition of vowel and consonants with an electrotactile aid (Alcantara, Cowan, Blaney, & Clark, 1990). Another study examined the ability to discriminate vowels with an eight-channel cochlear implant and with a vibration device, a tactile vocoder that provided vibratory patterns on a fingertip. This study found that vowel discrimination becomes possible with either device, when eight or more channels are used (Ifukube, 1989).

The sense of touch has long been used by persons who are blind to substitute for the visual impairment. Braille relies on the ability to discriminate raised dots on a page. Tactile mapping and graphs with raised lines have also been used to provide access to information. Using alternative senses when one sense is impaired has not yet been fully explored. For example, sound has only recently been studied as a way to convey graphical information for persons who are blind. Computer-generated sound patterns were used in a study to represent two-dimensional line graphs. This study determined that "mathematical concepts such as symmetry, monotonicity, and the slopes of lines could be determined quickly using sound" (Mansur, Blattner, & Joy, 1985).

For persons who are both deaf and blind, the sense of touch is extremely important. Zuckerman (1984) published one of the first papers exploring the use of a Morse code system with a vibrotactile device linked with a computer and used for communication. This approach makes it possible for a person who is deaf and blind to "sense" what he or she has typed—what is on the screen—through the vibrotactile device. It also serves as a communication device. A sighted person can see what is on the computer screen and type information back that is sent out to the person through the vibrotactile device.

The use of vibration offers a rich area for future research. Many questions remain unanswered. We have demonstrated that vibration can be used by persons with other sensory impairments. But what are the optimal vibration "conditions"? One study examined this question and determined "the optimum set of parameters for minimum power and minimum

sensitivity are 250 Hz frequency of stimulation, 2-second recovery time, 10 pulses per burst, and a 1/25 duty cycle" (Nunziata, Perez, Jarmul, Lipetz, & Weed, 1989, p. 423). These numbers may have little immediate value for the therapist who is interested in applying the technology, but they are a beginning in building new devices that will provide the optimal conditions for using vibration-based assistive devices.

Chapter 3 References

Alcantara, J.I., Cowan, R.S., Blaney, P.J., & Clark, G.M. (1990). A comparison of two training strategies for speech recognition with an electrotactile speech processor. *Journal of Speech and Hearing Research, 33*(1), 195–204.

Bureau of the Census. (1986). *Disability, functional limitation, and health insurance coverage: 1984–85 current population reports, series P-70, #8.* Washington, DC: U.S. Government Printing Office.

Cochlear Implant Project: Patient Information Booklet (Clinical Series). University of California, San Francisco, Department of Otolaryngology, San Francisco, CA 94143; Coleman and Eastern Laboratories; and Storz Instrument Co., 3365 Tree Court Industrial Blvd., St. Louis, MO 63122.

Cowan, R.S., Alcantara, J.I., Blaney, P.J., Whitford, L.A., & Clark, G.M. (1989). Speech perception studies using a multichannel electrotactile speech processor, residual hearing, and lip reading. *Journal of the Acoustical Society of America, 86*(6), 2593–2607.

Elliott, H. (1990). My experience with a cochlear implant. *International Journal of Technology and Aging 3*(2), 151–159.

Friel-Patti, S., & Roeser, R.J. (1983). Evaluating changes in the communication skills of deaf children using vibrotactile stimulation. *Ear and Hearing, 4*(1), 31–40.

Glass, L.E. (1986). Rehabilitation for deaf and hearing-impaired elderly. In S.J. Brody & G.E. Ruff (Eds.), *Aging and rehabilitation* (pp. 218–236). New York: Springer.

Hotchkiss, D. (1989). *The hearing-impaired elderly population: Estimation, projection, and assessment, monograph series A, #1.* Washington, DC: Gallaudet Research Institute.

Ifukube, T. (1989). Discrimination of synthetic vowels by using tactile vocoder and a comparison to that of an eight-channel cochlear implant. *Trans Biomedical Engineering, 36*, 1085–1091.

Jensema, C.J. (1990). Specialized audio, visual, and tactile alerting devices for deaf and hard-of-hearing people.

Gallaudet Research Institute Occasional Paper 90-2. Washington, DC: Gallaudet University.

Kirchner, C. (1988). *Data on blindness and visual impairment in the U.S.* New York: American Foundation for the Blind.

Mansur, D.L., Blattner, M.M., & Joy K.I. (1985). Sound graphs: A numerical data analysis method for the blind. *Journal of Medical Systems, 9*(3), 163–174.

Nunziata, E., Perez, C., Jarmul, E., Lipetz, L.E., & Weed H.R. (1989). Effect of tactile stimulation pulse characteristics on sensation threshold and power consumption. *Annals of Biomedical Engineering, 17,* 423–425.

Public Health Service. (1988). *Prevalence of selected chronic conditions, United States, 1983–1985, advance data from vital and health statistics, #155* (DHHS Publication No. PHS 88-1250). Hyattsville, MD: Author.

Trombly, C.A. (1989). *Occupational therapy for physical dysfunction* (3rd ed.). Baltimore: Williams & Wilkins.

Zuckerman, D. (1984). Use of personal computing technology by deaf-blind individuals. *Journal of Medical Systems, 8,* 431–436.

Chapter 3 Study Questions

1. List the three major types of hearing loss. Describe the kinds of environmental approaches you would take to enhance communication and the types of devices that might be appropriate for persons with each condition.

2. Contact three organizations that frequently host large numbers of people (e.g., church, movie theater, or concert hall) to determine the accommodations they make for persons with hearing impairments. Be prepared to describe to them possible options for large facilities.

3. List the four major causes of vision loss and describe the effect they have on vision.

4. List 10 "low-tech/no-tech" steps you can take to improve communication and help a person with a visual impairment interact with the environment.

5. Describe seven categories of assistive devices for persons with visual impairments.

6. Describe the importance of the sensations of pain, temperature, and touch.

Chapter 4:
Assistive Communication Technologies for Persons With Expressive Communication and Cognitive Disabilities

I. Communication and Communication Disorders
- A. Individuals With Severe Communication Disabilities
- B. Etiologies of Severe Communication Disorders
    1. Dysarthria
    2. Apraxia
    3. Aphasia
    4. Traumatic Brain Injury
    5. Degenerative Diseases
    6. Laryngectomy
    7. Specific Language Impairments
    8. Cognitive Challenges
    9. Physical Disabilities

II. Speech Production Aids and Augmentative Communication Technologies
- A. Speech Production Aids
    1. Speech Aids for Laryngectomies
    2. Speech Amplification Systems
    3. Speech Training Technologies
    4. Speech Recognition Systems
- B. Augmentative Communication Systems
    1. Physical Access to Augmentative Communication Technologies
    2. Symbol Systems
    3. Augmentative Communication Aids

III. Learning Tools
- A. Language Learning Tools
- B. Augmented Literacy Instruction
- C. Cognitive Aids

IV. Service Delivery for Augmentative Communication
- A. Augmentative Communication Assessment Protocol
    1. Background Information
    2. Needs Analysis
    3. Capabilities Assessment
    4. Observation
    5. Technology Access
    6. Cognitive Status
    7. Speech
    8. Language

V. Summary

4.

Assistive Communication Technologies for Persons With Expressive Communication and Cognitive Disabilities

D. Jeffery Higginbotham, PhD, Susan Lawrence-Dederich, MA, Rae M. Sonnenmeier, MA, and Kyung-Eun Kim, MA

Communication and Communication Disorders

Expressive communication is comprised of two distinct abilities or skills. In order for individuals to communicate their ideas in specific situations, they need to be able to select words and organize them into sentences. The rules governing such choices are referred to as *language and social communication skills.* The words and sentences need to be conveyed so that someone else may understand them. Most often this is accomplished through *speech,* although it may also occur through writing. An individual may have difficulties in either or both of these areas that result in a communication disorder. Such disorders are identified and treated by *speech–language pathologists.* If the communication disorder is so severe that the individual's speech is not understood by others, he or she may need to support communication attempts through other means, referred to as *augmentative communication.* Such support may include the use of sign language, communication boards, and electronic and computer technologies (see Figure 4.1).

This chapter will briefly review various etiologies that lead to communication disorders in individuals who may benefit from the use of augmentative communication technologies. It will also describe the types of devices and software available to develop and support communication, and outline service delivery strategies used by speech–language pathologists and other professionals involved in providing services to those with severe communication disabilities.

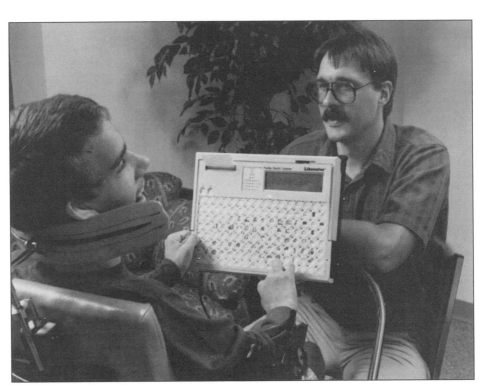

Figure 4.1. A conversational interaction using an augmentative communication device. Photograph courtesy of the Prentke Romich Co., Inc.

Individuals With Severe Communication Disabilities

It has been conservatively estimated that 1 to 2 million persons in the United States are unable to employ speech for communication purposes (ASHA, 1981; Blackstone, 1986). Between 0.3% and 0.6% of the total school-age population and from 3.5% to 7% of students receiving special education services have severe speech impairments and may benefit from the use of augmentative communication technologies (Shane, 1986). The inability to talk has been regarded as one of the most debilitative and socially stigmatizing of all disabling conditions—particularly by its victims (Beukelman & Mirenda, 1992; Brooks, 1986; Creech & Viggiano 1981; Higginbotham & Yoder, 1982).

Common to all individuals with severe communication disorders are the tremendous discrepancies between their communication competencies and their ability to express themselves. Augmentative communication device users Creech and Viggiano (1981) and Brooks (1986) speak of the years of loneliness, strained social relationships, and inappropriate educational interventions associated with their inability to speak. Pettygrove (1982) describes the psychosocial ramifications of being regarded as socially incompetent on the basis of one's unintelligible speech. Without appropriate technological and social-behavioral interventions, the results of this type of disability lead to increasing frustration on the part of the individual with severe communication disabilities, the diminishment of self-esteem, the erosion of communicative competence, and increasing stigmatization by society (Higginbotham & Yoder, 1982; Pettygrove, 1982). For children with severe communication disabilities, the lack of appropriate and effective means of communication can be particularly devastating because it denies them the means to actively engage in the educational process and condemns them to a life of dependency.

Etiologies of Severe Communication Disorders

A variety of diverse etiologies may affect an individual's communication skills to such an extent that he or she may benefit from the support of augmentative communication technologies. Some individuals acquire disabilities that affect speech production or the use of language due to an injury to the brain or a degenerative disease. Other individuals are born with disabilities that affect their ability to speak or use language effectively. Characteristics of various communication disorders are described below.

Dysarthria

Dysarthria refers to a group of speech disorders caused by weakness, paralysis, slowness, incoordination, or sensory loss in the muscle groups responsible for speech (Brookshire, 1992). Individuals born with cerebral palsy, as well as those who have had a traumatic brain injury or stroke, may exhibit dysarthria. Speech characteristics include difficulty having enough breath support, resulting in short, choppy sentences; imprecise articulation; and difficulty controlling pitch, intonation, and speech rate. In some cases, efficient communication can be achieved with the support of augmentative communication to clarify what the individual is attempting to say.

Apraxia

Apraxia is the term used to describe the deficiencies in the voluntary movements of the speech articulators in the absence of paralysis or sensory loss (Brookshire, 1992). Apraxia may be developmental or acquired due to an injury to the brain. Individuals who have apraxia are usually able to speak more clearly if they are spontaneously responding to something or giving an automatic response. Difficulties arise when they are asked to give a response on demand, such as when answering a specific question. Speech patterns observed in apraxia include substitutions of sounds due to imprecise placement of the articulators, errors where one sound is produced in anticipation of another sound, and overall inconsistency of the speech errors (Brookshire).

Aphasia

Aphasia refers to a communication disorder that affects language skills, resulting from a cerebral vascular accident (stroke). The four primary areas of language functioning (listening, speaking, reading, and writing) are frequently affected (Brookshire, 1992). Difficulties with the auditory comprehension of language are often central to aphasia, because an individual has trouble understanding what has been said. Speaking may be affected because sometimes an individual is only able to say a few words in a slow and halting fashion, as with Broca's aphasia, or may only be able to form sentences whose meaning is unclear, as with Werniche's aphasia. An individual's speech may present characteristics of dysarthria or apraxia following the stroke. For some individuals, the ability to comprehend or produce written language may also be impaired, due either to the inability to form meaningful sentences as a result of the language impairment, or to paralysis that affects the physical act of writing.

Traumatic Brain Injury

Accidents may also result in a communication disorder. A *traumatic brain injury* is caused by a sudden blow to the head, as when a rapidly moving object hits the head or when the head strikes a stationary object (Brookshire, 1992). Patients are usually unconscious during the initial stages following the accident. As the patient recovers, cognitive skills related to communication are often affected, including memory skills, abstract reasoning and judgment, and the ability to tolerate noise and distractions (Brookshire). These difficulties may lead to trouble following directions, poor organizational skills, and difficulties recalling newly acquired information. Dysarthria and apraxia, as well as reading and writing difficulties, may also be present.

Degenerative Diseases

Degenerative diseases such as dementia, Parkinson's disease, muscular dystrophy, amyotrophic lateral sclerosis (ALS), and so forth affect the central nervous system in one way or another. These diseases often result in dysarthria, leading to an eventual inability to speak at all. An early sign of dementia is poor memory. In these cases, the primary goal of intervention is to maintain an individual's quality of life, including effective and efficient communication.

Laryngectomy

Individuals may also lose their ability to talk due to cancer of the head and neck. In particular, cancer of the larynx, where the vocal folds are located, frequently results in a *laryngectomy,* in which the larynx is removed. This eliminates an individual's ability to adequately produce the sound needed for speech.

Specific Language Impairments

Many individuals are born with disabilities that affect their development of speech and language. Some children have *specific language impairments* in which they develop normally in all areas except communication skills. They acquire language more slowly than their peers and may always have difficulty with communication, including reading and writing. Some suggest that specific language impairments are a form of *learning disability* (Swisher, 1994). Individuals' abilities are affected in

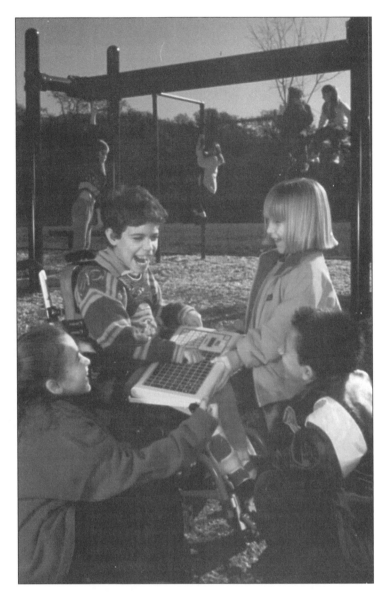

Figure 4.2. Children interacting using a Phonic Ear VOIS 160 communication device. Photograph courtesy of Phonic Ear, Inc.

one or more of the basic psychological processes involved in understanding or using spoken or written language that affect areas such as reading, spelling, and the ability to perform mathematical calculations (P.L. 94-142, The Education of All Handicapped Children Act).

Cognitive Challenges

Individuals may also experience difficulties with communication due to *cognitive challenges*. Swisher (1994) outlines a number of causes of cognitive challenges including chromosomal disorders (e.g., Down's syndrome, fragile-X syndrome), toxins experienced before birth (e.g., fetal alcohol syndrome, drug exposure), and trauma experienced before or during birth (e.g., anoxia that restricts the flow of oxygen to the brain at birth). Cerebral palsy and other motor disabilities may also be present, leading to dysarthria in addition to language difficulties. Autism and pervasive developmental disorders are characterized by difficulties in social interactions, delayed language development, and difficulties developing play and other imaginative activities (Swisher). Many individuals with these disabilities do not speak and must rely on other means of communication. Those who do speak may use language in unusual ways, including "echolalia," in which they repeat what others say, use unusual intonation patterns and phrasings, and repeat the same topics from one interaction to the next.

Physical Disabilities

Individuals with severe *physical disabilities* may not be able to control the movements of their bodies sufficiently to allow for spoken or written communication. These individuals may or may not have language impairments or cognitive challenges in addition to their physical needs. The physical disabilities may also affect an individual's ability to interact with his or her environment (e.g., by reaching for objects, walking, etc.), which may also require assistive technology. Those with severe physical challenges due to cerebral palsy, muscular dystrophy,

other neurological involvement, and so forth may not be able to use computer technologies through usual means (e.g., typing). Adapted access may need to be considered to allow for the use of augmentative communication technologies (see Figure 4.2).

As the etiologies associated with severe communication disabilities are diverse, so are the augmentative communication technologies that have been developed to support individuals' effective and efficient communication. The various types of technologies, as well as clinical considerations, are discussed below.

Speech Production Aids and Augmentative Communication Technologies

To date, more than 700 different technologies are commercially available to improve the expressive communication and cognitive functioning of persons with disabilities (Trace Research and Development Center, 1994). These assistive technologies fall into four general categories:

1. devices that are used to improve speech production,
2. augmentative communication systems that provide an alternative means to speak and write,

Table 4.1. Speech Production Aids.

Name	Description	Manufacturer	Price
Technologies for Laryngectomies	Artificial larynges substitute a mechanical vibration for natural laryngeal voice. Both hand-held and intraoral models are available.	Luminaud Artificial Speech Aids AT&T Health Concepts, Inc. Simens Hearing	$190–$400 $90 $130 $2,750 $560
Voice Amplification Systems	Voice amplifier systems increase the volume of the speech sound for individuals with weak voices. Microphones can be either hand-held or mounted on a lightweight headset.	Luminaud Crestwood Co. AT&T Williams Sound Corp. Park Surgical Co. Inc.	$80–$160 $15 $80 $300 $270–$320
Speech Training Aids	Computer technology designed to facilitate assessment and training of speech and voice problems.	Micro Video (APPLE II, DOS, MAC) IBM Corp.	$3,500 $900
Voice Recognition	Computer hardware and software "interprets" a user's speech patterns and responds by performing computer commands or typing the user's spoken words.	Articulate Systems (MAC) Dragon Systems (DOS) Apple Computer	$2,500 $9,000 free

3. computer software that supports the learning of basic skills and language concepts, and

4. cognitive training software to support the development and retraining of memory, organization, and reasoning skills.

In recent years each of these technology types has benefited greatly from developments in microelectronics and computer technologies. The following sections describe many of the current technologies used in each of the areas.

Speech Production Aids

Many individuals with communication disabilities have difficulties producing intelligible speech. Technological solutions to these problems include (a) devices that modify the communicator's own speech, (b) technology to assist in training intelligible speech, and (c) technologies that provide alternate means of communication by translating a user's keystrokes or switch selections into printed text or artificial speech. A summary of various speech production aids is presented in Table 4.1.

Speech Aids for Laryngectomies

For an individual whose larynx (voice box) is removed and who is unable to benefit from esophageal speech therapy or surgical procedures, an *electrolarynx* may be used to restore speech function. An electrolarynx consists of a portable vibrator that produces a noise. Several of these devices are shown in Figures 4.3 and 4.4. Some models are held against the neck. The vibration produced by the diaphragm at the end of the device produces a sound in the oral cavity that is articulated into human speech sounds. Other electrolarynges employ a plastic tube attached to the diaphragm and inserted into the mouth. This

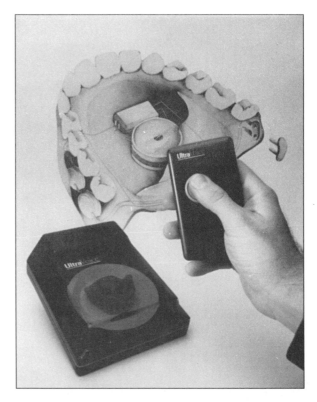

Figure 4.4. The Ultravoice dental electrolarynx. Photograph courtesy of Health Concepts, Inc.

type of intraoral electrolarynx can be used just after the operation or by individuals who are unable to achieve appropriate placement on the neck. The newest electrolarynx technology involves placing the vibratory mechanism into a dental prosthesis. Voicing is created by pressing a hand-held buzzer that operates the device via radio control.

Figure 4.3. Variety of artificial larynx devices. From J.B. Tomblin, H. Morris, & D.C. Spriestersbach, 1994. *Diagnosis in Speech-Language Pathology*, San Diego, CA: Singular Publishing Group Inc. Copyright © 1994; reprinted by permission.

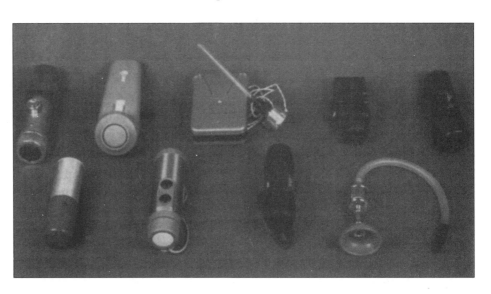

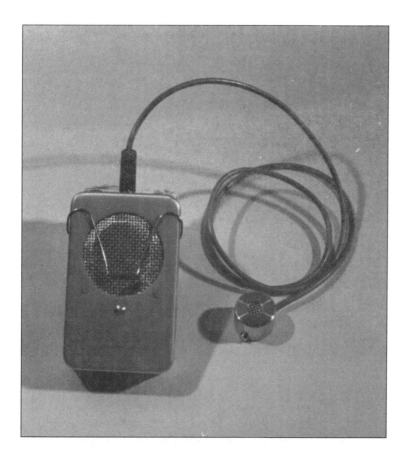

Figure 4.5a. The Rand Voice Amplifier. Photograph courtesy of Luminaud, Inc.

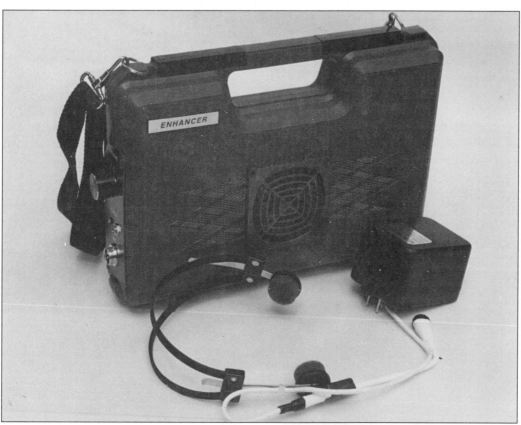

Figure 4.5b. The Speech Enhancer. Photograph courtesy of Luminaud, Inc.

Speech Amplification Systems

Individuals with weak voices due to injury or disease can benefit from voice amplification systems. These systems consist of a small microphone attached to a headset and a small amplifier that boosts the speaker's voice so that it can be clearly heard in noisy environments (e.g., a party) or on occasions in which a loud, clear-sounding voice is important (e.g., a lecture). Figures 4.5a and 4.5b present examples of these devices.

Speech Training Technologies

Over recent years, speech-language pathologists have begun to use computers to facilitate and document voice and speech production therapy. Computers can perform rapid and accurate acoustic analyses of the pitch, loudness, duration, voicing, and resonant characteristics of an individual's speech. By providing feedback to users regarding the accuracy of their speech production, computerized speech training systems can guide the individual in progressively approximating speech targets.

The IBM Speechviewer™ (Figure 4.6), for example, provides a game-like interface for motivation and visual feedback on the accuracy of an individual's speech production. The Speechviewer can also provide acoustic analysis of an individual's speech patterns and track his or her clinical performance.

Speech Recognition Systems

With recent technical advances in computer technology, many new computers are capable of recognizing and responding to human speech. *Speech recognition* systems are now found on many of today's off-the-shelf computer systems, for little or no extra cost. Apple computers has developed "Plaintalk™," which, with repeated exposure to someone's voice, can "learn" to respond to human voice commands by performing a variety of prespecified activities (e.g., "save file"). Comparable speech recognition systems are available for DOS and Windows-based micro-

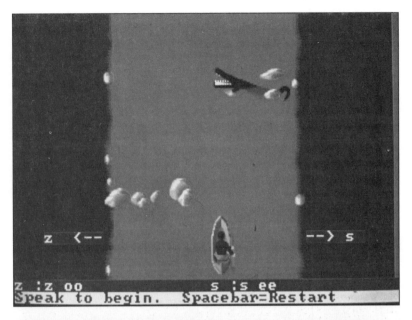
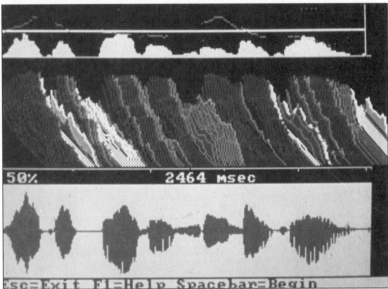

Figure 4.6. Screen dump of a speech training game and a speech spectrogram produced by the IBM Speechviewer. Photograph courtesy of IBM Corporation.

computers. More powerful speech recognition technologies are capable of recognizing up to 30,000 individual words when spoken at a rate of about 40 words per minute (150 wpm is average for normal speech production purposes). These technologies are used by persons with severe physical disabilities—but essentially normal speech—to vocally control a microcomputer and to generate text materials for word processing and database management.

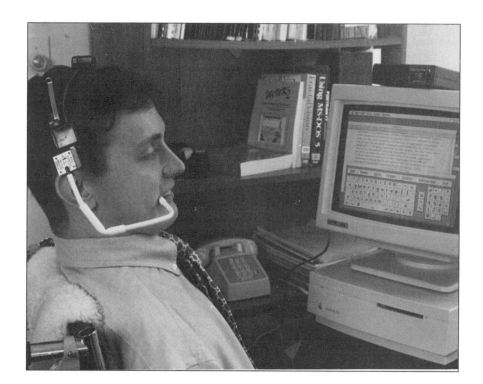

Figure 4.7. Individual using the Headmaster acoustic pointer for computer access Photograph courtesy of Prentke Romich Co., Inc.

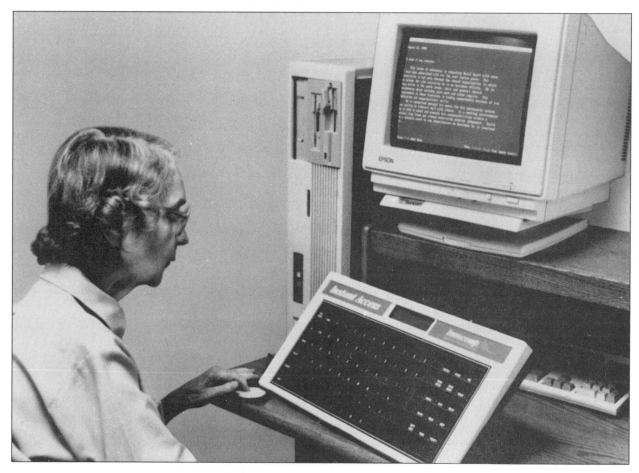

Figure 4.8. Individual using a switch with Innocomp Instant Access keyboard to operate a computer. Photograph courtesy of Innocomp, Inc.

Augmentative Communication Systems

For individuals who are unable to use speech as their primary means of communication, augmentative and alternative communication technologies can provide a means for spoken and written communication. Today, augmentative communication technologies consist of (a) nonelectronic and electronically enhanced methods to provide technology access for persons with physical disabilities, (b) symbol and code systems for use by persons with language learning difficulties and/or for efficient retrieval of stored information, and (c) printed text and artificial speech output to enhance intelligibility. Other persons with language learning difficulties can use these technologies to assist with written language.

Physical Access to Augmentative Communication Technologies

A wide range of technologies has been developed to help individuals who have problems controlling their movement patterns or making the movements necessary to access a computer or augmentative communication aid. The majority of these technologies consist of:

- modifiable keyboards,
- switches,
- joysticks, and
- long-range electronic pointers (acoustic, optical, laser), and software to adapt a standard computer for alternate access.

Figures 4.7 and 4.8 illustrate how such adapted access technologies are used by individuals. These access technologies are covered in depth by Sprigle and Lane (see Chapter 2).

Symbol Systems

A wide variety of graphic-based symbol systems are used on nonelectronic and electronic augmentative communication devices (see Table 4.2). These symbol systems range from photographs, to simple concrete representational line drawings, to more abstract and rule-based symbol sets. Figure 4.9 shows how several of these systems portray various vocabulary items. When using nonelectronic technologies, a user points to the symbol that represents a need or

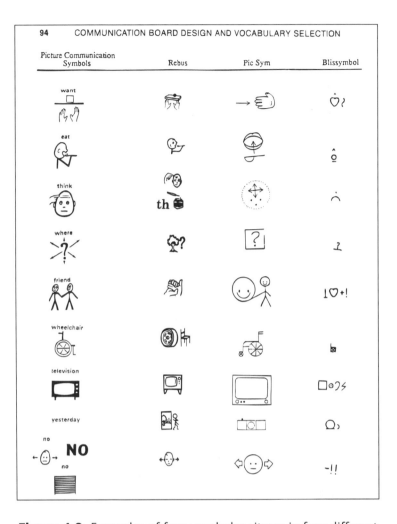

Figure 4.9. Examples of four vocabulary items in four different symbol systems. From S. Brandenburg, & G. Vanderheiden, 1988. Communication board design and vocabulary selection. In L. Bernstein (Ed.), *The vocally impaired: Clinical practice and research,* (p. 94). Copyright © 1988 by Allyn and Bacon; reprinted/adapted by permission.

thought. His or her communication partner then reads the text printed below the symbol and guesses the user's intended message based on the partner's relationship with the user and interpretation of the event.

Computer technology replaces the need for interpretation by the communication partner by translating the user's letter or symbol selections and producing printed text or artificial speech. In order to improve communication speed and efficiency, letters and symbols can serve as codes to access larger chunks of information stored in the computer system. For example, the user may type in a string of symbol codes (e.g., apple, car) or a letter-based abbreviation (e.g., BK) to produce a message such as "I want to

Table 4.2. Symbol Systems.

Name	Description	Manufacturer	Price
Technologies for Symbols	Photographs, line drawings, abstract symbols used on nonelectronic and electronic devices. They may be used by persons who are unable to read text, or serve as code elements for computerized technologies.	Blissymbolics Mayer-Johnson Crestwood Co. Baggeboda Press	$20–$260 $10–$50 $20–$130 $30
Computerized Symbol Databases	Database programs containing large numbers of symbols. Symbol vocabulary can be searched, organized, and printed using the included software programs.	Don Johnston (MAC) Mayer-Johnson 　(MAC, WIN)	$50–$650 $300–$400

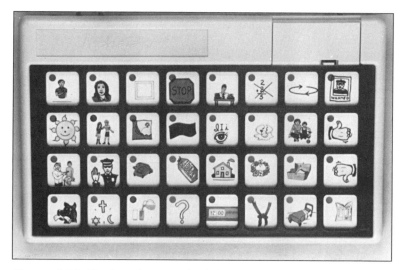

Figure 4.10. The Prentke Romich AlphaTalker digitized speech communication device with MiniSymbols. Photograph courtesy of Prentke Romich Co.

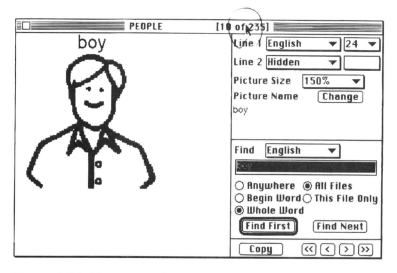

Figure 4.11. The Mayer-Johnson Boardmaker symbol database.

go to Burger King." Figure 4.10 shows a set of Minspeak™ symbols on a Prentke Romich AlphaTalker™. The vocabulary and codes are frequently programmed into the system by a communicator or his or her clinician. Recently, some large-scale vocabulary systems have been preprogrammed on the device or have become available for separate purchase. Preprogrammed vocabularies can save the user or specialist many hours of programming effort, but may require modification depending on the communicator's specific needs and capabilities.

Computerized symbol system databases and communication board layout tools have also been designed to facilitate the development of symbol boards and electronic communication aids. Instead of photocopying symbols from a book and cutting and pasting them onto communication boards, the clinician queries a database for the right symbol, then transfers it to a computerized layout of the communication device. When the symbols are arranged in the appropriate fashion, the communication board is printed out. A number of companies now provide symbol database software for their own equipment, as well as for other manufacturers' equipment (see Figure 4.11). Don Johnston Developmental Equipment Corporation recently released a CD-ROM containing several symbol sets and layout tools.

Augmentative Communication Aids

Letters and symbol systems are usually placed on various augmentative communication devices to allow communication. These technologies vary from common nonelectronic means of communication to sophisticated microcomputer-based systems. *Nonelectronic communication systems* incorporate letters, words, and/or symbols into communication boards and books, providing a highly portable and durable technology for interactive communication.

Other nonelectronic technologies rely on eye gaze. For example, an *Etran board* (as shown in Figure 4.12a) consists of a large square of Plexiglas mounted upright between the communicator and his or her partner. Pictures or graphic symbols are placed on the periphery of the plexiglass square. The partner can then determine what the communicator wants by tracking his or her eye gaze. The *Eye-Link board* (see Figure 4.12b) utilizes a similar approach. It consists of a thin, clear Mylar sheet with letters or pictures mounted on its surface, held by the communication partner. To communicate, the user looks at each letter or picture. The partner then slowly moves the Eye-Link until their eyes "link" or achieve a mutual gaze. The communicator then looks at the next picture or letter and the process continues.

Although nonelectronic technologies are very durable and often foster the intimacy needed for interpersonal exchanges, they require the immediate presence of a cooperative partner. *Electronic communication aids* allow the user to construct messages independent of other individuals and to express those messages through print, sound, and speech output. As presented in Table 4.3, these devices include both dedicated communication aids and adapted microcomputers. Dedicated communication aids utilize computer technologies and are designed specifically to facilitate the communication of disabled individuals. They typically:

- are portable,
- are durable,
- provide alternate methods of access,
- support text and/or graphic symbol communication,
- provide digitized and/or synthetic speech output, and
- interface with other computers and environmental controls.

Standard microcomputers are modified through software or utilize computer peripherals like an adapted keyboard. Although not as portable or durable as

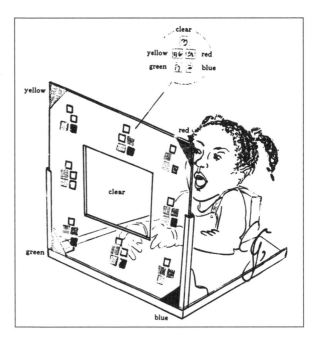

Figure 4.12a. Child using a transparent Etran communication board. Copyright © 1987, Decker Periodical; reprinted by permission.

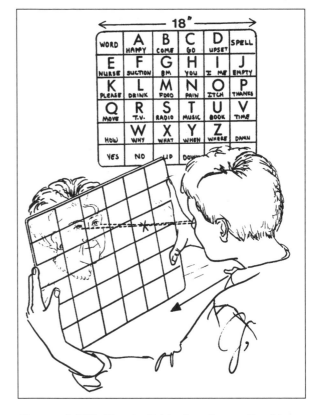

Figure 4.12b. Two individuals using an Eye-Link communication board. From C. Goosens' & S. Crain, 1987. Overview of nonelectronic eye-gaze communication techniques. *Augmentative and Alternative Communication, 3,* 77–89. Copyright © 1987, Decker Periodical; reprinted by permission.

Table 4.3. Electronic Communication Aids.

Name	Description	Manufacturer	Price
Lightweight Keyboard-Based Aids	Lightweight, hand-held communication aids. QWERTY/Alphabet keyboard layout with display, printed and/or spoken output.	Canon U.S.A. Brother Zygo	$800–$1,400 $160 $900–$3,730
Dedicated Voice Output Aids	Alphabetic and/or graphic symbol keyboard layout with synthetic and/or digitized speech. Printed output is available with some devices. Most devices are designed to be adapted to a wide variety of user needs (e.g., input methods, symbols, vocabularies).	Innocomp Words+ Phonic Ear Prentke Romich AbleNet	$2,000 $480–$950 $3,600–$4,130 $1,100–$7,350 $370
Dynamic Display Aids	Dynamic display technologies allow the user to navigate between different information screens or electronic pages. The content of the pages may be programmed by the user or specialist. Technologies come as computer software or a dedicated electronic device. Most dynamic display technologies utilize both synthetic speech and digitized sound.	Sentient Systems Words+ Don Johnston (MAC) Mayer-Johnson (MAC)	$4,000–$4,790 $5,880–$7,950 $780 $300
Word Prediction	Software using the techniques where the system "predicts" the user's possible next selection based on spelling, word frequency, recent use, and grammar. Some programs may be used with standard word processing software. Voice output options are available.	Don Johnston (MAC) Words+ (DOS) Madenta (MAC) Scetlandar Software (DOS) Institute of Applied Technology (DOS) BrownBag Software	$100–$1,020 $1,260 $300 $50 $150 $80

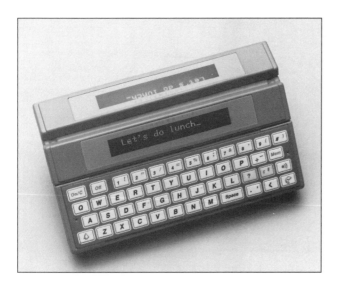

Figure 4.13. Zygo Lightwriter communication device. Photograph courtesy of Zygo, Inc.

some dedicated aids, adapted computers can provide a lower-cost alternative to dedicated devices without sacrificing function. Once the computer has been adapted for access, the user can also work with standard computer software (see Figures 4.7 & 4.20).

A number of communication aids consist of *lightweight keyboard-based devices* using a LCD screen or printed tape for message output. These devices range from personal organizers and label makers available from discount stores and electronic shops to specially designed systems. Some devices, like the Canon Communicator, come equipped with a keyguard, a printer, and printed message and recorded speech storage capabilities. The Lightwriter communicator (shown in Figure 4.13) features a two-sided display panel allowing the partner to read the communicator's message while engaging in face-to-face communication. This device also provides synthetic speech output.

Digitized sound communication aids provide the ability to "play back" medium- to high-quality recorded sounds or speech. Typically, the therapist or clinical staff will record messages on the device, then program specific keys to retrieve the speech message from the computer's memory. The advantages of digitized speech devices are that they are easy and quick to program, produce moderate- to high-quality human speech, and are available at relatively low prices. However, their capacity for storing sound and speech is limited to only a few minutes. Also, because the message elements consist of digitized rather than synthesized speech, the communicator is limited to using only those messages previously recorded on the device. The Prentke Romich AlphaTalker (see Figure 4.10) is a good example of a digitized speech device.

Another group of technologies provides alternate means of access (e.g., adapted keyboard, scanning, Morse code input, and remote pointing), support for symbol use, and speech and/or sound output. For example, the Say-It-All Simply™ (Innocomp) consists of a large touch-sensitive pad with synthetic speech output (see Figure 4.14). The device may be customized to accept graphic materials (e.g., photos, line drawings, symbols) of varying sizes. Messages can be programmed into the device so that when an item is touched, the message will be heard through the speech synthesizer.

Dedicated communication devices like the Say-It-All™ (Innocomp), the VOIS™ 160 (Phonic Ear®) and the TouchTalker™, LightTalker™, and Liberator™ (Prentke Romich Company) are equipped with a number of features including touch sensitivity, switch and long-range pointing access, printing capabilities, and high-quality speech synthesis. Large, preprogrammed vocabularies are also available for these devices. The vocabularies come with specialized symbol systems and are designed to serve specific groups of individuals. For example, Figure 4.15 shows VoiceShapes™ (Phonic Ear) for the VOIS 160, which utilizes sign language symbols. It is designed for non-text-literate individuals who have a background in sign language. The Power and Play™ vocabulary from Prentke Romich consists of requests, protests, nursery rhymes, and interaction games. It is aimed at the first-time device user who is just beginning to learn expressive language. In contrast, Words Strategy™ (Prentke Romich Company) consists of a 4,000-single-word and phrase vocabulary designed for adult language users with some literacy skills. Vocabulary items are represented by one or two Minspeak icons associated with the vocabu-

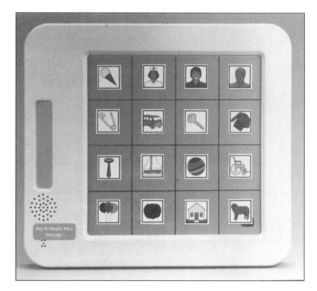

Figure 4.14. Innocomp Say-It-All Simply Plus. Photograph courtesy of Innocomp, Inc.

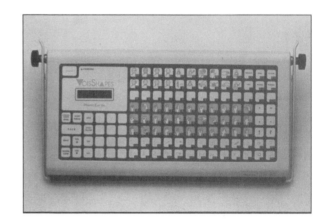

Figure 4.15. The VOIS 160 with VoiceShapes™ vocabulary software. Photograph courtesy of Phonic Ear, Inc.

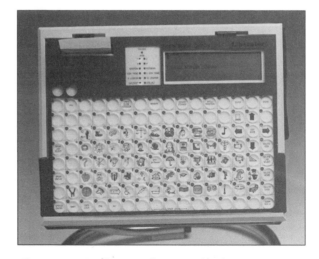

Figure 4.16. The Prentke Romich Liberator™. Photograph courtesy of Prentke Romich Co.

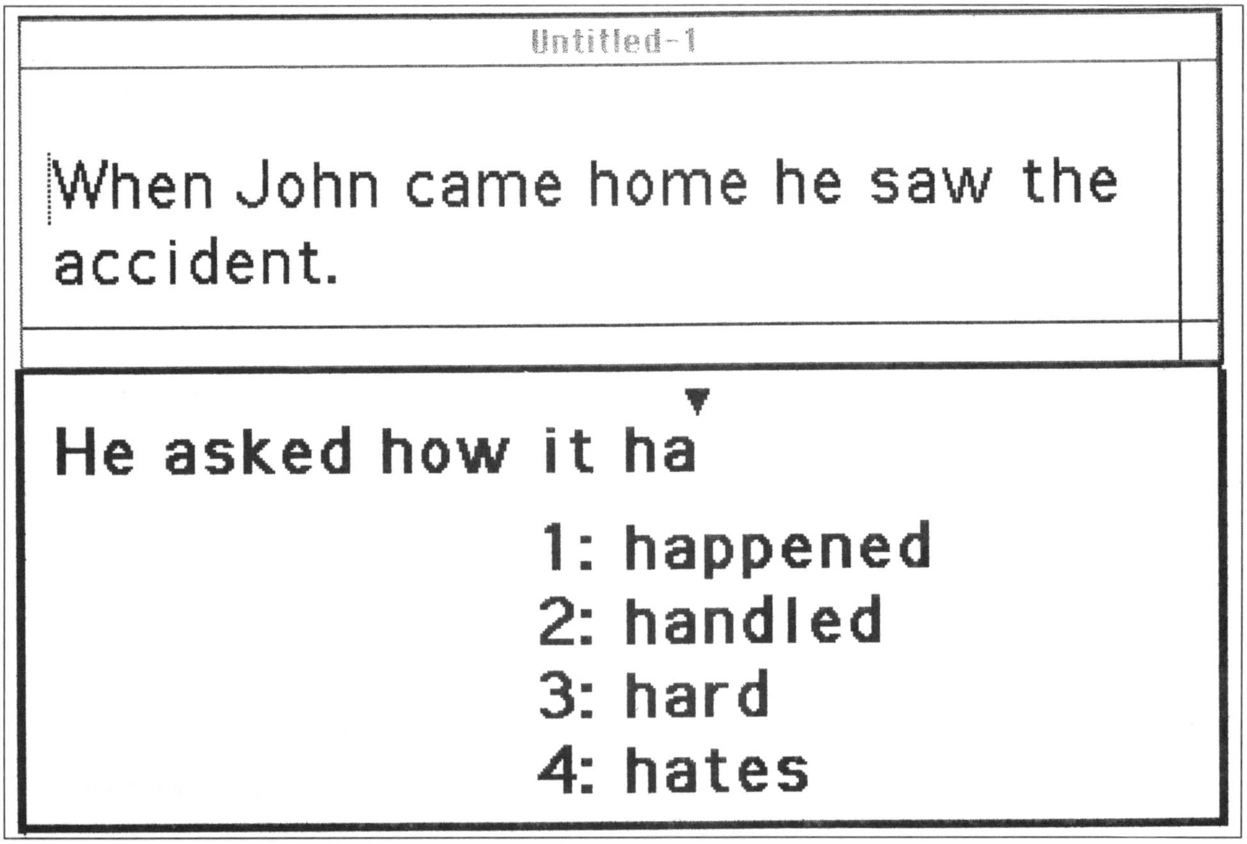

Figure 4.17. Don Johnston Co:Writer™ word prediction software.

lary concept plus a corresponding grammatical marker (see Figure 4.16). Finally, for individuals with adequate spelling skills, the PALS™ system (Phonic Ear) consists of the alphabet and the 75 most frequently used words, prefixes, and consonant blends. The strategic use of the letter sequences can result in considerable keystroke savings for the user (around 45%) and improved communication success (Higginbotham, 1992).

Dynamic display technologies employ a computer screen to display information for selection. Based on the user's choice, the content of the information screen may be changed or updated. One kind of dynamic display technology is word prediction. These programs are designed to reduce keystrokes as well as spelling and memory demands by continually trying to guess the full word or phrase being typed out by the user. As the user types out each letter of a word, the *word prediction* program displays a list of candidate words, based on the initial spelling sequence, word frequency, words recently used, and grammatical category information. Word prediction programs usually contain user-modifiable vocabularies (2,000 to 10,000 words) and are capable of

accepting new words. Most word prediction programs are made for microcomputers and can be used with regular software applications like word processors. Programs like EZYkeys™ (Words+) and Co:Writer™ (Don Johnston, shown in Figure 4.17) also can access speech synthesizers and can be used for conversational purposes. Recent research indicates that users can save up to 45% of their keystrokes using these programs; however, the amount of time needed to scan the prediction list may slow down communication output (Higginbotham, 1992; Mathy-Laikko, West, & Jones, 1993). In addition, Newell, Booth, Arnott, and Beattie (1993) found significant gains in the quality and quantity of work produced by individuals with severe physical and learning disabilities trained to use word prediction systems. They hypothesized that in addition to the significant keystroke savings, the word predictor decreased children's problems with the mechanics of spelling, thus allowing them to focus on the content of their writing assignments.

Other dynamic display devices employ a touchscreen, allowing users to directly interact with text and graphic symbols by selecting them from the computer screen. Once the selection is made, the computer may provide a new set of information related to the selection, or output an associated message. For instance, the Dynavox™ system is programmed like a book so that users may construct a message by selecting information from different electronic pages of the device. Several technologies including the Ke:nx™ (Don Johnston) and Speaking Dynamically™ (Mayer-Johnson, shown in Figure 4.18) turn the Macintosh computer into a reconfigurable dynamic display device equipped with high-quality Macintosh synthetic speech.

Learning Tools

Language Learning Tools

Computer software to support language and literacy learning has gained popularity in recent years. Beukelman and Mirenda (1992) cite a number of factors that may benefit children, including increased motivation, improved attention to tasks, decreased frustration levels, and increased opportunities for repeated practice. A summary of the types of software available and representative examples of products are presented in Table 4.4.

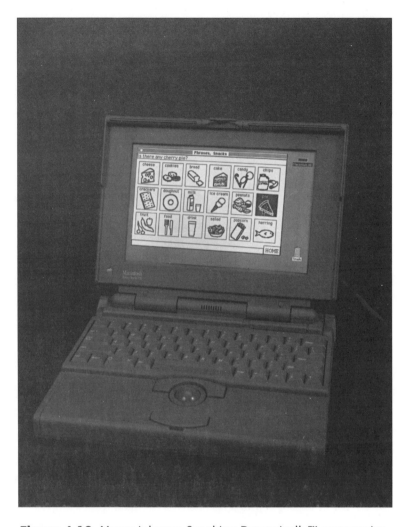

Figure 4.18. Mayer-Johnson Speaking Dynamically™ communication software on a Macintosh Powerbook. Photograph courtesy of Mayer-Johnson Co.

Some computer software programs have been specifically designed to incorporate speech output, adapted keyboard access, and graphic symbol displays in an interactive format. Also, certain skills are required for an individual to utilize augmentative communication technologies. Software programs are available to allow individuals to practice these skills in game and interactive formats. Programs support the development of skills relevant to single switch use, scanning control, and computer access. Other programs support the understanding of cause-and-effect relationships necessary for the development of technology-mediated communication.

Software programs have been developed to provide practice of specific perceptual skills needed to use augmentative communication technologies through games and drill activities. These skills include attending, figure–ground discrimination,

matching skills, and so forth. Emphasis on basic concepts that support language learning, such as categorization skills and understanding of size relations, opposites, colors, shapes, and so forth, are presented in motivating game formats. Children can develop their conceptual skills while learning about computer access and cause-and-effect relations.

Children with specific language impairments, as well as those who use augmentative communication, may develop their language skills through tutorials specifically designed to support language learning. Programs emphasize language skills such as following directions, understanding complex language, using various parts of speech, and constructing phrases and sentences using correct grammatical forms. Some programs also support language comprehension retraining for those with aphasia.

Table 4.4. Examples of Computer Software Programs for Language and Cognitive Learning.

Skill	Software Descriptions	Sample Products/Manufacturers*	Cost
Precursor Skills Such as Access, Motor Skills, and Cause-Effect	Provide practice in accessing single switch and scanning systems, developing motor skills for computer access, cause and effect, and switch control training. Some include speech feedback.	*Make it Happen; Learn to Scan; Motor Training Games; Interaction Games*/Don Johnston (Apple)	$35–$60
Perceptual Skills, Basic Concepts, and Cognitive Development	Games and drill activities that provide practice of perceptual skills, including attending, figure–ground discrimination, matching skills, etc.; basic concepts such as categories, size relations, opposites, colors, shapes, etc.	*Colors and Shapes*/Boston Educational Systems & Technology, Inc. (DOS) *Jokus Software: Toystore*/Don Johnston (MAC) *Understanding Attributes*/Parrot Software (Apple, DOS) *First Categories: Words and Concepts*/Laureate Learning Systems (Apple, DOS)	N/A $95 $99 $220–$225
Language Learning and Retraining	Tutorials that provide practice in receptive and expressive language skills, such as following directions, understanding complex language, use of nouns and verbs, phrase and sentence construction; many include speech feedback. Some programs support language comprehension retraining for those with aphasia.	*Talking Nouns I & II; Talking Verbs; Following Directions*/Laureate Learning Systems (Apple, DOS, MAC) *Word Order in Sentences; Aphasia Series*/Parrot (Apple, DOS) *Picture Sentence Key*/Mayer Johnson Co. (MAC) *Symbol Writer*/Don Johnston (Apple)	$115–$130 $175–$200 $235 $99 $89 $75
Literacy Development and Support	Provide opportunities for story reading and writing, including the use of symbols, pictures, and sounds to support the text. Many allow for adapted access (e.g., using Ke:nx); some read text using speech output technologies; others emphasize reading comprehension skills.	*Story-Ware; Gateway Stories*/Don Johnston (Apple, MAC); *Readable Stories*/Laureate Learning Systems (Apple)	$95 $125 $110
Cognitive Retraining	Tutorials designed to develop skills in the areas of attention, scanning, memory, word retrieval, sequencing, problem solving, reasoning, inferencing decision making, etc. Level of difficulty often changes based on the individual's performance.	*CogRehab*/Life Science Associates (Apple, DOS) *Inferential Naming for Cognitive & Language Disorders; Cognitive Disorders*/Parrot (Apple, DOS) *Rehab Software for Young Adults*/ComputAbility Corp (Apple) *Problem Solving*/ Psychological Software (Apple, DOS, Atari) *Contemporary Living: Decision Making*/Aquarius Instructional (Apple, DOS)	$95 $99 $150–$300 $175–$150 $39.95

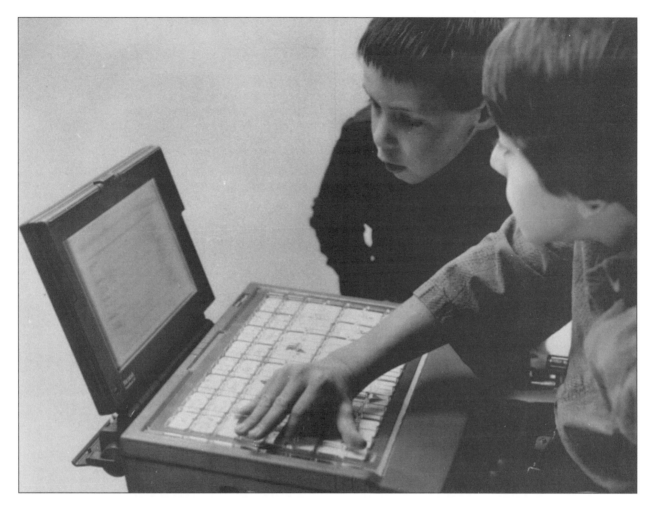

Figure 4.19. Two children sharing a computer activity using a Ke:nx On:Board alternative keyboard and Macintosh Powerbook computer. Photograph courtesy of Don Johnston, Inc.

Augmented Literacy Instruction

Individuals with learning disabilities may need assistance in developing and using their literacy skills. Beukelman and Mirenda (1992) note that computers should not take the place of books but should be used to expand the range of learning opportunities. Simple programs are available to encourage early drawing skills and to teach letter and number recognition, preliteracy concepts (e.g., matching), basic keyboarding skills, and other skills related to literacy development. Software is also available to teach basic reading skills, such as phonics and word recognition, and reading comprehension. These programs may be used with regular keyboards and those with alternative access and thus may be used by individuals with either physical or learning disabilities.

Software programs are available to support the development of storytelling skills as well. In addition to the word prediction programs described above,

several programs support story reading and writing by incorporating the use of symbols, pictures, and sounds. These programs provide children with repeated opportunities to learn how to use print or symbols for expressive communication. Many programs allow for adapted access (e.g., using Ke:nx as shown in Figure 4.19) so that those with physical disabilities may utilize the programs as well.

Writing is closely linked to reading. Early learning should emphasize having children focus on the process of writing, including translating their ideas, feelings, and insights into written form. There should be less concern for the mechanics of writing such as spelling, punctuation, grammatical form, and organization. The advantage of using a computer is that it allows students with learning disabilities the opportunity to write without worrying about handwriting and to revise without crossouts and revisions being present on their drafts.

Table 4.5. Components of an Augmentative Communication Assessment.

Assessment Sections	Rationale
Background Information: 1. Questionnaire 2. Reports 3. Video	1. To understand client expectations and present/future communication needs. 2. Collect related reports: educational, OT, PT, ST, medical, etc. 3. Observe seating and positioning. Review social interaction skills with familiar partners in various contexts.
Observations	To observe the client within natural contexts, interacting with family, peers, and educators/other professionals. To document the needs of the client within various environments.
Needs Analysis	To determine communication needs with respect to seating and positioning in different social contexts across various communication partners, etc.
Capability Assessment: 1. Access 2. Cognition 3. Speech 4. Language 5. Symbol 6. Literacy 7. Sensory/Perceptual: Visual, Tactile, Hearing	1. Explores the fine, voluntary, and gross motor control of the individual. 2. Investigates the individual's conceptual and world knowledge. 3. Determines the structure and function of the oral mechanism. 4. Determines the social interaction skills, and receptive and expressive language skills of the individual. 5. Determines comprehension of symbol representation of objects, actions, and events. 6. Determines the individual's ability to understand written language. 7. Determines the individual's ability to receive and discriminate spoken language and visual and tactile stimuli.
Customization, Training, and Selection of Equipment	Trial period of use to determine whether the system meets the individual's capabilities and future needs.

Cognitive Aids

Cognitive aids can be viewed from two perspectives: (a) to remediate the cognitive impairment and (b) to compensate for the functional difficulties that are related to a cognitive impairment. A number of factors must be considered when determining the type of technology that will be beneficial to an individual: (a) age, including the age at the onset of the disability and the current age of the individual; (b) severity and type of cognitive impairment; and (c) whether other impairments, such as visual or motor difficulties, are present.

Cognitive retraining software primarily focuses on providing practice of those cognitive skills that may be affected by a head injury, degenerative disease, or stroke. These skills include those that are necessary to sustain communicative interactions such as attention to a task, memory, word retrieval, problem solving, and decision making. Often the difficulty level of the program increases based on the individual's performance.

Service Delivery for Augmentative Communication

Providing appropriate communication technologies for severely disabled individuals can be a complex and long-term process. Due to their disabilities, many individuals may not be able to provide the clinical team with the information necessary for valid clinical decisions. Sometimes the individuals' responses may be slow and ambiguous, increasing the evaluation time. In order to determine an individual's communication status and eligibility for assistive communication technology, specialists have developed a variety of clinical approaches (Beukelman & Mirenda, 1992, Goossens' & Crain, 1992; Goossens', Crain, & Elder, 1992). Determination of present communication needs and capabilities, along with information about current communication technologies, is used to develop the individual's communication system and intervention plan.

Collection of this information frequently draws

from multiple perspectives because few augmentative communication specialists are able to provide assessment and intervention in all of the areas needed to understand an individual's communication needs. It is often necessary to work with a collaboration among client, family, and a variety of professionals, including the following:

- Speech-Language Pathologists
- Occupational Therapists
- Physical Therapists
- Rehabilitation Engineers
- Regular Education Teachers
- Psychologists
- Special Education Teachers
- Social Workers
- Resource Room Teachers
- Vocational Counselors
- Classroom Aides
- Physicians
- Visual Specialists
- Audiologists
- Manufacturers' Representatives
- Computer Technologists

When determining the appropriate augmentative communication system, the speech-language pathologist usually orchestrates the collaborative efforts on behalf of the individual and family. At the onset of the process, the speech-language pathologist may refer the individual for specific evaluations (e.g., vision or hearing). During the augmentative communication assessment, the speech-language pathologist works with various professionals (e.g., occupational therapists, physical therapists, and rehabilitation engineers) to determine appropriate seating, positioning, and physical access to the device. Other professionals who participate in the augmentative communication assessment may be part of the individual's educational or vocational team (e.g., teachers, agency support staff, case management workers).

Augmentative Communication Assessment Protocol

Beukelman, Yorkston, and Dowden (1985) present a service delivery approach for the determination of assistive communication technology for individuals with spoken and written communication needs. The augmentative communication assessment examines the individual's social interaction and physical, cognitive, language, and sensory capacities to discern an appropriate communication system that meets present and future communication requirements. Table 4.5 contains a list of the components typically involved in an augmentative communication assessment based on a model presented by Lee and Thomas (1990).

Background Information

One of the first steps in the assessment process is to collect background information about the individual with a disability. This information may include pertinent historical data (e.g., medical, developmental, educational, vocational), current assessment reports (e.g., psychological, speech and language, physical therapy, occupational therapy), and descriptions of communication performance.

These data may be collected from questionnaires and videos completed prior to the augmentative assessment, or during the initial interview period. The information collected is then used to frame the individual's current situation and to structure the assessment approach.

Needs Analysis

Along with the background information, questionnaire, and video, the needs assessment focuses on determining the individual's future communication needs within a variety of social contexts. For example, does the individual's present means of communication fulfill all the communication requirements of the school or work context? A needs assessment also pinpoints the need for particular augmentative communication components, such as speech output or printer support, that would meet specific communication requirements (e.g., answering questions in school). An example of a needs assessment is presented in Table 4.6.

Capabilities Assessment

A capabilities assessment documents the individual's current abilities to communicate and use an augmentative communication system. Assessment components may include evaluation of the following areas: physical access of technology, cognitive development and processing, speech production, language and social communication, symbol system use, literacy skills, and sensory/perceptual considerations. The components of the capabilities assessment are listed in Table 4.6 and are described in detail below.

Observation

Observations are made as the individual communicates within various daily living contexts (e.g., home, school, work). These data can be used to document communication skills and problems, verify results from testing, and confirm hypotheses generated dur-

Table 4.6. Needs Assessment.

Area of need:

1. What physical positions does the individual need to be in while using an augmentative or alternative communication (AAC) system?
   - Lying supine
   - Lying prone
   - Sitting in bed
   - In arm restraints
   - In a variety of positions

2. During what activities does the AAC system need to be available?
   - Moving from room to room
   - Carrying the device while walking
   - Independently positioning the device
   - Communicating within a manual/electric wheelchair
   - Simultaneously accessing the device & wheelchair controls
   - Accessing the device while using a lap tray
   - Accessing the device while the chair is tilted at ____%
   - Communicating while being transported

3. With what other equipment use will the AAC system be employed?
   - While orally intubated
   - While using a tracheostomy tube (a tube that goes into the airway below the larynx)
   - While using an oxygen mask
   - While using environmental control units

4. Within what environments will the AAC system be used?
   - Noisy or quiet room
   - Movie theater
   - Restaurant
   - Dimly lit room

5. With whom does the individual communicate?
   - Anyone visually or hearing impaired
   - More than one listener
   - An unfamiliar partner

6. What will the AAC system be used for?
   - To answer questions
   - To ask questions
   - To provide unique information
   - To convey basic medical needs

7. What output modes are important to the individual?
   - Produce a printed copy
   - Take notes
   - Use a telephone
   - Volley from writing to speaking

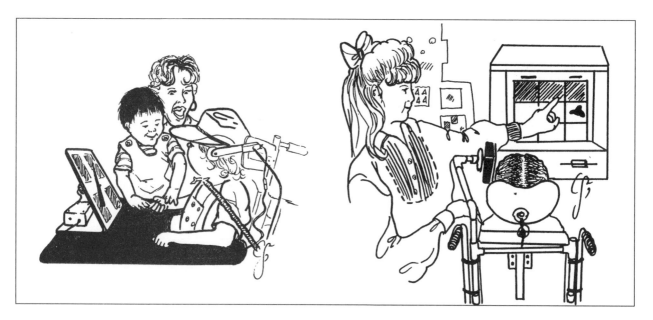

Figure 4.20. Two children using scanning systems to interact with their friends and computers. From C. Goossens' & S. Crain, 1992. *Utilizing switch interfaces with children who are severely physically challenged.* Austin, TX: PRO-ED. Copyright © 1992; reprinted by permission.

ing the initial phases of the assessment process. Observational data can be collected online using organized checklists or event recording techniques, or by making audio and video recordings that are later transcribed and analyzed.

Technology Access

A fundamental goal of a capabilities assessment is to determine the best way for the individual to physically access a communication aid. The clinician usually begins an access assessment by observing the individual's natural body movements during communication. For example, if the person can accurately point to picture books or letter boards, then pointing may be a viable means of technological access. The investigation also determines the size and number of items the individual can physically access through pointing. The smaller the target size, the more items the individual can access on his or her communication device.

If the individual's physical limitations preclude pointing, then the clinician systematically evaluates specific body parts, such as head, face, mouth, upper and lower limbs, trunk, and so forth, as potential sites for switch access (see Figure 4.20). The clinician may also investigate the benefit of assistive devices for stabilizing or controlling movements. Straps, dowels, or head or mouthsticks may be appropriate devices to enable access. The goal here is to determine the most appropriate means through

which the individual can select a message with the least fatigue and resistance for the longest time.

Cognitive Status

Cognitive assessments are performed to determine what an individual understands about the world and the integrity of the psychological processes associated with learning. With respect to augmentative communication, cognitive assessments can provide information about an individual's ability to use technology, as well as his or her learning style. Most standardized assessment procedures cannot be used with individuals with severe disabilities, because the responses frequently rely on physical and speech skills. Rather, reliance is often placed on the clinician's observations of the individual's cognitive skills underlying play and other naturally occurring activities (Uzgiris & Hunt, 1975; Westby, 1988).

Beukelman and Mirenda (1992) propose a set of basic cognitive skills needed to use an augmentative communication device. These include the ability to:

- remain alert and attend to the task,
- visually or auditorily track events in the environment,
- comprehend physical cause-and-effect relationships,
- express preferences and make choices through existing means of communication,

- remember objects, people, and events, and
- associate graphic symbols with an object, person, or event.

Using structured tasks or observational techniques, the team collects data on the individual's cognitive skills to determine how the individual's cognitive abilities may affect communication device learning and use.

Speech

The speech assessment examines the individual's speech, voice, and articulatory and respiratory functions to determine candidacy for an oral communication approach. The speech-language pathologist conducts an *oral facial exam* to investigate the structural and functional integrity of the articulators during various speech and nonspeech tasks. A *voice exam* provides information about the presence and extent of any abnormalities of the voice that may impede intelligibility. Voice problems include hoarseness, vocal weakness, excessively high or low pitch, or a breathy voice that impedes speech. These voice problems may be due to vocal fold abnormalities, breathing problems, or nervous system dysfunction related to the individual's disability. Also, the individual may have had his or her larynx removed due to cancer, leaving a lack of laryngeal speech ability.

Assessment of respiratory function evaluates the integrity of the individual's breathing patterns (inhalation and exhalation) as they relate to speech capability. Insufficient breath support, or problems with the coordination of breath during speech tasks, can seriously impede speech intelligibility. Accurate determination of speech function problems is fundamental to choosing the appropriate course of treatment. Collectively, the assessment of speech function can be used to determine whether to recommend speech therapy as an alternative to, or as part of, the augmentative communication approach.

Language

Language assessments investigate the individual's understanding and expression of meaning, use of sentence structures, and social interaction skills. This is accomplished by observing the individual within his or her natural environments, taking language samples, and completing formal language tests. For those individuals who do not have a formal means of communication, the clinical team may request that the family, or individuals at the educational or employment site, keep a diary of the words, sentences, and concepts the individual understands. Based on the information collected, the speech-lan-guage pathologist documents the individual's knowledge and use of language and social communication. This language assessment information is used to determine appropriate device and vocabulary software selection, as well as intervention targets. Such information also provides a starting point for assessing the individual's graphic symbol skills.

Symbol Representation

Symbol assessment is completed to determine the symbol form (e.g., photographs, line drawings, abstract symbols, traditional orthography), symbol size, and types of information to be represented by the selected symbol set on the augmentative communication device. Although abstract symbols such as Blissymbolics™, Minspeak™, and letters provide for larger vocabularies and more complex messages, they can be harder to understand by individuals with certain cognitive disabilities, These individuals may benefit from the use of photographs or line drawings (Vanderheiden & Lloyd, 1986). For example, Elder, Goossens', and Bray (1989) reported on the developmental differences in children's abilities to use different symbol association strategies and to use symbol sequences to represent words. Such skills need to be considered when determining the symbol set to be used.

A symbol assessment typically consists of identification tasks in which the individual is asked to indicate the name of the symbol spoken by the clinician by pointing or other gestures (e.g., head nod). The clinician may also have the individual point to symbols in response to questions or instructions of varying complexity (e.g., *What did you eat for lunch?, Show me "big."*) in order to determine what abstract aspects of the symbol set are being comprehended. Based on such an evaluation, the most appropriate symbol set is chosen to meet the individual's cognitive and communicative needs.

Literacy

Literacy skills are assessed to determine the presence of and potential for spelling and reading capabilities. Recently, literacy acquisition has been shown to be a lifelong process beginning in infancy (Koppenhaver, Coleman, Kalman, & Yoder, 1991). Because literacy is an important component of augmentative communication, many specialists now focus on determining text literacy potential and fostering its development at young ages.

Literacy assessments determine the individual's ability to recognize letters and words, spontaneous spelling skills, and the ability to comprehend printed materials. Results of literacy assessments can be used to determine the individual's candidacy for text-based augmentative communication systems, such as word prediction or advanced vocabulary software (e.g., Words Strategy™). These data can also be used to plan how the individual's augmentative communication system may be integrated into the school curriculum.

Sensory/Perceptual Skills

Investigation of the individual's visual, hearing, and tactile function will provide information regarding the kinds of augmentative equipment that may be used to meet his or her spoken and written communication needs.

Most augmentative communication systems require adequate *visual acuity* and *discrimination skills* for their use. If an individual's vision is in question, visual function may be evaluated by an ophthalmologist or functional vision specialist. Based on the results, the clinical team may continue to evaluate the individual's functional vision skills to determine the potential use of various communication devices and symbol materials.

Hearing ability is fundamental to most communication approaches, in terms of both social interaction and device use. For individuals with vision impairments, adequate hearing abilities may provide the only viable method to receive feedback from their communication device. Hearing assessments may be carried out by an otolaryngologist or audiologist.

Evaluations of *tactile sensitivity* are usually carried out by occupational therapists. An individual who is tactile defensive may not be able to tolerate touching certain surfaces or using the requisite amount of physical pressure to operate a communication device. Such problems can be dealt with effectively with therapy.

Device Selection and Evaluation

Based on the results of the assessments, the clinical team determines the type of augmentative communication system that will address the communication needs and capabilities of the individual. Once the system is acquired and configured, the individual may then engage in a series of performance trials. The results of these trials will be used to make further modifications to the proposed system, or to select another system if necessary. Upon successful completion of the trial usage period, final recommendations are made for device selection.

Augmentative Communication Intervention

Implementing augmentative communication technologies varies greatly per individual and is dependent on the individual's abilities, which are determined during the assessment. Different training strategies may be employed to teach the individual to communicate using an augmentative communication device. The following information profiles several training strategies commonly used with individuals who present different communication needs.

Basic Skill Training

As discussed above, certain basic skills are needed to use augmentative communication devices, including attention, understanding of cause–effect relationships, the ability to make choices, and so forth.

From a functional perspective, use of predictable routines and adaptive play may encourage the development of these basic skills. Many times individuals with motor involvement have not had the opportunity to learn these skills, given their difficulties engaging in manipulative play. The clinical team may arrange for the individual to use battery-operated toys with adapted switch access in order to foster sustained attention and the understanding of cause and effect. To foster choice making, the individual may be encouraged to choose from a variety of activities such as adapted appliances, play boxes, and adjustable easels. Switch training games also promote basic cognitive skills by providing immediate auditory and visual feedback of the individual's actions.

Aided Language Stimulation

Aided language stimulation is a complete language immersion approach that trains individuals to understand and use picture symbols to communicate (Goossens' & Crain, 1992). The purpose is to provide individuals with opportunities to use symbols in a versatile manner. Training is conducted in organized natural environments with support personnel who can provide the individual with ongoing language stimulation using picture communication symbols. Routines are designed to structure the augmentative communication training so that the individual is provided opportunities for natural communicative interaction. For example, if the clinician is going to encourage communication during a music activity, he or she might say, "Let's turn on the music," while pointing to the symbols "Let's," "turn on," "music." In time the individual not only associates the action or object with the picture communication symbol, but learns to use the item as a means of expression. Such comprehensive environmental adaptation of daily activities and routines provides the educator with readily available picture communication symbols to constantly promote language and social interaction skills.

Literacy

A physically disabled individual just learning to read will have different training strategies from an individual with an acquired disability who has already learned these skills, but needs retraining.

Koppenhaver et al. (1991) suggest that literacy should be learned through functional daily activities involving spoken and written language. For example, placing print in the child's line of vision within the environment, providing opportunities for child-to-child interaction during storytelling through the use of interactive software, repeated storytelling, and independent access to storybooks enhance the potential for the individual using augmentative communication to engage socially and increase literacy skills.

An individual with an acquired disability who has learned to read and write may be retrained to use a keyboard with word prediction to promote spoken and written communication. However, it may be difficult for the individual to relearn old skills and may require time and practice. For others, using a graphic symbol-based communication aid with preprogrammed messages may be easier.

Summary

This chapter has presented an overview of the assistive communication technologies and related service delivery approaches currently used by speech-language pathologists and augmentative communication specialists. As one can deduce from this chapter, the technical innovations in this field are significant in their impact, and are developing at a rapid pace. By the end of the decade we may expect to find many communication technologies to be so small that they are unobtrusive or invisible. Augmentative communication aids will become increasingly easier to use and more intelligible, and will contain an almost unlimited store of text materials. One may also expect that virtual reality applications will be used to create computer generated assessment and intervention environments, and to serve as a computer communication tool to compensate for different disabling conditions.

However, as we pointed out above, technology is limited in its ability to provide solutions for the communication problems faced by individuals with disabilities. Substantial effort will need to be put into developing therapeutic approaches to assist these persons, as well as finding ways of integrating new and existing technologies into peoples' lives. This chapter has shown both the innovations and the intricacies involved in the therapeutic application of assistive communication technologies.

Chapter 4 References

American Speech-Language-Hearing Association. (1981). Position statement on nonspeech communication. *ASHA, 23,* 577–581.

Beukelman, D., & Mirenda, P. (1992). *Augmentative and alternative communication: Management of severe communication disorders in children and adults.* Baltimore, MD: Paul H. Brookes.

Beukelman, D., Yorkston, K. & Dowden, P. (1985). *Communication augmentation: A casebook of clinical management.* Austin, TX: PRO-ED.

Blackstone, S. (1986). *Augmentative communication: An introduction.* Rockville, MD: American Speech-Language-Hearing Association.

Brooks, J. (1986, April 23). *A study in conversational protocol between communication aid users and non-users.* Presentation to Nonspeaking Person's Consumer Group, Kalamazoo, MI.

Brookshire, R. (1992). *An introduction to neurogenic communication disorders* (4th ed.). St. Louis, MO: Mosby.

Creech, R., & Viggiano, J. (1981). Consumers speak out on the life of a non-speaker. *ASHA, 23,* 550–555.

Elder, P., Goossens', C., & Bray, N. (1989). *Semantic compaction competency in normally developing preschool and school-age children.* Presented at the 4th Annual Minspeak Conference, St. Louis, MO.

Goossens', C., & Crain, S. (1992). *Utilizing switch interfaces with children who are severely physically challenged.* Austin, TX: PRO-ED.

Goossens', C., Crain, S., & Elder, P. (1992). *Engineering the preschool environment: 18 months to 5 years.* Birmingham, AL: Southeast Augmentative Communication Conference.

Higginbotham, D.J. (1992). Evaluation of keystroke savings across five assistive communication technologies. *Augmentative and Alternative Communication, 8,* 258–272.

Higginbotham, D.J., & Yoder, D. (1982). Communication within natural conversational interaction: Implications for severe communicatively impaired persons. *Topics in Language Disorders, 2,* 1–19.

Koppenhaver, D., Coleman, P., Kalman, S., & Yoder, D. (1991). The implications of emergent literacy research for children with developmental disabilities. *American Journal of Speech Language Pathology, 1,* 38–44.

Lee, K., & Thomas, D. (1990). *Control of computer-based technology for people with physical disabilities: An assessment manual.* Toronto: University of Toronto Press.

Mathy-Laikko, P., West, C., & Jones, R. (1993). Development and assessment of a rate acceleration keyboard for direct-selection augmentative and alternative communication users. *Technology and Disability, 2,* 57–67.

Newell, A., Booth, L., Arnott, J., & Beattie, W. (1993). Increasing literacy levels by the use of linguistic prediction. *Journal of Child Language Teaching and Therapy,* 138–187.

Pettygrove, W. (1982). A psychosocial perspective on the glossectomy experience. *Journal of Speech and Hearing Disorders, 50,* 107–108.

Shane H. (1986). Goals and uses. In S. Blackstone (Ed.), *Augmentative communication: An introduction* (pp. 29–47). Rockville, MD: American Speech-Language-Hearing Association.

Swisher, L. (1994). Language disorders in children. In F. Minifie (Ed.), *Introduction to communication sciences and disorders* (pp. 237–278). San Diego, CA: Singular Publishing Group.

Trace Research and Development Center. (1994). HyperAbledata. *Co-Net: Cooperative database distribution network for assistive technology.* Madison, WI: University of Wisconsin.

Uzgiris, I., & Hunt, J. McV. (1975). *Assessment in infancy: Ordinal scales of psychological development.* Chicago: University of Illinois Press.

Vanderheiden, G., & Lloyd, L. (1986). Communication systems and their components. In S. Blackstone (Ed.), *Augmentative communication: An introduction* (pp. 49–161). Rockville, MD: American Speech-Language-Hearing Association.

Westby, C. (1988). Children's play: Reflections of social competence. *Seminars in Speech and Language, 9,* 1–13.

Chapter 4 Study Questions

1. List and describe the major disorders that impact communication.

2. What is a "speech production aid?" Provide examples.

3. Describe augmentative communication technology.

4. Describe methods of access of an augmentative communication device for a person with quadriplegia who also requires augmentative communication.

5. What are dynamic display technologies?

6. Define each of the following terms:
   a. Language Learning Tool
   b. Augmented Literacy Instruction
   c. Cognitive Aids

7. Describe each of the components of an augmentative communication assessment.

Unit III: Assistive Technology Applications

Introduction to Unit III

Unit III discusses the use of assistive technology by people in different life roles. People of different ages may have the same categories of functional limitations, but these limitations combine with other factors for different outcomes. People of different ages also interact with their environments in different ways. The child in a family attending school draws upon a different set of functions than does and elderly person living alone. Unit III illustrates the nearly endless combination of assistive technology that is useful to people of all ages and with all types of functional limitations.

The four chapters present assistive technology applications for life roles that correspond closely to age. Chapter 5 discusses devices for preschool and school-aged children. Chapter 6 covers assistive technology in higher education and in transition to work. Chapter 7 presents applications for adults in the workplace, and their impact on employees and employers alike. Chapter 8 looks at assistive technology for older persons, particularly for those trying to maintain their independence.

All four chapters place these life roles in the context of current thinking as represented in the literature, available support systems as implemented through laws and regulations, and the evolving nature of interactions between people and technology. Each chapter includes case studies that describe how assistive technology was applied in the lives of actual people. The cases start from the initial contact with service programs, and follow through assessment, recommendation, delivery, implementation, and use.

Unit III and the case studies in particular, are included to ground the book in the complexities of daily life. They should remind the reader that people continually grow and their needs change. Any assistive technology intervention is designed to be optimal, given the known conditions. However, all conditions can never be known and they change, so these interventions cannot be expected to remain optimal over time. The chapters in the following section (Unit IV) emphasize the need for a thorough assessment and regular follow-up.

Chapter 5:
Using Assistive Technology for Play and Learning: Children, From Birth to Ten Years of Age

I.   Introduction

II.   Play, Learning, and Development for Typical Children
   A.   Stage One: Sensorimotor
   B.   Stage Two: Preoperational
   C.   Stage Three: Concrete (Logical) Operations

III.   Barriers to Play, Learning, and Development for Children with Disabilities
   A.   Assistive Technology Potential
   B.   Assistive Technology Devices and Services
   C.   Categories of Assistive Technology Use
       1.   High and Low Technology
           a.   Positioning/Mobility
           b.   Manipulation
           c.   Communication
           d.   Learning
       2.   Assessing Assistive Technology Need
       3.   Customized and Commercial Technology
           a.   Commercial Items
           b.   Devices that Adapt Commercial Items
           c.   Specialized Devices

IV.   Selecting and Using Assistive Technology Solutions
   A.   Infant and Toddlers: Potential of Assistive Technology to Facilitate Play
   B.   Preschoolers: Potential of Assistive Technology for Communication, Socialization, and Participation
       1.   Standard Computer Input
       2.   Keyboard Alternatives
       3.   Mouse Movement Controllers
       4.   Choosing Software for Young Children
           a.   Selection Criteria
           b.   Categories of Software Use
   C.   Elementary Student: Potential of Assistive Technology to Assist Learning

V.   Benefits of Technology for Students with Disabilities
   A.   Modifying Computer Input
       1.   Utilities
       2.   Keyboards
   B.   Software
       1.   Beginning Word Processors
       2.   Special Features

VI. Success Stories

A. Case Study: Michael, 11 Months of Age
1. Child's Abilities
2. Child's Needs/Functional Objectives
3. Barriers to Participation
4. Assistive Technology Assessment and Solutions
5. Implementation and Reevaluation

B. Case Study: Andy, 4 Years of Age
1. Child's Abilities
2. Child's Needs/Functional Objectives
3. Barriers to Participation
4. Assistive Technology Assessment and Solutions
5. Implementation and Reevaluation

C. Case Study: Amanda, 7 Years of Age
1. Child's Abilities
2. Child's Needs/Functional Tasks
3. Barriers to Participation
4. Assistive Technology Assessment and Solutions
5. Intervention and Reevaluation

5.

Using Assistive Technology for Play and Learning: Children, From Birth to 10 Years of Age

Susan G. Mistrett, MS Ed, and Shelly J. Lane, PhD, OTR/L, FAOTA

Introduction

This chapter examines the use of assistive technology with children with disabilities from birth to 10 years of age. Technology is making a dramatic impact on all of our lives and affects how we work, play, and learn. We change television channels by speaking into a remote control unit, we cook food in microwave ovens, and we listen to radios fitted into the earpiece of a headset. Our access to information is accelerating as the information superhighway adds a million new users each month. Eighty-five percent of U.S. homes with boys 8 to 16 years of age own a videogame player, and the number of classroom computers has increased by 150% since 1986. Technology is more compact, portable, and affordable than ever and is being used by everyone from infants to elderly persons.

Technology helps us do things more efficiently, from keeping up with the news to baking a cake. For persons with disabilities, technology provides the freedom to accomplish what was once thought impossible. Assistive technology helps children and youths participate in the mainstream of life (Heward & Orlansky, 1992). It gives voice to nonverbal children (Biklin & Schubert, 1991), provides movement for children with physical disabilities (Moore, Yin, & Lahm, 1986), talks to visually impaired children, enhances communication for children with hearing impairments (Mahshie, 1988), and furnishes learning opportunities for children with mental impairments and learning disabilities (Carnine, 1989; Higgins, 1988). Its effective use in homes, classrooms, therapy rooms, and community settings is becoming more pronounced. These trends show no sign of abating; in fact, they are expected to accelerate.

Although all children can benefit from the use of technology, there are particular benefits for children with disabilities. Technology holds unique attributes for teaching and advancing the life choices of persons with disabilities (Lahm, 1989). Exciting developments in the field of technology are providing ways for children to learn to take active control over decisions about what they would like to have, say, and do in their lives. Because of this, parents and professionals who interact with children with disabilities must develop greater sensitivity to technology issues. Even more important, they must learn to think about technology in independent and creative ways that will enable them to use technology to meet the present and future needs of their children.

Parents, educators, and related service providers require more than an awareness of available devices and software programs. They must know how to use the technology to enhance learning (Cates & McNaull, 1993); what options exist to expand the child's potential to interact, learn, and develop (Male, 1994); where assistive technology activities are used; how technology is integrated into the current interests and abilities of the child's life; the role of peers and adults; and the contextual design of the environment. These issues will determine how often and how well children with disabilities participate in home and community settings.

Technology is now an essential tool for persons with disabilities for achievement in education, employment, and participation in the world. The early use of assistive technology with children provides an independent means to interact with objects and people, the functions that provide the building blocks to learning and acceptance. In this chapter, we will first examine the various roles of children in three stages of life: birth to infant/toddler (3 years of age), early childhood (4 to 6 years of age), and school age (7 to 10 years of age). Next, we will investigate the effects of disability on the growth and development of young children, and begin to identify specific barriers to participation that disabilities present. As the child develops, the use of assistive technology will change and take on different supporting roles as dictated by the child. For example, using assistive technology to provide independent toy selection at 18 months can lay the foundation for written communication skills at 9 years of age. We conclude by examining success stories of assistive technology solutions for three children with disabilities.

Play, Learning, and Development for Typical Children

The primary role of the child is to grow and develop; he or she begins this role immediately after birth through playful interactions with objects and persons in first the immediate and then the broader environment. Recent research focuses on the play behaviors of children and the critical impact of play on their total development. Play has a significant role in promoting the social/emotional, cognitive, motor, and language development of very young children.

Many professionals have attempted to define play. Play should be intrinsically motivating, engaged in because one wants to, and most of all fun (Musselwhite, 1986)! Play, often described as the "work of children" is far more than a job. Play starts and stops when the player wants it to. Its self-initiated, self-directed quality offers a flexibility not found in work. A player can do what he or she wants to do, including changing play at any time, restructuring it, or restarting it as the player wants (Florey, 1971; Takata, 1971). As the result of natural and spontaneous actions, play provides a way to also develop problem-solving skills through the continuous acquisition of new skills springing from the mastery of older ones (Fewell & Kaminski, 1988).

Piaget (1962) divides development into four chronological stages. These stages include:

- sensorimotor (0–2 years of age)
- preoperational (2–7 years of age)
- concrete operations (7–11 years of age)
- formal operations (11–15 years of age or older)

The sensorimotor stage involves the infant's use of senses and motor abilities to understand and explore the world. Babies engage in repetitive motor movements with an object, such as shaking a rattle. As children develop, they begin to apply several actions to objects (e.g., placing objects in and out of containers, or adding other toys to increase the complexity of their initial function). This symbolic or preoperational stage of play typically begins to emerge around 2 years of age and continues to promote the development of more elaborate play skills as the child's ability to make believe becomes more adept. By a child's 7th year, he or she demonstrates the ability to carry out concrete operations. In this third stage, the child becomes involved with games with rules that are played through cooperation with others; with intellectual maturity that results in more complex play rules. As children's thoughts become more logical and orderly, they learn to understand basic concepts of classification, number, and other processes. Reading, writing, and computation skills are the result of higher-order cognitive processing that is developed throughout the school-age years, where the child moves from concrete to abstract operations. The last stage, which occurs around the 12th year, is the formal operational stage where the adolescent is able to use abstract reasoning to theorize opinion based on past experience. In this chapter, the first three stages of development will be addressed as they relate to the role of the child.

Stage One: Sensorimotor

As babies and young children playfully interact with the people and objects in their immediate surroundings, they become increasingly aware of their existence and their ability to affect their world. However, before a child can interact and play "with" toys, a child must engage in exploration of them. The infant's role is to become increasingly aware of his or her environment through the use of the senses and to begin physically exploring objects. Looking, grasping, holding, and mouthing are exploratory actions (Figure 5.1). These actions result in rudimentary knowledge of objects' distinctive characteristics such as color, size, shape, response, and function. Attributes take on increased definition as the child explores more objects and finds common characteristics. He or she begins to develop preferences for objects and to find different ways to interact with them. Through active participation in this exploration process, a young child is provided with sensory information that leads to further development.

Reaching, grasping, banging, and manipulating objects further adds to the child's repertoire of skills in manipulating and controlling toys. Concepts are tested and retested to ensure their reliability. For example, young children begin to realize that blocks are stacked and always fall down when hit with an arm, that mom will come to pick them up if they cry enough, and that kicking their legs makes the mobile over the crib shake and move. The very young child's growing awareness that he or she causes these effects is the foundation of learning.

The toddler extends these actions into larger, more purposeful movements. Rolling over, creeping, and crawling soon give way to toddling, walking, running, climbing, jumping, and using vehicles. Toys are explored beyond shaking, batting, and dropping; they are held, examined, opened, picked up and placed with other toys. Within play activities, infants and toddlers use their emerging physical abilities to further explore their environment, which leads to more diversity in play activities. Play behaviors increasingly mimic real life situations as the child begins to demonstrate symbolic play attributes. Characteristics of toys may influence their selection at different stages of development. Young children begin to simulate daily routines by pretending to drink, eat, or sleep. By learning the use of play materials, the child manipulates objects to construct or create something (i.e., making clay pies, filling water containers, scribbling). Children begin playing with more than one object at a time, often using the objects in ways that begin to develop spatial relations (putting the spoon on top of the block), causal relations (objects pushed beyond a certain point fall from the table), and categorical relations (size and texture). Eventually, the child takes on different roles, pretends to be someone else, and uses objects as props. However, a young child's total concern for self and his or her needs is gradually is succeeded by an awareness of others and, beginning in the preschool years, an increasing ability for reciprocal social interaction (Smilansky, 1968).

Stage Two: Preoperational

During this stage, the young child continues to learn more about his or her surroundings; he or she moves away from self-focused activities and increasingly interacts with people and objects in ever-expanding environments. The child begins to move more, displaying coordination and increasingly developed gross motor skills (Kerr, 1985): He or she learns to hop and skip and progresses from standing and

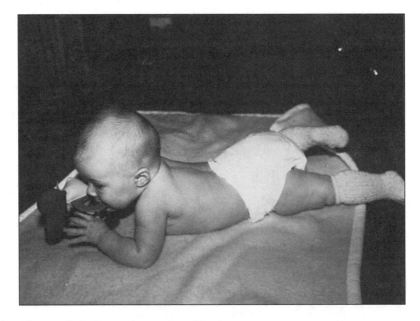

Figure 5.1. Sensorimotor exploration.

climbing to riding first a tricycle, then a bicycle. Preschool children learn basic motor skills by teaching themselves and by watching other children (Berger, 1994). Other learning skills become more developed. Mastery motivation in play emerges, through a spontaneous, internal incentive to develop skills by adjusting to new situations, problem solving, persisting, trying out new ways, and generalizing solutions (Messer, Rachfor, McCarthey, & Yarrow, 1987). During this stage, play continues as the primary mode of growth; through play physical and cognitive skills are expanded. Play provides opportunities for young children to develop social skills and roles. Fine motor skills that require increased muscle control, judgment, and persistence develop during this stage. Eye–hand coordination is required for prewriting and reading skills such as drawing, clay work, and puzzle completion.

Between the 3rd and 6th years, children begin to see themselves as part of a group and accept and adjust to prearranged rules. The child controls actions and reactions within given limits. During the beginning of the preoperational stage, children continue to explore their environment, develop their creativity, and therefore enhance their feelings of self-reliance and self-worth. More complex play activities promote social skills though the emergence of pretend (dramatic) play and games with rules (Figure 5.2). As active participants, children learn more about the properties of objects, relationships with persons in various environments, and their impact on

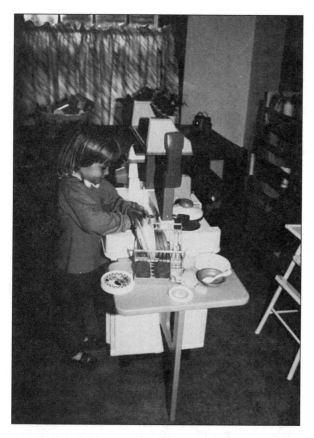

Figure 5.2. Pretend/dramatic play.

their environment by combining and generalizing skills. Vertical block towers expand to represent towns with specific areas of use, paintings depict actual people and situations, and shape puzzles are completed with relative ease. The communicative abilities of children increase at an amazing rate; no other period of growth is as rapid (Jones, Smith, & Landau, 1991).

The number of environments in which a child participates also expands from the home to the neighborhood, community, and school. Social development is closely allied with cognition. As a child becomes more aware of the world, he or she begins to participate in more complex play. Children develop problem-solving and critical-thinking skills through socialized play.

Stage Three: Concrete (Logical) Operations

During this stage, the child refines existing skills. He or she grows more slowly during this period than in early childhood or adolescence. As skills are mastered, they are used to develop higher-level skills. The role of the child entering elementary school changes from play initiator and partner to student. The child's roles become increasingly social; athletics, arts and crafts, social groups, lessons, and recreation take up much of the child's day. The concrete operations stage unfolds to where a child can logically reason about objects and events, and begins to understand principles that can be applied to real and observable examples. With the understanding of concrete operations comes the ability to simultaneously remember and compare various characteristics of people, objects, or situations (Case, 1985). During this operational stage, the ability to use ideas and symbols to develop principles about combined experiences is developed. Children now acquire not only new factual information, but also new ways to organize and assemble facts (Flavell, 1985). The role of the student includes the development of skills to expand his or her knowledge base (i.e., to listen, attend, concentrate/memorize, read, write, and compute). Social and cognitive skills combine in the classroom as children work together in large and small groups. This promotes active learning experiences and active discussion. Learning tasks become specific and are often directed or facilitated by an adult. However, children continue to be active learners. They rely on questioning, exploring, and doing for discovery learning.

Barriers to Play, Learning, and Development for Children With Disabilities

This complex process of child development requires active participation by the child. Children with physical, sensory, or communicative disabilities appear to have less control over and participation in this learning and development process. Impairments in motor, language, and sensory processes hinder spontaneous exploration and social development. Attending skills are often not developed because young children with disabilities respond only to gross changes in visual and auditory stimuli. This lack of sensory awareness and limitations in exploratory behavior drastically reduce the emergence of typical play activity (Wehman, 1979). If a child is unaware of objects and activities in his or her surroundings, he or she is unable to gather new information about the environment and is therefore inhibited in the development of more advanced and complex play activities.

Another threat to the development of children with disabilities is the lack of sustained interaction during an activity. Some children with disabilities require greater and more frequent amounts of reinforcement to continue their interactions (Landry & Chapieski, 1989). Such external supports are required to promote play because the child may not pursue play for the intrinsic pleasure that results from his initiations, and thus, the natural curiosity to explore diminishes.

Limited interaction with play materials or the lack of control over life events can be detrimental for several reasons. The inability to gain access to objects eliminates opportunities to explore, manipulate, and combine materials. This may lead to developmental delays. Children with disabilities appear to be more resigned, less persistent, and less motivated than their nondisabled peers (Jennings, Connors, Stegman, Sankaranaryan, & Mendelesohn, 1985; Newson & Head, 1979). Diminished motivation can result in passivity and learned helplessness. Play behaviors of children with disabilities are generally less complex when the children are less engaged in play. They tend to prefer solitary play to social play with their peers (Field, 1980). Children with disabilities also display a lack of social skill development; they are less able to engage in mutually satisfying interactions with their parents, peers, and teachers than their nondisabled peers (Rosenberg & Robinson, 1988).

Parents, a child's first play partners, may unwittingly promote play deficits in their children. Research suggests that mothers of children with disabilities play less with and are more controlling of their children (Hanzlik, 1989; Kogan & Tyler, 1973). Their role of parent as play partner often shifts to that of a medical overseer/coordinator by acting as an in-home therapy "aide" for their child.

Children who have disabilities that restrict them from active play need alternatives to experience the sense of freedom, spontaneity and accomplishment that comes from play. Play is the foundation for cognitive, social, language, and motor development. Play promotes a child's alertness and thus extends the development of an attention span. Play depends on choice making, which develops a future ability to make decisions and a sense of identity. Opportunities to develop these skills through play are, therefore, critical to the child's development and future well-being.

Assistive Technology Potential

What happens to the development of the child if he or she, because of physical, sensory, communicative, or cognitive barriers, is unable to participate in typical play behaviors? Can the child be taught compensatory behaviors to accommodate the attributes of play? Because play requires movement, it is obvious that the child with physical disabilities is precluded from participation in many play activities unless the activities or play equipment are modified. Similarly, youngsters with sensory or cognitive impairments may be unable to engage, or sustain involvement in typical opportunities for play.

When children with disabilities fail to interact with the persons and objects in their surroundings, they fall behind in reaching developmental milestones. Compensatory activities that maximize the active involvement of all children are needed; those in which participants interact with each other, where materials are used, and where all are engaged for the same purpose (Rosenberg, Clark, Filer, Hupp, & Finkler, 1992). Parents and professionals need to develop activities that will promote their child's interaction, maximize their involvement, and extend their competence and natural curiosity. Assistive technology strategies are one solution that has the potential to increase independence, decrease passivity, and promote participation. Assistive technology can help to create play environments that are increasingly complex, yet accessible, and enhance the overall development of the child. Providing play activities that meet the needs of children with disabilities may require additional thought and effort to use traditional and nontraditional play materials in novel ways.

Technology offers opportunities for all children to extend control to new environments. For children with disabilities, assistive technology gives them access to untried experiences. Research demonstrates strategies to augment existing play abilities or compensate for limitations imposed by disabilities by using assistive technology applications. Assistive technology extends the play repertoires and interactivity of young children with disabilities (Behrman, 1984; Brinker & Lewis, 1982; Swinth, Anson, & Deitz, 1993). In other words, the early use of adaptive toys, switches, computers, and powered mobility is effective in forestalling the development of learned helplessness and learning deficits (Behrman & Lahm, 1984; Bradley, 1994; Hanson & Hanline, 1985; Langley, 1990; Van Tatenhove, 1987) and may lay the foundation for transition to the use of other adaptive devices such as computers and augmentative communication devices (Wilds, 1989). In fact, assistive technology may be the only means by which some children with significant disabilities can be engaged in a physically and socially responsive environment. Technology can make it possible for the child to act on and receive a response from the environment (Wilds).

Other reports of assistive technology use with children with disabilities agree that assistive technology has the potential to increase social interaction skills of young children with disabilities (Mistrett, Constantino, & Pomerantz, 1994), that prerequisite abilities are not required (Sloan-Armstrong & Jones, 1994), and that the best solutions are those that are the least restrictive for each activity. Realistic solutions that promote active participation result from first identifying the functional participatory tasks required within the natural environment (i.e., grasp a toy with two hands, draw a picture, or indicate the answer) and then extending the abilities of the child with technology devices and strategies. However, care is required to select appropriate technology and to identify strategies that promote the child's independence. The technology itself is not a panacea. It must be applied so that the children actively participate in daily routines.

Assistive Technology Devices and Services

Recent legislation, both in civil rights (Americans With Disabilities Act of 1990) and education (Individuals With Disabilities Education Act of 1990), promote the use of assistive technology for children and students with disabilities to "increase, maintain, or improve functional capabilities of individuals with disabilities" (20 U.S.C. Chapter 33, Section 1401[25]). Both assistive technology devices and services, defined by law, must be made available to children when determined to be appropriate by their parents and the professionals who provide their early intervention, special education, and related services. For infants and toddlers birth to 2 years of age, each state's lead agency for the early intervention program is responsible for the provision of such items. The identification and use of specific items and related support services are described on the individual family service plan (IFSP) developed for each child's family.

For students with disabilities who are 3 to 21 years of age, the school district is responsible for providing the assistive technology devices and services identified by the student's transdisciplinary team. The team recommends devices and services identified as necessary to ensure the student's attainment of a "free and appropriate public education" (IDEA, 1990). Ongoing clarifications by the U.S. Department of Education state that assistive technology devices and services are the responsibility of the school district and must be provided to the student at no cost to the parents. These devices and services are identified on the student's individual education program (IEP) as either special education, related services, or support to the student in an inclusive educational setting.

Assistive technology services are defined as "any service that directly assists a person with a disability in the selection, acquisition, or use of an assistive technology device" (Individuals With Disabilities Education Act, 1990; Technology Related Assistance for Individuals with Disabilities, 1988). Such services include evaluating the child's assistive technology needs in his or her natural environment; acquiring, customizing, maintaining, or repairing the device; and training in device use for the person, the family, and the team members who provide coordinated services to the child. Both assistive technology devices and services must be included in each child's program. Training is necessary to ensure that the recommended device is used to increase the child's independence and participation in daily activities.

Categories of Assistive Technology Use

Given these broad federal definitions, there have been several attempts to categorize uses and types of available assistive technology, as they change based on the individual differences in children. Categorizing by use, Cavalier, Ferretti, and Okolo (1994) suggest that assistive technologies can be separated into two major areas. First, as a *prosthesis,* technology provides a function that would otherwise be absent or impaired. This area includes productive tools such as hearing aids, calculators, and portable devices for communication. A second area of use is that of *scaffolding,* where technology acts to temporarily support the acquisition of a new skill. This can include the creation of individualized software activities, or designing a means to stabilize a toy for play.

High and Low Technology

Categorizing the types of assistive technology by complexity allows us to examine the varying characteristics of low and high technology. Both high and low assistive technology solutions should be considered; one is not preferred over the other. A variety of environmental factors will influence the selection of the devices, including the availability of personnel, ease of device use, adaptability of device, and fre-

Table 5.1. Primary Uses of Assistive Technology.

Primary Use	Low Tech	High Tech
Mobility		
▪ Help a child sit	chair inserts: towels, telephone books	customized seating system, floor sitters
▪ Help a child move	scooters, walkers, pedal blocks	motorized cars, wheelchairs
Manipulation		
▪ Hold things steady	Velcro®, Dycem®	customized support
▪ Make things easier to work	large knobs, extenders, adapted utensils	environmental control systems, electric feeders
▪ Help a child play	switch toys, built up tools, (i.e. crayons, scissors), beeping balls	robotics, computer drawing programs, Nintendo®
Communication		
▪ Help a child interact	loop tapes/tape recorders, call systems, picture boards	IntroTalker®, Liberator®, speech synthesizers
▪ Help a child make choices	pointers—penlights	communication software
Learning		
▪ Help a child to see or hear better	magnifiers	CCTV
▪ Help a child discover	big books, large pegs, blocks	storybook software

quency of child's activity change. Low-technology items generally are more available and less costly, and require less training for use. High-technology items usually employ more complex electronics and require individualized setup and training, yet they may provide a more customized and responsive system. Both types help a child play, move, communicate, and learn, in different ways. The primary categories of assistive technology use for children with disabilities, from birth to 10 years of age, follow.

Positioning/Mobility. In the home, community center, or classroom, children with physical disabilities may need assistance with positioning (i.e., sitting, standing, lying down) so that they can participate more effectively. Assistive technology devices such as wedges, seating inserts/supports, and floor tables should be used to provide stable yet comfortable positioning while promoting interactions with peers. Mobility devices such as scooters, adapted tricycles, and motorized cars help a child with physical or sensory impairments travel within various environments and participate in activities.

Manipulation. Some children may need assistance with self-care activities such as feeding, dressing, and toileting. Adapting existing utensils/tools or substituting them with electronic devices can help. All children want to play and socially interact with their peers. Devices that provide successful opportunities for play and recreation such as switches, built-up utensils, and adapted toys and games are included in this category.

Communication. Every child needs a means to communicate or interact with others in a variety of situations. Devices should be flexible and easy to program and understand, and incorporate conversational phrases and pertinent vocabulary identified by peers and family members. Communication systems are available that are portable and programmable with the touch of a button. These systems address the variety of responses required for each activity in which a child participates.

Learning. Learning tasks can be individualized with the help of assistive technology devices. Materials such as puzzles, pegs, blocks, and number lines can be adapted to meet the needs of the user. These adaptations include larger pegs and puzzle pieces and three-dimensional number lines. Computer software programs can provide independent access to music, art, reading, writing, and math activities for children with disabilities. Both computer input (how the program is controlled) and output (sound, Braille printout) devices can be selected from a wide range of options.

Developing children use a variety of strategies in their play and learning, and it is most likely that a child with a disability will use a combination of low- and high-technology solutions. Table 5.1 depicts the primary uses of technology for children with disabilities and gives examples of both low- and high-technology solutions.

Assessing Assistive Technology Need

A child's functional strengths and needs should be clearly defined before considering any assistive technology device or service. What he or she needs to do to actively participate in daily activities should drive the selection of the technology, not the other way around. Families and the people who assist the child in daily activities are vital participants in determining which assistive technologies fit best into their lives. A complex, sophisticated system may be intimidating to a family or team of service providers, and it may require training and practice for its most effective use. A complex system may make the child appear to have a more significant disability than the parents and child perceive. Conversely, another child may have such significant limitations that a complex system is the only feasible option for increasing independence. Assistive technology decisions must be made on a case-by-case basis and reflect the uniqueness of each child.

An evaluation is the first step in identifying first the child's functional skills and then the child's assistive technology needs. An evaluation of the child's status is carried out by a multidisciplinary team that includes professionals knowledgeable in all areas related to the child's suspected disability. Child data come from a variety of sources including "aptitude and achievement tests, teacher recommendations, physical condition, social or cultural background and adaptive behavior" (Individuals With Disabilities Education Act, 1990). The extensive nature of the evaluation process provides information needed to determine an appropriate program for the child. All special education and related services must be listed in the IFSP or IEP, which then serves as a written commitment for delivery of services to meet a child's needs.

The child, the family, and the persons who provide the identified special education and related services comprise the child's IFSP/IEP team and are responsible for implementing the child's prescribed program.

When the IFSP/IEP of a child with a disability is being developed or reviewed, the child's need for assistive technology devices and services must be included in the evaluation. If the IFSP/IEP team members are not sufficiently trained in the selection, acquisition, or use of assistive technology devices, then a supplemental evaluation by an assistive technology team is warranted. This specialized group works with the child's IFSP/IEP team to identify appropriate assistive technology solutions.

Determining assistive technology solutions is dependent on two important factors: the evaluation must take place in the natural environment and the child's IFSP/IEP team, including the family, should be present. The natural environment is where the technology will be used. This natural environment includes not only the home, but also the preschool center, school, and other places in the community. Input from the child's family and professional team members who provide special services is available within the natural environment. This approach provides a more accurate picture of the child's abilities and the factors that will influence the use of the technology.

A child's IFSP/IEP team can best identify the child's functional needs. The assistive technology team works with them to identify potential assistive technology solutions for the child. Assistive technology evaluation tasks include:

- assessing the abilities of the child,
- identifying the child's needs, the functional objectives for participation, and interaction in the setting in which the technology will be used,
- identifying the barriers limiting the participation of the child,
- developing potential assistive technology intervention solutions, and
- implementing and reevaluating the interventions.

After the child's needs, abilities, and barriers to participation are assessed, assistive technology devices and services can be identified, justified, and recommended as the child's team explores possible solutions with the guidance of the assistive technology team. By matching the child's participatory tasks and his or her current abilities with both high- and low-technology solutions, a variety of techniques and strategies are identified to be used across environments and service provisions. Typically, developing children use a variety of strategies to learn, and this requires that flexible assistive technology solutions be selected to best meet the needs of the child in specific environments.

The involvement of the child's IFSP/IEP team, with primary direction provided by the child and family, results in effective functional use of assistive technology. By including input from all members of the child's team, the integration of assistive technology devices into natural environments is enhanced. Often, the occupational therapist can suggest assistive technology solutions because professionals in this discipline often use special equipment to extend daily function (Hopkins & Smith, 1988). The educator or parent, as team leaders in home and school environments, can guide the use of the equipment to best achieve their stated goals. Reevaluation of assistive technology solutions for the child should be constant.

Customized and Commercial Technology

There is a wide range of assistive technology devices for children. Three general categories of appropriate assistive technology devices should be considered as potential assistive technology resources.

Commercial Items. Many families look to this source first to find toys and other items that have general appeal to children. Certain design features of particular toys or commercially available devices may make them more accessible to a child. For example, selecting an item with large buttons, picture symbols, or nonslip grips may provide better access for a child with physical, sensory, or cognitive disabilities (see Figure 5.3).

Devices That Adapt Commercial Items. This category includes not only materials that can extend or stabilize commercial items (e.g., Dycem®, Velcro®, longer handles), but also those that act as an interface between the user and the product. Examples include alternative keyboards and pointing devices to more effectively use a computer, switches that can activate

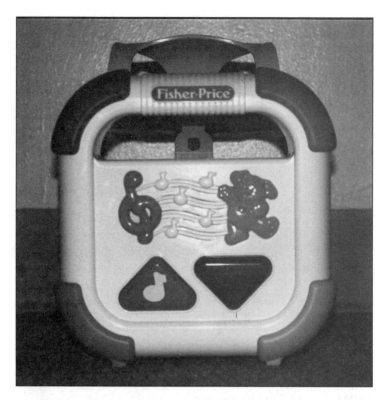

Figure 5.3. Commercial toy.

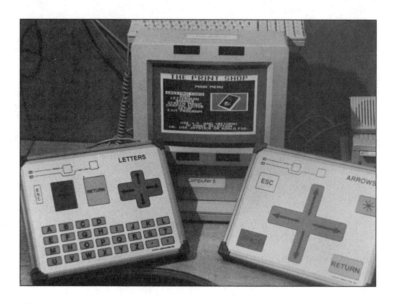

Figure 5.4. Adaptations to standard computer.

any battery-operated toy, and seating supports on a bicycle (see Figure 5.4).

Specialized Devices. These items are designed specifically for a child with a disability, including dedicated augmentative communication devices, computer screen readers, Braille notetakers, and wheelchairs.

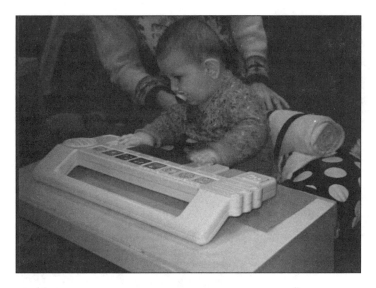

Figure 5.5. Low-tech play supports.

Selecting and Using Assistive Technology Solutions

Infants and Toddlers: Potential of Assistive Technology to Facilitate Play

Assistive technology provides access to play settings. When a young child with a disability is successful in starting a toy in motion, this initiation encourages him or her to watch with interest what he or she has started. Often this results in increased animation, attention, and enjoyment. This initial control of the environment can be extended by the use of accessible toys in a variety of ways. Robots and radio-controlled cars may promote more interactive play for children in wheelchairs, while switch-activated tape recorders and toys allow a child with physical disabilities to examine and manipulate features of the toys.

Toys are selected based on several characteristics that include their sensory feedback, means of access, and physical attributes (Lane & Mistrett, 1994). Sensory feedback relates to how the toy responds when it is used (i.e., the visual, auditory, or vibrating reactions of a toy). Most children will indicate a preference for a certain type of feedback. A toy with high visual and auditory responsivity may be selected for a child who responds best to novel, stimulating objects. Another child may be most responsive to soft musical sounds, whereas loud sounds may cause the child to stop attending or playing. Careful observation of the child's focus on and reaction to specific toys will provide cues as to his or her play choices.

The toy's access features (the size of the parts,

the sequence of actions, and the motor movements required) determine how a toy can be manipulated; the size of the parts, the sequence of actions, and the motor movements required. Often a toy can be made more accessible by stabilizing it or by extending or building up different parts. Several materials can assist with adapting a toy, such as Dycem®, Velcro®, extenders, and build-up material. Watching a child interact with a toy will provide clues for toy and positioning adaptations.

The toy's physical attributes include the size, color, or shape of the toy. Toys may be too large for use on a table at home or on a desk. In addition, an unusual shape may make it difficult to fit a toy on a child's lap tray. It is important to acknowledge the child's preferences and to recognize particular elements that must be present for maximized play performance when selecting a toy.

When identifying potential assistive technology solutions, the selection of the toy or access to a toy is only one element. Developing children move frequently during play; they squat, turn, crawl, and sit, all within a short amount of time. Children with disabilities may require assistance to reposition themselves or the toy during play. For example, an infant lying on his or her back views the world from a different perspective than when sitting upright. When supine, the infant may be able to use both hands to reach up and manipulate toys. However, when sitting, he or she may be able to visually track the movement of people and objects, interact with a greater number of toy choices, and use toys in more complex ways. Devices that provide trunk support may be indicated to increase play options for children with disabilities (see Figure 5.5). All positions should be considered for play, including sitting, supine, and prone. These positions can be supported with assistive technology devices such as wedges, corner chairs, pillows, towels, or donut-shaped holders (Boppys®).

For children who have difficulty initiating or sustaining interactions, battery-operated switch toys are effective to promote and extend their play skills. Because any battery-operated toy can be used with a switch by interfacing the toy with a switch–battery interrupter, a variety of commercial toys can be successfully adapted for use by children with disabilities. The switch for a particular child will be selected based on his or her ability to control specific movements. Table 5.2 depicts the switches most frequently

Table 5.2. Commonly Used Switches.

Name/Example	Activation	Comments	Vendors
Flat Switch	Small low-force movement of arms, hands, legs, head, etc.	• flatness allows placement under many objects • notebook switch provides larger surface area	Don Johnston TASH
Leaf Switch	Flexible switch that is activated when bent or pressed gently.	• requires mounting • can improve head control and fine motor skills	Don Johnston TASH Enabling Devices
Mercury (Tilt) Switch	Gravity-sensitive switch activates when tilted beyond a certain point.	• can improve head or other posture control • attaches easily with Velcro® strap	HCTS TASH Enabling Devices
Plate Switch - Rectangular	Downward pressure on plate by hand, foot, arm, leg, or other reliable movement.	• most common • can be covered with various textures • some offer light, music, vibration, vertical position	Don Johnston TASH Enabling Devices
Plate Switch - Circular	Light touch anywhere on the top surface.	• recommended for young children • click provides auditory feedback • 5" diameter and smaller size available	Ablenet TASH
Voice Activated	Significant vocalizations (1–2 seconds) required.	• can improve vocalizations • sound sensitivity control	Enabling Devices
Wobble Switch	Requires slight press to midline for activation; audible click.	• versatile and multi-faceted • available with gooseneck positioner • sturdy	Prentke-Romich Enabling Devices
Puzzle Switch	Pieces must be properly inserted to activate toy.	• ideal for introducing children to basic cognitive concepts • can improve fine motor skills • complexity of task can be varied	Enabling Devices

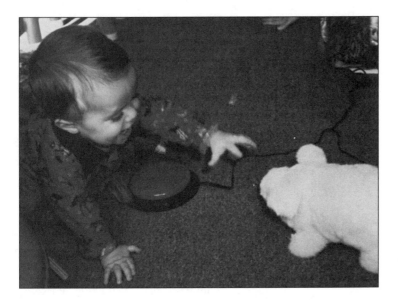

Figure 5.6. Switch-activated toy.

Table 5.3. Sequence for Selection and Use of Switch Toys.

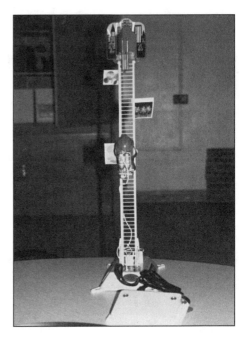

Figure 5.7. Promoting communication through switch toy use.

Toy Type	Example
Stationary	*Bear with Drum tape recorder
Horizontal movement	*Pudgy Piglet
Vertical movement	*Baby Biff Bear Climber *Fireman ladder
Three dimensional	*Penguins Roller Coaster
Random movement: Bump and Go	*Police Car

*Toy examples from Enabling Devices Catalog.

used by children with disabilities. Chapter 2 contains additional information on switches. By activating a single switch, the child can make the toy go. This is the first and most important feature of controlling the toy. This controlled movement can be simply used to elicit a response from the toy. In this way, a small movement from the child results in large response.

In selecting a particular switch toy, the toy's characteristics are matched with the abilities and preferences of the child. During initial use of a toy, the child may react to any movement and delight in

controlling its starting and stopping. As control over cause and effect develops, a child will activate the switch and immediately look to the toy (Figure 5.6) for a response or will respond to directional cues. In using switch toys, the "manipulation" ability depends on the movement of the toy after it is activated. To ensure that the movement response of the toy is appropriate for the child and reflects the child's ability to anticipate, follow, and direct the movement of the toy, switch toys must be carefully chosen. Table 5.3 describes a progression of switch-toy selections based on visual motor skills required by the user, along with specific toy examples. Note that "Bump and Go" toys are listed last. Because of the random movements of these toys, they may require highly skilled visual motor control.

As the child develops skill with switch activation of a battery-operated toy, his or her play partner should look toward adding complexity to the activity. The partner can add toy people or cars to an existing block structure and model a drive-through restaurant with nondisabled children to change and extend the purpose of the initial play activity. Likewise, the movement of a switch toy can be made more complex by modifying the result of the switch use. For example, suggesting that a child make the battery-operated dinosaur (which moves horizontally) move toward the blocks to knock down the block tower gives a purpose to the switch use and encourages a purposeful sustained press. These means-ends activi-

Table 5.4. Switch Interfaces.

Name/Example	Action it Modifies	Comments	Vendors
Battery Device Adapter	Allows a battery-operated device to be activated by a switch.	• nonpermanent • can be used with most on/off toys, radios, and tape recorders	Ablenet Don Johnston Enabling Devices
Computer Switch Interface	Allows single-switch access to an Apple computer.	• accepts one or two switches • sustitutes switches for joysticks	Ablenet Don Johnston TASH
Control Unit	Enables electrical devices to be activated by a switch.	• allows children to participate with peers • used with continuous closure or on/off • timer can be set from 2–90 seconds	Ablenet Don Johnston TASH
Series Adapter	Connects two switches and one toy. Both switches must be activated at the same time.	• encourages bilateral movement • promotes cooperation between two children	Don Johnston HCTS Enabling Devices
Switch Latch Interface	Turns the device on and off with each switch activation.	• good for children who are unable to maintain switch closure for any length of time	Ablenet Don Johnston HCTS Enabling Devices
Timer Module	When switch is closed, a toy is activated for a preset time.	• the toy activates for 1–90 seconds, depending on the vendor	Ablenet HCTS Enabling Devices
Jack Adapter	Works to convert the size of the jack to the size required by the toy or device.	• must be mono to work with switches	Radio Shack

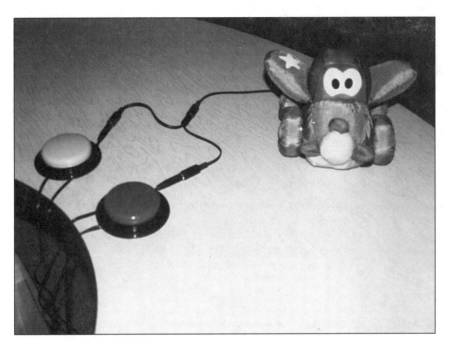

Figure 5.8. Toy with series adapter interface.

Table 5.5. Activity: Circletime.

Expected Child Tasks	Modifications
Get to circle area	Aide wheels child to new area
Sit on floor	Aide positions child; corner chair used for independent seating
Identify children present	Picture board with photos; penlight for pointing
Answer questions: calendar, weather	Penlight for pointing
Raise hand	No modifications
Select storybook	Penlight to point to book or related object
Say refrain with group recorder	Prerecorded loop tape
Move to next activity	Aide repositions child and moves to new area

ties provide more challenging opportunities and build on the child's capacity to "do." Other activities may include pictures of communication choices set up in the path of the toy (see Figure 5.7) or the use of spatial concepts (go under the chair, off the table, stop at the edge, etc.). Races toward a common area with several children using switch-operated toy are is an effective way to promote cooperative, social play. Incorporating other toys and players in the child's play encourages the development of more complex play skills.

Extending the outcome of the switch press has the potential to increase the child's play level. Adapting the complexity of how the switch is used with the toy can also provide new challenges for the child with disabilities. Table 5.4 illustrates several commonly used switch-interface devices. These can be creatively applied to play situations to extend interactions. For example, when a series adapter (Figure 5.8) is used between the switch and the toy, *both* switches must be activated for the toy to function. This interface is used to promote bilateral hand movement. It is also used as a cooperative peer activity where two children are required to press their switches at the same time.

Preschoolers: Potential of Assistive Technology for Communication, Socialization, and Participation

As a child becomes older, he or she is expected to interact within a broader environment and with a larger number of people. Participation for the preschooler includes playing with toys and space exploration, as well as communication and social skill development. The family and child's IFSP/IEP team must develop strategies to ensure that children with disabilities are able to play and participate in activities with nondisabled peers. Professionals who work with children should analyze the activities present in the environment to identify what the child is expected to do to participate. The team will examine factors such as purpose of activity, required device setup time, number and types of support, length of activity, movement required, and so on. Participation begins with acknowledging the importance of physical inclusion. If an activity calls for children to be on the floor, then all children should be on the floor. Identifying the functional tasks expected of the children for each activity will result in naming the specific tasks to be modified. Table 5.5 breaks down the functional tasks required by children participating in Circletime, an activity time (i.e., Social Studies) in Early Childhood programs. The example includes modifications suggested for increased interactions by young children whose barriers to participation include the inability to speak, walk, and reposition themselves.

Because many of the tasks associated with Circletime include a need for communication, a programmable augmentative communication device can be used that "speaks" certain messages when activated. However, this device requires setup time to program responses for each part of the activity. The use of a low-technology device (penlight) results in similar participatory outcomes, and minimizes setup time. The penlight is the least restrictive solution because it allows the child to participate independently with no interruption for device adjustment.

Using computers with young children is effective in promoting participation in preschool activities (Mistrett, Constantino, & Pomerantz, 1994). In fact, computers may be the only means for participation for children with disabilities. High-technology devices, although requiring setup and customization, are used to provide the most independent access. For example, for a preschool child who is nonambulatory and nonverbal to best participate in the game "Duck, Duck, Goose," one team designed a talking board by using a PowerPad® keyboard connected to a computer with a speech synthesizer. The PowerPad®, with its 12" x 12" surface, was divided in half, with a picture of a duck on one side and a goose on the other. The user selected a classmate as a "pinch-hitter" to go around the circle while touching children on the head. The child with the PowerPad® was able to verbally designate who was a "duck" and who was a "goose" by pressing the pictures on the pad. In this way, all children participated as fully as possible in the game.

Computer technology is being seen more frequently in the preschool classroom. Using the computer for communication is an obvious means of participation for nonverbal children. However, when used as a tool for discovery-oriented activities, computers expand the opportunities for exploration and learning available to children with disabilities.

Computers provide a flexible learning and play environment in two ways: (a) through the selection of different software programs and (b) through the use of different computer-input devices. Software programs are available to help children develop basic cause-and-effect responses, make choices, problem-solve, draw pictures, create music, construct new items, play games, and even sing. The computer is a way for children of varying abilities to play together on an equal basis; it provides a place to begin. However, care must be taken in selecting appropriate software programs and devices that ensure a child-controlled environment.

The way software is used can facilitate specific child outcomes. For example, putting children in pairs or small groups for computer activities encourages social interactions, group problem solving, and cooperative learning. Highly motivating programs promote the acquisition of computer-literacy skills by encouraging children to navigate and control this new interactive environment.

Standard Computer Input

Standard computer input devices, the keyboard and mouse, must be modified for use by children with disabilities. Neither method is suitable for young children. The standard keyboard presents a problem with its large number of small keys that are spaced closely together, which makes access difficult for a child's small hands. Because young children are nonreaders, letters and symbols on the keys create additional barriers to the use of a standard keyboard. Solutions to these problems include alternative and customizable expanded keyboards that limit the number of key choices and provide larger press areas. The keys can be labeled with pictures and symbols more meaningful to a young child. Software programs are increasingly controlled by mouse movements that require the user to "point and click" on their selection. Alternatives that provide more concrete learning experiences should be investigated. By replacing the keyboard or mouse with a more developmentally appropriate and motorically successful input device, young children independently operate programs and learn to share, create, and solve problems together. In giving the child opportunities to control the computer on his or her own developmental level, interactive ability is promoted. The child focuses on the changes his or her actions have made to the screen instead of emphasizing the mechanics of moving the mouse to direct the on-screen pointer or the selection of the correct key.

Table 5.6. Keyboard Alternatives for Young Children.

Keyboard	Description	Vendor	Cost
PowerPad	Touch-sensitive membrane keyboard uses picture overlays for large key selection	Dunamis, Inc.	$230
Muppet Learning Keys	Redesigned keyboard for young children; letters and numbers arranged in sequence; graphics depict key functions	Sunburst Communications	$129
IntelliKeys (with Overlay Maker)	Alternative keyboard with ability to create customized overlays for any program with special software	Overlay Maker IntelliTools	$70 $395
Concept Keyboard	Customizable keyboard; overlays illustrate cooperative use	Hach Associates	$495–$595
Key Largo	Customizable keyboard; requires Ke:nx interface	Don Johnston Inc.	$320 Ke:nx: $780

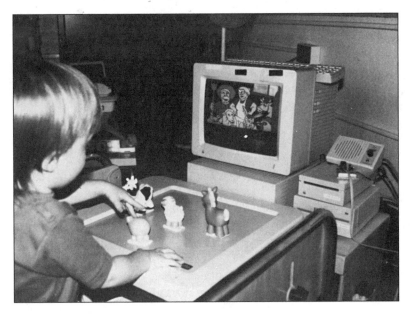

Figure 5.9. PowerPad® adapted with three-dimensional figures to work with *Old MacDonald's Farm* (UCLA).

Keyboard Alternatives

There are several sources of keyboard alternatives. Access methods that give a child control offer large key selections with fewer key choices, and use objects, pictures, or symbols directly associated with changes on the computer screen. Offering only those keys necessary to interact with a software program eliminates distractions and promotes independent use. Table 5.6 depicts several alternative keyboards designed specifically for children. Prerequisite skills are not required for computer use, because children develop skills through the use of the technology.

Software programs can be used to extend a child's developmental level or to reinforce existing skills. For example, if a child shows interest in farm animal sounds, a software program such as *Old MacDonald's Farm* (UCLA) designed for the PowerPad® (Dunamis) is used to promote this interest. The overlay that accompanies the software program includes pictures of the farmer and six common farm animals. In the first level of the software program, the child simply presses a picture of an animal on the pad and an animated picture appears on the screen and a voice says, "the cow says moo-moo." For children unable to relate to a picture of an animal, objects (i.e., Fisher-Price farm animals) are used. The animals are attached to the board's surface with Velcro®, on the corresponding areas of the pictured overlay (Figure 5.9). As the child grabs the toy cow, his or her touch activates the key area and the computer responds with "the cow says moo-moo" while showing a picture of the cow. The development of object-representation skills can be promoted with such exercises.

Table 5.7. Pointing Devices for Young Children.

Name	Description	Manufacturer	Cost
KidzMouse	Designed for small hands; "ears" are controller buttons	Logitech	$40
Computer Crayon	Designed to be held and used as a crayon	Appoint	$40
Trackball	An "upside-down" mouse; the large roller ball controls the movement of the pointer	Kensington, Logitech, ProHance	$40–$150
TouchWindow	Touch screen that attaches to the monitor; provides the most direct selection method	Edmark Corp.	$270–$350

Table 5.8. Computer Switch Interfaces.

Name	Description	Manufacturer	Cost
Apple switch interface	Connects one or two switches to run software, connects to the Apple II nine-pin joystick port	Don Johnston, Inc.	$42
Macintosh switch interface	Plugs into an ADB connector on the keyboard; contains five switch options, including mouse click	Don Johnston, Inc.	$135
BEST switch interface	For DOS computers; assigns any key or string of keys to one, two; or three switches; connects to the serial port	BEST, Inc.	$99

Mouse Movement Controllers

Many current software programs require the use of a mouse. Using the mouse to control software programs is too abstract for children with disabilities because the movement is controlled by an unseen rollerball. By using alternative pointing devices, the child controls the pointer on the screen.

The most direct alternative input method is the TouchWindow® (Edmark Corp.), which affixes to the computer monitor with Velcro® strips. Any mouse-driven program designed for Macintosh or IBM-compatible computers can be used with the TouchWindow. A child simply touches the screen to make a selection. In this way all visual, language, motor, and cognitive abilities are focused on the same area. The device works well with a finger or stylus. Other mouse alternatives that may be successful with children are depicted in Table 5.7.

For young children unable to control computer software with the aforementioned standard or alterna-tive methods, the use of switches should be investigated. The same switches that activate battery operated toys are used to interact with software programs with the use of a computer-switch interface. Many software programs are available for immediate switch use, and others can be adapted for use by a single switch. Beyond providing computer access to children with physical disabilities, switches can be used to reduce software control to a single key or switch. This is helpful in introducing computers to young children by focusing their attention on the changes on the screen instead of on which key to press.

Computer-switch interfaces are also used to translate the mouse click into a single-switch press, which provides a structure for cooperative learning activities. For example, one child can maneuver the mouse pointer to a chosen area with any pointing device, and the child using the switch can press to click to select it. Table 5.8 lists the switch interfaces for various computer platforms.

Different input devices are used to develop skills. For example, software designed for mouse control can be initially used with a TouchWindow. After independence with the software is achieved by the child, an alternative keyboard that shows mouse arrow movement can be used with the same software. In time, a trackball may be introduced. Care should be taken to change only one variable at a time (software, positioning, or device) as the child experiences success. If the input device is changed, the software and child positioning should remain the same.

Choosing Software for Young Children

Selection Criteria. In the past few years, the amount of software designed for young children has grown dramatically. Making the right selection will depend on the abilities of the children as well as the adult's approach to learning interests. Five criteria emerge in identifying software features appropriate for young children. A program does not need to include all criteria to qualify as useful.

1. *Easy to Use.* After initial use of the software, the child should be able to manipulate it independently. Software with a limited number of keys for input is recommended so that the mechanics involved in using the software are secondary to the manipulation of the program itself.

2. *Several Levels of Difficulty.* Software should support the growth and development of the young child. As the child begins to explore and manipulate the software, skills required are low. Software that provides several levels of difficulty is able to expand as the child explores and teach skills as he or she is ready to learn. Editing features help monitor several expansion features.

3. *High Child Interest.* Young children are motivated by graphics and sound that represent and reinforce concepts that relate to their experiences in the real world. Music and sound should be used to make information relevant, and response to a key press should be immediate. There should be many opportunities for discovery that enhance the child's natural curiosity.

4. *Independent Control.* The software should promote active participation by the child in creating change in the screen. The child should be able to initiate change, not simply respond to computer instructions. The purpose of the software should be clear to the child after minimal directions.

Direction should be spoken or graphically illustrated so that the nonreader can interact.

5. *Appropriate Responses.* A correct response should be reinforced through sound and animation. Responses to wrong answers should be polite and not signal errors with irritating noises. Software that provides cues to facilitate the answer is recommended.

Categories of Software Use. Computers play many roles in the education and development of children. Software can be categorized into five different categories of use (Mistrett, 1992). Although the categories are treated as discrete in the descriptions below, they in fact overlap. Examples of various software programs are included to illustrate the different categories.

1. *Exploratory.* Programs that allow the child to play and explore the different press areas, which cause something to happen on the screen. There is no correct answer or sequence of key presses required. The purpose is to provide an environment in which children can learn by experimentation.
   - *StickyBear Series* (Optimum Resource)
   - *McGee Series* (Lawrence Productions)
   - *Millie's Math House, Sammy's Science House, Bailey's Book House, Thinking Things* (Edmark)

2. *Drill and Practice.* These programs provide opportunities for guided practice. Information is presented, the child responds, and then the child receives immediate feedback about the accuracy of the answer. These programs should be used to practice known skills and concepts, not to introduce new ideas. These programs present information in a variety of ways; many of the game programs are cleverly disguised drill-and-practice programs.
   - *KidsMath* (Great Wave)
   - *Writer and Reader Rabbit* (Learning Co.)
   - *The Playroom* (Broderbund)

3. *Constructive.* Programs that provide for the graphical creation of new objects, designs, or layouts. Children are able to work together to produce an original picture, mask, or storybook. The majority of these programs provide for picture printout.
   - *Big Book Maker* (Toucan)
   - *KidPix* (Broderbund)
   - *KidCad* (Davidson)

4. *Word Processing.* These programs are designed to develop early writing and lan-

guage skills. They are motivationally appealing with the use of graphics for rebus writing, large letters, talking words, and sound effects.

- *KidWorks* (Davidson)
- *IntelliTalk* (IntelliTools)
- *StoryBook Weaver* (MECC)

5. *StoryBooks.* These programs, often called lapware, provide opportunities to read a story. Many programs are interactive in that the child can turn the pages, determine the course of the story, or interact with objects on the screen.

- *Reading Magic: Jack and the Beanstalk and Flodd the Bad Guy* (Tom Snyder)
- *Grandma and Me* (Broderbund)
- *Thomas' Snowsuit* (Discis)

Many software publishers include different kinds of software programs within a single package. Often, exploratory programs are packaged with drill and practice programs or provide various levels of interaction. A complete review by a knowledgeable member of the child's team is necessary before the child is introduced to the program.

Elementary Student: Potential of Assistive Technology to Assist in Learning

Consistent with current trends, technology affects the lives of students with disabilities, 7 to 10 years of age, at home, in the community, and at school. With increasing numbers of computers used for instructional, recreational, and exploration purposes, accessibility becomes an issue so that all students can participate. As addressed previously, federal legislation is supporting the use of assistive technology for the inclusion of persons with disabilities in everyday life, with specific mandates on its use by students with disabilities. Under the Individuals With Disabilities Education Act (IDEA of 1990), school districts must help persons with disabilities select and acquire appropriate assistive technology devices and then train them to use them. Consistent with the IDEA mandate, assistive technology has been added to the continuum of related services it provides for individuals with disabilities. As a result, the specific student use and intended outcomes of the assistive technology must be added to the IEP. America's Education Goals, endorsed by Presidents Bush and Clinton, promotes the improvement of our education system and directs each state to begin to prepare its students "to meet the demands of a new century." In New York, for example, the Board of Regents and the State Education Department have affirmed that:

> The goals and desired learning outcomes will apply to all pupils. All pupils are entitled to programs which make it possible for them to learn the skills and acquire the knowledge needed to function effectively in society. An instructional program derived from the goals and desired learning outcomes is not just a requirement, but an entitlement (*A New Compact for Learning*, 1991, p. 4).

In addition, to specifically address technology-related issues, the *Regents Long Range Plan for Technology in Elementary and Secondary Education in New York State* (1990) addresses the need to integrate technology into all school-related operations. Specifically, instructional applications of technology must directly support the teaching/learning environment and enhance the interactions between students and resources. The implementation of this technology plan will ensure the availability of computers in the schools.

Computers are increasingly used in elementary and secondary classrooms. The U.S. Congress Office of Technology Assessment's (1995) report to Congress finds that technology can assist teachers with different parts of their job:

1. To enhance instruction, technology can
   - bring new resources into the curriculum,
   - develop new forms of instruction,
   - motivate learners,
   - individualize student learning,
   - redefine teachers' roles.

2. To simplify administrative tasks, technology can
   - keep records,
   - assess student learning,
   - prepare curriculum materials,
   - improve communication.

3. To foster professional growth, technology can
   - expand opportunities for continuing education,
   - foster collegial work with other professionals.

Technology must be integrated into traditional learning methodologies, not only to give students access to current information, but also to provide skills to use this communication, research, and presentation tool to its maximum effort.

Benefits of Technology for Students With Disabilities

Children like computers. Computer use by students with and without disabilities results in increased attention, motivation, and time on task (Lindsey, 1993). This may be due to several factors that are inherent in today's computer environments.

- *Visual Organization.* Computer screens reflect a graphical user interface where the student points to an icon or pulls down a menu for a computer command. Because the commands are hidden under pictures, less physical and cognitive skill is required for control. Windows can be resized and repositioned to emphasize what is to be done next.
- *Singular Focus Area.* Because all key responses are reflected on the computer screen, usually in close proximity to the input system, the student's focus is directed to a small, manageable area. This assists in eliminating distractibility.
- *Motivation.* With the recent explosion of software designed with sound, animation, and music, students are encouraged to interact with and guide the software process. Immediate reaction by the computer to a click or key press encourages a student to continue to interact with the computer. Features can be adjusted for the different visual, auditory, and sensory aspects of different learners.
- *Consistent Commands.* Control procedures for a software program, once learned, stay the same. Menu bar location of certain commands (or their parallel keyboard combinations) are often the same in most programs. For example, "New," "Open," "Save," and "Print" commands can be found under the "File" option on the menu bar. This universal consistency supports the development of memory, sequence, and direction-following skills in students.
- *Self-Paced Learning.* Computer activities can provide opportunities for success in that they allow a student to proceed at his or her own pace; the screen does not change unless directed by the user. Students with disabilities often need more time to explore and complete assignments. Computers give a student time to problem-solve and make decisions without the pressure of time constraints.

- *Legible Output.* Because printers provide readable output, handwriting problems are eliminated. In addition, the ability of a student to proofread work is easier because the text is more legible. Rewrites are no longer necessary due to the file saving and editing capabilities of the computer.

Providing successful self-directed technology experiences can result in an increase in self-esteem and self-worth. Families are able to see what their children can do in an environment that supports their abilities and provides a productive tool.

Modifying Computer Input

Utilities

With the increased use of computers in America's classrooms and reports of its positive effect on learning, students of all abilities need access to this educational tool. Minor adjustments to the computer environment may provide immediate successful access for some students with disabilities. These "utilities" adjust key access, keyboard sound, and other aspects of the environment. They are included with Macintosh system software, or can be obtained free of charge for IBM-compatible computers (see *AccessDOS* and *AccessWin* information). A computer's owner's manual provides more complete information. The following options are often used with students to increase their control and decrease frustration with input and output of computer information.

- *StickyKeys.* This provides a way for single-finger typists to press two keys at once, for example, pressing "SHIFT" and the "4" to make a dollar sign ($). StickyKeys solves this problem by letting the user type first the modifier key and then another.
- *MouseKeys.* Because mouse control can be difficult for some people, MouseKeys provides a way for users who can not handle the mouse but who can press keys on the keyboard, to perform all the functions of the mouse. The keys on the numeric keypad are used to control all of the mouse functions.
- *RepeatKeys.* Most keyboards have an autorepeat feature; when a key is held down, the computer repeats that key over and over again. RepeatKeys allows the user to adjust how fast the autorepeat works or to turn it completely off.
- *SlowKeys.* Some users may accidentally touch keys while they are moving their fin-

gers toward the key they want. SlowKeys provides a way to adjust the length of time a key must be held before the computer interprets a press as input.

- *ShowSounds.* The computer signals errors or warnings to the user with beeping sounds. Users with hearing impairments or who work in noisy environments may be unable to hear these sounds. ShowSounds gives a visual indicator (screen or menu bar flash) of when the computer has beeped.

Keyboards

Keyboards that make the introduction to the standard keyboard easier should be used during the elementary grades. For instance, those which provide slightly larger key areas, or that are organized into like groups by color, are useful. Several recent keyboards address the needs of the beginner user by offering an alphabetical key layout that links the child's past experience with letters to this new experience (see Figure 5.10).

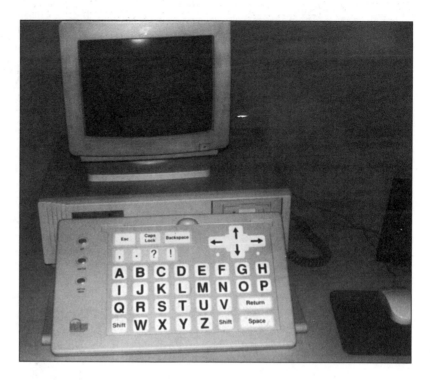

Figure 5.10. Alphabetical key layout.

- *Low-Technology Modifications.* Keyboard introduction and use is further eased by the use of several low-technology adaptations that act to either highlight the keyboard keys to be used, or cover those that are distractable or not required for a particular program. These include the use of key labels, stickers, key guards, and masks. Often the combined use of computer utilities with low-technology modifications on the keyboard results in the most effective solution.
- *Customizable Expanded Keyboards.* Because of individual limitations, even these "introductory" keyboards may not be accessible to all children. Larger key areas with several commands under a single key may be needed to accommodate independent use. Keyboards are available that provide a means to customize both the layout and size of the keys as well as the function of the key. Overlays can be designed for use by anyone with the ability to directly select a key choice. For students

with disabilities, customization activities provide individualized learning activities, communication boards and participation in recreation pursuits.

Software

Software in the primary grades is used to address specific skill and content areas that reflect curricular goals. Technology is integrated into daily activities as an instructive and practice tool. It can also be used as a means of participation. The curriculum dictates the type and use of technology that promotes independent participation. The software needs vary with content and activity. However, because reading, writing, and computation skills are those that are developed during this stage, software selection most often reflects those interests.

Beginning Word Processors

Because computers are frequently used to address the writing, reading, and comprehension skills of children, several software programs have features that can be used to provide better, more independent interactions by young students beginning to write. Most programs have limited commands, often in picture format. See Table 5.9 for special features of word processors.

Table 5.9. Special Features of Word Processors for Beginners.

Software Feature	Software Example
Large Text	Any software with font size options
Rebus Writing (combining text and pictures)	*Muppet Slate* (Sunburst) *KidWorks 2* (Davidson)
Talking Words/Letters	*IntelliTalk* (IntelliTools) *Write:OutLoud* (Don Johnston)
Sound effects	*My Words* (Hartley) *StoryBook Weaver* (MECC)

Special Features

Other software features assist with the mechanics of correct word production. These are often included as options within a standard word processor. They include spell checkers, grammar checkers, and thesauruses. Look for features such as glossaries and macro capabilities, because these can be used to provide efficient key use. For example, by using the glossary feature, a student can type "HDG" with a special command key, and a complete heading for social studies class will appear on the screen with the correct date. This helps the student to focus on the material to be newly created and not on the mechanics required to produce a standard page label.

Another helpful alternative is the use of word-prediction programs. These programs reduce the number of keystrokes a student must make by predicting the text that will be typed next. A window appears on the screen (see Figure 5.11) with word choices available; the student simply chooses the desired word. Word prediction programs often have a dictionary that can be modified to meet the vocabulary needs of the user.

Success Stories

The following success stories illustrate the impact of the selection of appropriate assistive technology applications on the performance outcomes of three children with differing needs. The selection and suggested use of the described solutions address the needs of each child at a certain point in development. It is important to continue to provide guidance to their families and education teams on the use of other technologies that may provide better access, both as the needs of the child change and as newer technology becomes available.

Case Study: Michael, 11 Months of Age

Child's Abilities

Michael is an 11-month-old child with Down's syndrome. He is socially responsive in attending to his siblings and parents, and watches and smiles as they talk and interact with him. Michael's abilities include focusing attention on a toy—or person as long as something is happening—grasping and holding toys—and demonstrating a definite preference for colorful toys. He is beginning to sit independently with the support of his hands and prefers grabbing toys with his right hand.

Child's Needs/Functional Objectives

Michael's parents requested an assistive technology evaluation due to concern over lags in developmental milestones. They felt that assistive technology might

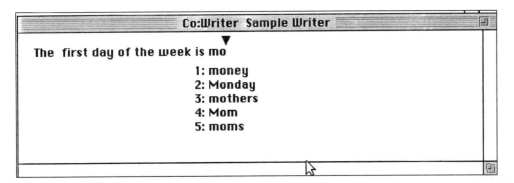

Figure 5.11. Screen with word prediction.

be beneficial to promote and extend Michael's abilities. Michael's parents noticed his lack of independence in changing positions and his inability to extend his arms to reach for and grasp objects with both hands when he was sitting. These movements are necessary to thoroughly explore objects and interact with them by banging or mouthing. It is a critical step for further development of hand-to-hand exchange, combining toys in play, and choice making.

Barriers to Participation

Michael's Down's syndrome resulted in overall low muscle tone, which caused difficulty in Michael's freely moving about. Although his trunk was becoming more stable in sitting (with hand and arm support), he did not roll over, creep, or get himself into or out of a sitting position. He also needed to free his hands in sitting to explore objects. His ability to communicate was restricted to facial animation and limited sound making. These factors were considered to be his barriers to playful interactions with objects and people in his environment.

Assistive Technology Assessment and Solutions

Michael was referred to a special project in the department of occupational therapy. Project staff included a pediatric occupational therapist, an early intervention assistive technology specialist, and a pediatric physical therapist. A telephone interview with Michael's mother was conducted to identify her goals and needs in regard to Michael. It was determined that Michael's assistive technology team would include the occupational therapist and early intervention assistive technology specialist. The evaluation took place in Michael's home. Michael's IFSP team included his parents and siblings, an occupational therapist, physical therapist, a speech therapist, and an early interventionist. Although only the family members were present during the assistive technology evaluation, the results were shared with his complete IFSP team. During the evaluation, Michael's family members were observed talking and interacting consistently with him, enthusiastically supporting any attempts to interact. A variety of colorful toys were available in his home that he reached for and held. Because repositioning would give him wider access to play materials (affecting his muscle strength, motor development, and visual/motor coordination) assistive technology solutions to support several positions were tried. One of his mother's concerns was the development of reach-

ing skills from sitting; she tried to encourage that movement by tugging on his arms to pull them forward. However, this resulted in him pulling back and resisting this movement. The occupational therapist suggested that she position him on her lap facing out and gently guide his upper arm from behind toward the toy, thereby supporting the development of the desired movement.

Michael used both hands together when he was lying supine. A jungle gym was used to increase his motivation and encourage him to use this movement. To bring the overhead toys within range of reach and grasp, links were added between jungle gym and toys to lower the toys. Toys and other household items were interchanged to increase the variety of materials. With these adaptations, Michael was immediately motivated to grab and manipulate the toys and objects hanging from the jungle gym.

Although Michael was beginning to sit independently, he was unable to use his hands to explore toys in this position because they were needed for support. By stabilizing his seated position with the use of a Boppy® (Figure 5.5) and placing toys on a table in front of him, the therapist freed his hands to reach for the toys. This seating position allowed Michael to watch and respond to other activities in the room. It also allowed his mother to play in front of him and respond to and encourage other play and communication skills. The early interventionist suggested that Michael's mother hold up two different toys for Michael to choose from to elicit toy-preference indicators.

In determining Michael's existing toy preferences, it became apparent that he was interested in a variety of toys with different responses, physical attributes, and access designs. Michael interacted most frequently with toys that incorporated high color contrast and were easy to grasp. He was able to hold, hit, and sometimes bring them to his mouth. Although he immediately responded to toys with sounds by looking in the direction of the toy, he preferred musical sounds to more startling noises, such as those from several electronic toys. When given a toy with sound he did not reach for it, but rather sat and watched. Toys with different tactile effects were also examined. Michael responded with great visual interest to a Koosh® ball but immediately withdrew his hand when he touched it. This element was new to Michael, and he needed further opportunities for interaction. The assistive technology team put a vibrating toy crab that was activated by sound or touch on the table. Although he did not use his

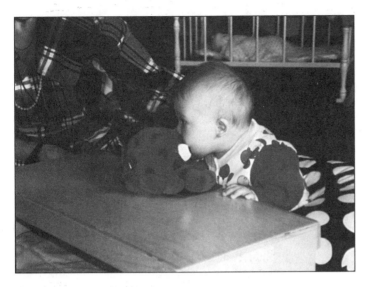

Figure 5.12. Michael with crab.

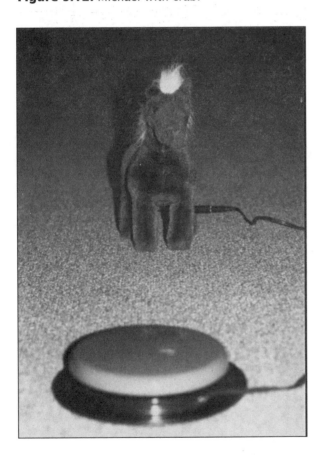

Figure 5.13. Big Red® and horse.

hands to reach for the crab, Michael was able to activate the toy with his mouth (Figure 5.12).

Play in a prone position is not easily tolerated for extended periods of time, yet it can help to develop strength in the shoulders and upper trunk and neck.

Michael maintained this new position longer when a switch toy was incorporated into the play activity. The occupational therapist showed Michael's mother how to place him on a narrow wedge to provide some upper trunk support. Michael was able to do some weight bearing on one hand while reaching with the other. A single switch (Big Red® by Ablenet) was attached to a battery-operated toy and placed in front of him on the floor (Figure 5.13). As Michael pressed the switch, the horse moved in a slow, horizontal motion in front of him. To include Michael as part of the play scenario, the toy was aimed toward him. As he pressed the switch again, the toy came closer to him. He then released the switch and grabbed for the horse. In this way, a single press resulted in a large response from the toy with Michael's role being integral to the play process.

Implemention and Reevaluation

As a result of the assessment, a play plan was developed by the assistive technology team and Michael's family. Michael's parents were to continue to encourage Michael's abilities to play by providing physical support to new play positions, following his play lead, and continuing to verbally identify what was happening when he was playing. The play plan (see Table 5.10) addressed the specific play goals and certain elements of the proposed solution (toys to be used and modifications, positions and modifications, and parent comments). Through the special university project, the assistive technology team was able to loan the assistive technology items (Boppy®, table, links, switch, and switch toy) used during the evaluation to the family for use at home.

Since this initial assessment, his parents have reported that Michael is sitting independently and is reaching for and better manipulating toys. He is beginning to roll over, and is particularly motivated to do so when the Koosh® ball is an available toy item. Colorful toys with tactile feedback are Michael's preference and his parents take care to change his positions more frequently. Michael has recently started to use an Exersaucer® (Evenflo) to support him in an upright position, which allows opportunities to use his legs more frequently. As part of the assistive technology evaluation process, a team member contacts his parents bimonthly to discuss progress in and changes to the jointly developed play plan.

Table 5.10. Play Plan: Michael.

What I want my child to do, and what we are working on.	Position.	What I need to make it work (positioning adaptations).	Toy or toys.	Toy modifications.	Strategies.	Comments.
sit without my help	sitting on the floor	using Boppy® with opening in the front; and tray	vibrating switch, jelly bean switch with horse, vibrating crab	put switch or toy on center of tray, if he needs help guide his arms to the toy or switch by pushing gently from the elbows		
			jungle gym with interesting rattles hanging from it	put jungle gym in front of him, close enough that he can reach, grab and bring some things to his mouth, shake other rattles		
play on his tummy	on his tummy with a towel roll under his arms for support	roll towel to about 3" thick and put it under his arms and across his chest to give him support	vibrating switch, lights go round, horse with jelly bean switch	make sure he is comfortable, arms forward, pay attention to when he becomes tired		
play on his back	in Boppy® with head on one 'arm' and legs on other	nothing special	jungle gym, bottle, teethers, rattles	give him things to play with with both hands; be there to pick things up for him when he begins this game; talk with him and encourage him to make sounds and faces, imitate those		

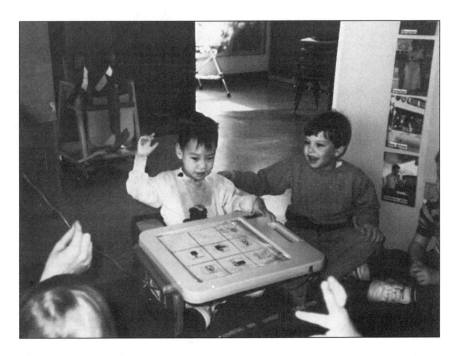

Figure 5.14. Andy in group.

Case Study: Andy, 4 Years of Age

Child's Abilities

Andy, a 4-year-old with cerebral palsy and spastic quadreparesis, is unable to walk or talk and demonstrates notable limitations in all motor abilities. Although his physical and communicative impairments are significant, his cognitive abilities were evaluated to be above average. Andy has used many assistive technology devices since he was very young. These devices include adaptive seating (powered wheelchair and adapted chair), modified eating and drawing tools, and a picture-board communication system. He demonstrated computer competence at a young age, beginning with switch and Touch Window® computer use, followed by a gradual introduction to alternative keyboards. His abilities include accurately pointing and pressing within a 2" area and the capacity to recognize and relate to pictures and symbols that represent a variety of functions and objects in his computer and life environments.

Child's Needs/Functional Objectives

Andy attended a community preschool center. He understood all activities in the classroom but was often restricted from full participation. His IEP team requested an assistive technology evaluation for additional assistance in the use of assistive technology to modify daily activities so that Andy could more

fully participate. This capability was most crucial because Andy was newly attending a community preschool center with nondisabled peers. The new environment had to be closely scrutinized to determine the functional tasks required of all children for involvement in each activity.

Barriers to Participation

Andy's primary barriers to participation were his lack of mobility and inability to speak. His IEP goals and objectives addressed methods of increased independence and participation in all aspects of the preschool program. Integrating these goals into the daily curriculum was of primary concern to his IEP team.

Assistive Technology Assessment and Solutions

Andy's IEP team consisted of his parents, two early educators, a special educator, an occupational therapist, physical therapist, and speech therapist. The special educator, as the IEP team leader, contacted the Center for Assistive Technology (CAT) to request an assistive technology evaluation. On receipt of background information from Andy's education team and family members, an assistive technology team was designated for his needs that included an occupational therapist and early education assistive technology specialist. This assistive technology team worked in conjunction with Andy's IEP team to develop appropriate assistive technology solutions. The evaluation took place at the integrated preschool center. Because of the high activity level in the early childhood classroom, the solutions focused around three general need areas: positioning, use of play materials, and communication.

1. *Positioning.* Although Andy was learning to use a powered wheelchair for independent mobility, he was unable to be positioned at the tables that the other children were using. Because the overriding goal for Andy was to participate in all aspects of the program, he needed to be at the same level as the others for various activities. To address this need, a

variety of positioning solutions were identified. A Rifton chair, fitted with appropriate inserts, was mounted onto a dolly. The chair was adapted so that it would fit at the tables, and a brake system on the dolly provided stability. Andy used his powered chair for outside walks but otherwise was pushed by his friends to the various activities throughout the day. In addition, because children tend to play on the floor, a corner chair was used. For several activities, small groups of children focused on language development, math and science concepts, and so on. For these activities, a table was available to be used with the floor sitter. This table provided a means for objects to be placed within Andy's reach and to hold his communication system (Figure 5.14).

2. *Use of Play Materials.* A wide range of play materials existed in the preschool classroom to encourage manipulation, construction, and pretend play. The staff received training on the selection of available materials that provide successful interactions for Andy. For example, puzzles with larger pieces or knobs, larger pegs, and blocks with Velcro® were used. Activities such as finger painting helped to build up Andy's hand skills. Paintbrushes and markers were modified for better grasp, and loop scissors encouraged independent cutting. For snack and lunch, Andy's aide cut up his food into small pieces that he could pick up and thus feed himself independently.

Computer activities were integrated throughout the program, specifically during "free time," where the children could select a favorite activity. Computer use during this time promoted the development of social and cooperative skills. Its use provided an opportunity for Andy to play on a more equal level with his peers, because he was proficient in controlling the computer. The assistive technology team chose software with an exploratory or constructive focus so that dyads of children could play and create together. Andy's prior computer skills allowed him to tutor many of his new friends in the workings of the software programs. An Apple IIgs with a speech synthesizer was available in the classroom. The children used it with a variety of input devices (i.e., switches, Touch Window®, PowerPad®, Muppet Learning Keys®).

3. *Communication.* Although Andy was unable to verbally interact, he communicated efficiently with facial gestures, sounds, and arm movements. Training was provided to the staff on methods of adapting questioning techniques so that Andy could participate in small group sessions. Communication boards were designed by the educators, with input from his therapists, and programmed into the PowerPad® by his aide for several activities each day. The computer's speech synthesizer and special software allowed Andy to respond to, initiate, and interact in the group activities. Special extenders made it possible for the PowerPad® and speech synthesizer to be used in different areas of the room without being noticeably attached to the computer. Velcro® strips ensured the PowerPad's® stability on the floor sitter table. By using this flexible communication system, Andy could initiate conversation and participate in a wide variety of activities.

Because Andy was a nonreader, symbols that represented story and activity content were used for communication, including photos, pictures, outlined drawings, and objects. Andy first explored each new board so that he could locate pertinent information.

Implementation and Reevaluation

Because Andy's IEP team maintained ongoing contact with the assistive technology team throughout the year, they reported increased proficiency in finding new uses for the communication system. It was used with groups of children for story sequencing, letting the computer say parts of the story, and for participation in gross motor (i.e., Simon Says, Hokey Pokey, Red Light/Green Light) and card and board games (i.e., Go Fish, BlockHead®, Candyland®). The assistive technology team continued to suggest software programs to encourage social development during free-time activities.

The assistive technology solutions developed by Andy's IEP team with the support of the assistive technology team were found to be responsive to Andy's needs within the early childhood center. Solutions were integrated into the daily activities by modifying or substituting materials and the presentation of information. Through work with the team and assessment within the natural environment, assistive technology solutions that addressed Andy's barriers to real participation were found and further expanded by the team members themselves.

Case Study: Amanda, 7 Years of Age

Child's Abilities

Amanda is 7 years of age—the youngest in a family of three children. Amanda was born with a neurological disorder that causes difficulties in all motor areas. Specifically, this condition produced significant delays in her fine, gross, and visuomotor development, which affects her ability to develop reading and written language and related skills. Amanda's auditory discrimination and perceptual abilities were within normal range.

Child's Needs/Functional Tasks

Amanda was unable to participate in many activities of the second grade curriculum due to motor control, balance, and speed and dexterity difficulties. These limitations created barriers to independent reading and writing. Her inability to take notes and write tests, stories, and homework assignments needed to be addressed. For written work, the classroom aide broke down the task to be done by prompting Amanda with questions such as, "Who is the story about?" and, "What happened next?" Amanda then entered her responses into the computer and printed out her story. Because her ability to read text was nonexistent, classroom accommodations for testing included rewording and rereading questions and recording her responses. Her IEP goals reflected the need to develop methods for increased independence and learning skills.

Barriers to Participation

Amanda was unable to participate in activities that incorporated reading or writing. With increasing dependence on the classroom aide, the IEP team requested an assistive technology assessment to identify solutions for more independent learning. Activities were needed that would promote the use of existing skills to experience successful learning opportunities.

Assistive Technology Assessment and Solutions

In Amanda's case, the school district's director of special education contacted CAT to request an assistive technology evaluation. When background forms indicating Amanda's needs and abilities were completed and returned to CAT by her education team and family, an assistive technology team was identified. The assistive technology team (an occupational therapist and education assistive technology specialist) worked with Amanda's IEP team members to identify both high- and low-technology solutions. Amanda's IEP team consisted of her parents, the second grade teacher, a consultant teacher, an aide, an occupational therapist, a physical therapist, and a speech therapist. The consultant teacher had modified several activities for Amanda that had some degree of success. These included larger, simpler worksheet figures; the use of concrete manipulatives in place of symbols/letters; and modified questioning techniques. The IEP team identified a need to continue these curricular modifications and added the option of providing separate yet related activities for small groups of children (including Amanda) to better address specific skill building. The assistive technology team suggested positioning and adapted tool use, such as a weighted pen to provide more sensory feedback during writing and, therefore, a better "connection" to the writing surface.

Because Amanda demonstrated a high interest in computer activities, the assistive technology team viewed this as a way to promote independent work skills. By incorporating the sound capabilities of the computer with a "talking" word processor (*IntelliTalk®*), her auditory and receptive language skills were maximized. Sound capabilities were used to reinforce typed letters, words, and sentences, as well as to read aloud text displayed on the screen. Amanda was most successful participating in activities that employed all learning modes including vision (seeing words and pictures on the screen), audition (hearing words spoken), and tactile/kinesthetic (typing words and making selections on the keyboard). Computer activities provided opportunities for Amanda to interact with the special talking software, which promoted the use of her existing capabilities and interests.

To address Amanda's motor limitations, an expanded keyboard (IntelliKeys®) was selected for use because it provided several different overlays that could be used with available software programs for easier access. An overlay with an alphabetical key layout (such as that shown in Figure 5.10) was included. Amanda stated that she could find letters better because she could find them by using her previous knowledge of alphabet sequencing.

To address the development of writing skills, IntelliTalk® was again used, this time to provide opportunities for Amanda to develop sight word recognition and to apply the use of words in written context. The assistive technology team encouraged Amanda to use whole words in various activities to build sight word, initial consonant, and rhyming

Figure 5.15.
Customized overlay.

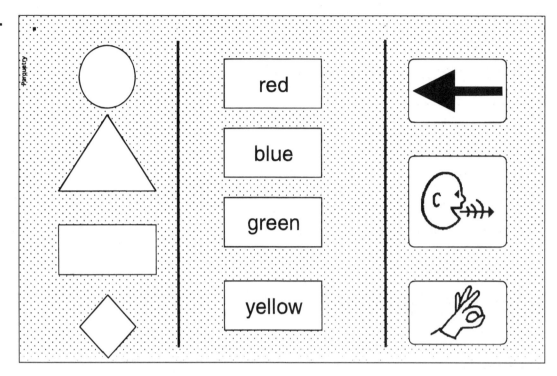

skills. The software is also capable of rereading certain words and stories so that Amanda could check and edit her work independently.

Although this method looked promising, Amanda needed independent activities to promote her use of words in context. The IEP and assistive technology teams worked together to design several activities on the basis of Amanda's interests that would use the capabilities of the computer. To further develop reading skills, overlays were designed with a software program, *Overlay Maker* (IntelliTools), that uses words and concepts that Amanda had mastery over (i.e., colors, numbers, family names). Overlays were designed to be used with the talking word processor that would promote sentence building, word choice, and the ability to self-correct. Each overlay also included several function keys that allowed Amanda to (a) accept her response as correct, (b) delete a response, (c) reread the current sentence, and (d) print. These functions were depicted with the use of symbols representing the different functions. In this way, Amanda could focus on the use of the whole word, and spelling skills were unnecessary. Amanda was able to begin writing and editing sentences. Figure 5.15 shows an overlay was used in conjunction with parquetry blocks. Amanda was given several blocks and told to identify them by using the overlay. When she was finished, she printed out her work.

Intervention and Reevaluation

Amanda worked independently with these customized overlays. The overlay was visually well organized. Tasks were based on prior knowledge and her ability to hear the word, make a choice, and choose to accept it as correct or to edit her answer. She used this activity with a variety of different objects (by editing the second column), even with popular toys (Power Rangers). Because Amanda easily identified colors, using related sight words as descriptors of these familiar objects helped to ensure interest and the generalization of color descriptors. The flexibility of the assistive technology solutions provided a means for modifications across the curriculum.

As these success stories show, assistive technology helps to increase the child's independence and access to learning and doing. For teachers, it provides the means to successful inclusion by adapting access to the curriculum itself.

Technology has come of age. These success stories illustrate how technology is used to provide a way for children to bypass or compensate for limitations imposed by disabilities. Technology is useful to extend the abilities of children with disabilities within their various life roles. It promotes autonomy and provides ways to increase participation in the home, community, and school environments.

Appendix

Vendors of Computer Peripherals for Young Children

BEST, Inc.

63 Forest Street
Chestnut Hill, MA 02167
(617) 277-0179

Don Johnston, Inc.

1000 North Rand Road., Bldg. 115
P.O. Box 639
Wauconda, IL 60084
(800) 999-4660

Dunamis, Inc.

3629 Highway 317
Suwanee, GA 30174
(800) 828-2443

Edmark Corporation

P.O. Box 3218
Redmond, WA 98073
(800) 426-0856

Hach Associates

P.O. Box 10849
Winston-Salem, NC 27108
(800) 624-7968

IntelliTools

55 Leveroni Ct., Ste. 9
Novato, CA 94949
(800) 899-6687
(415) 382-5959

Sunburst

101 Castleton Street
P.O. Box 100
Pleasantville, NY 10570
(800) 321-7511

Chapter 5 References

A New Compact for Learning: Improving public elementary, middle and secondary education results in the 1990's. (1991, Nov.). The University of the State of New York, State Education Department.

Americans with Disabilities Act of 1990, P.L. 101–336.

Behrman, M.M. (1984). A brighter future for early learning through high tech. *The Pointer, 28*(2), 23–26.

Behrman, M., & Lahm, E. (1984). Babies and robots: Technology to assist learning. *Rehabilitation Literature, 45*(7), 194–201.

Berger, K.S. (1994). *The developing person through the lifespan* (3rd ed.). New York: Worth.

Biklin, D., & Schubert, A. (1991). New words: The communication of students with autism. *Remedial and Special Education, 12*(6), 46–57.

Bradley, M.P. (1994). Computers for the very young: From the ridiculous to the sublime. *Closing the Gap, 13*(2), 15.

Brinker, R.P., & Lewis, M. (1982). Making the world work with microcomputers: A learning prosthesis for handicapped infants. *Exceptional Children, 49*(2), 163–170.

Carnine, D. (1989). Teaching complex content to learning disabled students: The role of technology. *Exceptional Children, 55,* 524–533.

Case, R. (1985). *Intellectual development: Birth to adulthood.* Orlando, FL: Academic Press.

Cates, W.M., & McNaull, P.A. (1993). Inservice training and university coursework: Its influence on computer use and attitudes among teachers of learning disabled students. *Journal of Research on Computing in Education, 25*(4), 447–463.

Cavalier, A.R., Ferretti, R.P., & Okolo, C. (1994). Technology and individual differences. *Journal of Special Education Technology, XII*(3), 175–181.

Fewell, R.R. & Kaminski, R. (1988). Play skills development and instruction for young children with handicaps. In S.L. Odom & M.B. Karnes (Eds.) *Early intervention of infants and children with handicaps: An empirical base.* Baltimore, MD: Paul Brookes, pp. 145–158.

Field, T. (1980). Self, teacher, toy and peer-directed behaviors of handicapped preschool children. In T. Field, S. Goldberg, D. Stern, & A. Sostek (Eds.), *High-risk infants and children: Adult and peer interactions.* New York: Academic Press.

Flavell, J.H. (1985). *Cognitive development* (2nd ed.). Englewood Cliffs, NJ: Prentice Hall.

Florey, L. (1971). An approach to play and play development. *American Journal of Occupational Therapy, 15*(6), 275–280.

Hanson, M.J., & Hanline, M.F. (1985). An analysis of response-contingent learning experiences for young children. *Journal of the Association for Persons with Severe Handicaps, 10*(1), 31–40.

Hanzlik, J.R. (1989). The effect of intervention on the free-play experience for mothers and their infants with developmental delay and cerebral palsy. *Physical & Occupational Therapy in Pediatrics, 9*(2), 33–51.

Heward, W.L., & Orlansky, M.D. (1992). *Exceptional children: An introductory survey of special education.* New York: Merrill.

Higgins, K.K. (1988). Hypertext computer assisted instruction and the social studies achievement of learning disabled, remedial, and regular education high school students. Unpublished doctoral dissertation, University of New Mexico, Albuquerque.

Hopkins, H.L., & Smith, H.D. (eds). (1988). *Willard and Spackman's occupational therapy* (7th ed.). Philadelphia: Lippincott.

Individuals with Disabilities Education Act of 1990, P.L. 101–476.

Jennings, K., Connors, R., Stegman, C., Sankaranaryan, P., & Mendelesohn, S. (1985). Mastery motivation in young preschoolers: Effect of a physical handicap and implications for educational programming. *Journal of Division for Early Childhood, 9,* 162–169.

Jones, S., Smith, L.B. & Landau, B. (1991). Object properties and knowledge in early lexical learning. *Child Development, 62,* 499–516.

Kerr, R. (1985). Fitts' law and motor control in children. In J.E. Clark & J.H. Humphrey (Eds.), *Motor development: Current selected research.* Princeton, NJ: Princeton Book Company.

Kogan, K.L., & Tyler, N. (1973). Mother-child interaction in young physically handicapped children. *American Journal of Mental Deficiency, 77*(5), 492–497.

Lahm, E.A. (ed.). (1989). *Technology with low incidence populations: Promoting access to education and learning.* Reston, VA: Center for Special Education Technology.

Landry, S.H., & Chapieski, M.L. (1989). Joint attention and infant toy exploration: Effects of Down syndrome and prematurity. *Child Development, 60,* 103–118.

Lane, S.J., & Mistrett, S.G. (1994). *Toy characteristics. 10*(2). Workshop conducted for NEOSERRC, Warren, Ohio.

Langley, M.B. (1990). A developmental approach to the use of toys for facilitation of environmental control. *Rehabilitation Technology,* 69–91.

Lindsey, J.D. (1993). *Computers and exceptional individuals.* Austin, TX: Pro-Ed.

Mahshie, J. (1988). Making strides: Speech training aids take a quantum leap with advanced computer technology. *Gallaudet Today, 18,* 14–17.

Male, M. (1994). *Technology for inclusion.* Needham Heights, MA: Allyn & Bacon.

Messer, D.J., Rachfor, D., McCarthey, M.E., & Yarrow, L.J. (1987). Assessment of mastery behavior at 30 months: Analysis of task-directed activities. *Developmental Psychology, 23,* 771–781.

Mistrett, S.G., Constantino, S.L., & Pomerantz, D. (1994). Using computers to increase the social interactions of preschoolers with disabilities at community-based sites. *Technology and Disability 3*(2), 148–157.

Mistrett, S.G. (1992). *Preschool integration through technology systems* (training kit). Buffalo, NY: UCPA.

Moore, G.B., Yin, R.K., & Lahm, E.A. (1986). Robotics, artificial intelligence, computer simulation: Future applications in special education. *Technological Horizons in Special Education, 14*(1), 74–76.

Musselwhite, C.R. (1986). *Adaptive play for special needs children.* San Diego, CA: College-Hill Press.

Newson, E., & Head, J. (1979). Play and playthings for the handicapped child. In J. Head & E. Newson, (Eds.), *Toys and playthings.* London: George, Allen and Bacon.

Piaget, J. (1962). *Play, dreams and limitation in childhood.* New York: Norton.

Regents long range plan for technology in elementary and secondary education in New York State. (1990, June). The University of the State of New York, the State Education Department.

Rosenberg, S., Clark, M., Filer, J., Hupp, S., & Finkler, D. (1992). Facilitating active learner participation. *Journal of Early Intervention, 16*(3), 262–274.

Rosenberg, S., & Robinson, C. (1988). *Interactions of parents with their young handicapped children.* In S. Odom & M. Karns (Eds.), *Research in early childhood special education.* pp. 139–177. Baltimore: Brookes.

Sloan-Armstrong, J., & Jones, K. (1994). Assistive technology and young children: Getting off to a great start! *Closing the Gap, 1,* 31–32.

Smilansky, S. (1968). *The effects of sociodramatic play on disadvantaged preschool children.* New York: Wiley.

Swinth, Y., & Case-Smith, J. (1993). Assistive technology in early intervention: Theory and practice. In J. Case-Smith (Ed.), *Pediatric occupational therapy and early intervention.* Boston: Andover Medical.

Swinth, Y., Anson, D., & Deitz, J. (1993). Single switch computer access for infants and toddlers. *American Journal of Occupational Therapy, 47*(11), 1031–1038.

Takata, N. (1971). The play milieu—A preliminary appraisal. *American Journal of Occupational Therapy, 15*(6), 281–284.

Technology Related Assistance for Individuals With Disabilities Act of 1988. P.L. 100–407.

U.S. Congress Office of Technology Assessment. (1995). *Teachers and technology: Making the connection, OTA-EHR-616.* Washington, DC: U.S. Government Printing Office.

Van Tatenhove, G. (1987). Teaching power through augmentative communication: Guidelines for early intervention. *Journal of Childhood Communication Disorders, 10*(2), 185–199.

Wehman, P. (1979). *Recreation programming for developmentally delayed persons.* Baltimore: University Park Press.

Wilds, M.L. (1989). Effective use of technology with young children. *NICHCY News Digest, 13*, 6–7.

Chapter 5 Study Questions

1. List and describe each of the four chronological stages of development as outlined by Piaget.

2. Give several examples of "barriers" to play, learning, and development faced by children with disabilities.

3. List four primary uses of assistive technology for children from birth to 10 years of age, and give examples of low-tech and high-tech interventions for each of the four primary uses.

4. List six commonly used types of switches. What is the activation mechanism for each switch?

5. Describe the selection and use of assistive technology with infants and toddlers.

6. Describe the selection and use of assistive technology with preschoolers.

7. Describe the selection and use of assistive technology with elementary school children.

8. List and describe four keyboard alternatives for young children.

9. List and describe three computer pointing devices for young children.

10. List and describe four special features of word processors useful for children with disabilities.

Chapter 6:
Technology and Higher Education

I. Introduction
   A. Impact of Legislation
   B. Transition Issues

II. Assistive Technology in Higher Education
   A. Technology for Hearing Impairments
   B. Technology for Visual Impairments
   C. Technology for Mobility Impairments
   D. Technology for Neurological Impairments
   E. Technology for Learning Disabilities

III. Computer Accessibility on College Campuses

IV. Assistive Technology Provision for Use in Higher Education
   A. Referral
   B. Assessment
   C. Procurement of Equipment
   D. Equipment Setup
   E. Training
   F. Follow-up
   G. Maintenance and Repair of Devices

V. Case Studies
   A. Case Study 1
      1. Background
      2. Assessment
      3. Intervention
      4. Outcome
      5. Conclusion
   B. Case Study 2
      1. Background
      2. Assessment
      3. Intervention
      4. Outcome
      5. Conclusion

6.

Technology and Higher Education

Christine R. Oddo, MS, OTR/L

Introduction

Impact of Legislation

Over the past several years, the advances in technology, especially computer technology, have created numerous opportunities for students with disabilities. This is evident in higher education, where students use devices for access to information and computers, for mobility around campuses, for communication, and for control of the environment. This use of technology has contributed to an increase in the number of students with disabilities participating in higher education programs.

The increasing number of students with disabilities on campus is supported by federal legislation that was enacted to end discrimination against persons with disabilities. Section 504 of the Rehabilitation Act of 1973 mandates that reasonable accommodations be made by institutions of higher education receiving federal funds to allow full participation by students with disabilities in educational programs and activities available to nondisabled students (College Consortium of Disability Advocates, 1993). This includes "appropriate academic adjustments and reasonable modifications to policies and practices" (College Consortium of Disability Advocates, p. 2). Initially, legislation largely addressed accessibility to buildings and physical barriers. Colleges soon determined that there is a strong need for access to classrooms, class materials, computers, and electronic information in addition to the need for campuses, buildings, and programs to be accessible. This legislation, along with varied student needs, has helped to provide accessibility and to develop support services for students with disabilities on college campuses and universities. More recent legislation, the Americans With Disabilities Act (ADA) of 1990, supports previous legislation and extends Section 504 to both the private and public sectors, regardless of whether federal financial assistance is received (Rubenstein & Milestein, 1993). This mandates equal opportunity in employment, public accommodation, transportation, state and local government services, and telecommunications.

Transition planning is now mandated for students with disabilities at the secondary level who receive special education under the Individuals With Disabilities Education Act (Pub. L. No. 101-476). This legislation defines transition services as:

a coordinated set of activities for a student, designed within an outcome-oriented process, which promotes movement from school to post-school activities, including post-secondary education, vocational training, integrated employment (including supported employment), continuing and adult education, adult services, independent living and/or community participation (20 U.S.C. Chapter 33, 1401 [a] [19]).

Transition Issues

Studies have indicated that persons with disabilities have poor postschool employment, residential independence, and participation in postsecondary education (Hasazi, Hock, & Cravedi-Cheng, 1992). Transition services are necessary to guide student choices. Planning is the combined effort of student, parents, school personnel, and other agencies or service providers involved in a student's future activities, and the individualized education program directs the types of services and educational accommodations made within the school. This differs from the

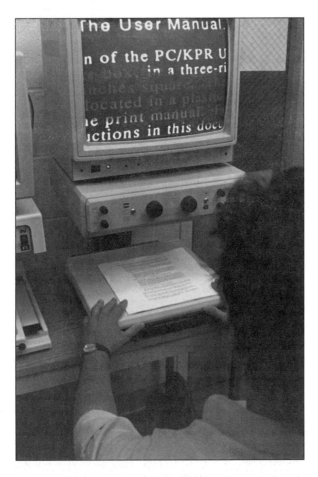

Figure 6.1. Closed-caption television.

postsecondary setting where students assume the main responsibility for procuring accommodations for full access to education. This planning process is important because it assists the secondary student who pursues postsecondary education and facilitates a smooth transition to college (Wagner, Blackorby, Cameto, & Newman, 1993).

To make this transition process successful, awareness of the range of education issues is necessary. These issues include the need for case coordination, direct experiences by the student, and outcome-oriented planning (Nochajski, 1993). Coordinated services of the educational agency, vocational rehabilitation and/or adult services agencies, and the student help to ensure access to needed services. Student participation in a variety of situations is necessary to increase awareness of available employment, education, and independent living options and to help make more informed choices. In addition, families and students have concerns related to student performance and success, independence, and self-advocacy that need to be addressed (Arnold & Czamanske, 1991). Outcome-oriented planning

focuses on both long-range and life goals.

Transition planning for postsecondary education is useful to resolve issues of student support, assistance with class-related needs, technology available and modifications implemented, and other procedures associated with a student's needs. The provision and training in use of assistive devices prior to college enrollment prepares the student for more optimal performance and equips him or her with skills to maintain pace and perform necessary tasks with more independence.

The awareness of available assistive technology and its use facilitates a student's progress in the pursuit of higher education and in transition to work. Educators, students, and those assisting students with the transition to postsecondary education or to work require information and updates on current devices and how they support educational endeavors. In addition, development of self-advocacy skills during the transition process facilitates student performance at the postsecondary level (College Consortium of Disability Advocates, 1993; Yuditsky, 1991). Strategies necessary to helping students learn about their needs, what accommodations will help, and how to advocate for modifications, include (a) identifying student strengths and weaknesses, (b) developing relevant questions concerning accommodations and procedures, and (c) identifying available assistive devices and resources for community support.

Transition from the postsecondary experience to work also requires planning (Deykes & Anthony, 1994). This planning continues throughout the postsecondary experience to assist with college requirements. It promotes a smooth and successful transition from postsecondary activities and the education environment to gainful employment and the workplace environment. College personnel who assist students with disabilities must be directed toward finding ways to expand the students' capabilities. This also requires helping students to educate employers, and identifying innovative ways to make students marketable and competitive for jobs by using current advances in technology.

Services, accommodations, and devices that assist students with disabilities are offered either through offices known as disabled student services, or through a coordinator designated to provide assistance to these students. Assistance includes alternative testing arrangements where examination time, testing method, or location is modified; use of special equipment, including a variety of assistive technology; adapted computer access; flexibility in course requirements; and extended time to complete course-work (Heath Resource Center, 1994). These accommodations and services also include notetakers to assist in class lectures; readers to assist with tests or assignments; sign language interpreters; special help or tutoring; and physical access to campus classrooms, the library, and other student-related activities. Yuditsky (1991) emphasizes that each student's experience is unique and should be considered in making accommodations. Accommodations, services, and adaptations vary depending on student needs.

Students typically initiate the process for receiving special services and accommodations. They identify themselves to the educational institution as having a disability. Accommodations, services, or adaptations needed for academic performance are determined in meetings with college personnel. Interaction with specific faculty members or instructors provides critical information exchange about class formats, expectations, and requirements, and student needs. This also helps to accurately inform and eliminate myths about a student's abilities and disabilities, thus facilitating more opportunities for a successful college experience.

This chapter focuses on the use of assistive technology in higher education. It presents issues related to students with disabilities and assistive technology. Assistive technology is examined through case studies.

Assistive Technology in Higher Education

An extensive range of assistive technology allows students to access computers, classroom activities, and the overall higher education environment (Beaver & Mann, 1994; Brown, 1987; Castorina, 1994; Church & Glennen, 1992; Coombs & Cartwright, 1994; Lazzaro, 1993; Mann & Lane, 1991; Murphy, 1991). Devices assist all ages and ranges of persons with disabilities. Many such devices are customized to meet individual needs to promote more active participation in the learning process and in performing coursework (Brown).

For example, colleges frequently provide reading machines in centralized locations for students with poor vision who are unable to read standard-size print. Figure 6.1 shows a closed-caption television.

This device enlarges printed text and can be adjusted for letter size, contrast, and other visual presentation options to meet the user's specific needs. It permits the student to read class-related materials

and complete reading assignments. Murphy (1991) suggests that the majority of technology use by college students with disabilities is computer-related and focuses on several higher education sites that provide technology services or programs. These programs address computer access and technology devices for students with various disabilities, including visual and hearing impairments, learning disabilities, and communication impairments. These and other exemplary technology programs have provided assistive technology services to both students and institutions to promote education.

Institutions of higher education are increasingly proactive in helping students with disabilities to identify and address their needs and to access the resources to successfully complete their education (Murphy, 1991). Together, students and colleges identify ways to assist students in the education process. Interventions and options include modifying the physical environment, altering the way information is presented, adapting the educational methods used, and improving the awareness of peer students and instructors. Many adaptations offered to students with disabilities in the postsecondary setting include assistive technology (Heath Resource Center, 1994; Spiers, 1992; Yuditsky, 1991)—the use of adapted workstations within computer laboratories. College advocacy programs encourage students with disabilities to request information about assistive devices and campus accommodations—especially when a student requires the use of assistive technology to complete course requirements (College Consortium of Disability Advocates, 1993; Spiers). Assistive technology has been shown to improve learning and productivity among students with disabilities (Lenker, 1993).

Coombs and Cartwright (1994) describe on-line support for students with disabilities, including electronic discussion lists, an electronic journal, and a "gopher" to assist with accessible technology use. The electronic discussion lists enable users to discuss relevant issues related to technology and education over the Internet. The electronic journal provides articles on-line that can be viewed on a monitor, read with screen-reading software, or printed in standard print or Braille. A gopher permits users to browse, search for, and retrieve information on specific topics or areas of interest. It is used to assist the user with a more selective way to locate information on disability issues. These on-line features provide a mechanism for disabled students to resolve problems, interact with others, search for more information, and

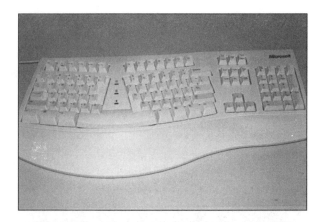

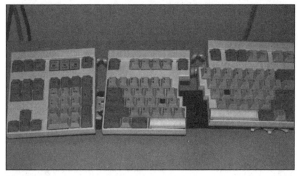

Figure 6.2. Alternative keyboards.

promote active participation and independence by using assistive technology.

Continued advances in information technology applications in the educational environment require students to access information from a variety of sources and create a means for producing high-quality assignments. Devices are used to assist students in the areas of oral and written communication, mobility, education, and learning (Castorina, 1994). For example, a variety of augmentative communication devices with speech output provide assistance with communication for nonverbal students or for students whose speech is not understandable. Students use these devices to interact with others and to actively participate in course tasks that involve speaking. Mobility devices such as wheelchairs, walkers, and canes assist students with moving around a campus and within buildings. Travel aids provide information about the environment to students with sensory impairments. Assistive technology enables students with a wide range of disabilities to write papers, access electronic information and technology for research, and perform other tasks to meet the demands of college courses.

Assistive technology is also related to proper positioning, computer access, assistive listening, com-

puter-based instruction, and visual aids (RESNA Technical Assistance Project, 1992). Adapted computer use enables students to access the computer for instruction programs, assignments, telecommunications, and library research. A variety of alternative input devices and methods permit students who are unable to use the standard keyboard or mouse to input information into the computer (Lau & O'Leary, 1993).

For example, as shown in Figure 6.2, there are multiple alternative keyboards that vary in size and key layout and are customizable for direct access to the computer. A student uses the alternative device to input keystrokes and commands and to produce necessary written work. Devices provide ways for students to perform tasks they are unable to do as a result of a disability.

Many students with disabilities use alternative methods to complete educational requirements by using assistive technology. For example, some students perform written tasks and assignments better by using auditory feedback to listen to work they have produced. Computer hardware and software programs such as screen readers or talking word processors read text on the screen. Students can listen to words or sentences as they compose. This strategy is also used for test taking, where the test is presented in electronic format on a computer screen and read to the student by using voice output from a computer.

Various strategies and a variety of assistive devices are used by students with specific impairments. The devices discussed below are often used across disabilities and for a variety of purposes. This discussion highlights devices used for students with hearing and visual impairments, mobility impairments, neurological impairments, and learning disabilities. Other chapters address in detail assistive technology for persons with hearing impairments, visual impairments, and physical disabilities.

Technology for Hearing Impairments

Hearing impairments in students, from deafness to partial hearing loss, affect the student's ability to communicate. These impairments often contribute to additional deficits in speaking and reading. Personal interactions and communication within a group is affected along with a student's participation in and contribution to class activities. Independence in tasks and performance in a variety of college activities are affected, such as access to the content of lectures, recordings, videotapes, and other instructional materials. Assistive devices often used are hearing aids, frequency modulation (FM) amplification systems, written captions to visual aids, and electronic and carbon notepaper. Students also use telecommunication devices and e-mail to facilitate communication with other students and instructors. Figure 6.3 depicts a TTY device.

A hearing impairment also affects the way a student accesses the computer. Students may not be able to interpret auditory feedback from software programs or from hardware. Adaptations to the computer include assistive software and hardware that provide visual flashes or vibratory output as alternatives to auditory beeps or signals.

Technology for Visual Impairments

Impairments in vision range from partial vision loss due to a distortion in part of the visual field to total blindness. These impairments result in difficulty with mobility and orientation around campuses and buildings; inability to access printed materials, lecture notes, and books; inability to access the computer; and increased dependence in educational and life activities.

Assistive technology plays a large role in compensating for visual loss. Devices include low-technology adaptations that provide color or tactile contrast and variation in size. For example, adaptations include a computer keyboard layout adapted with a high contrast of white letters on a black background together with enlarged letter size and raised dot symbols located on the home keys. A white-on-black keyboard is shown in Figure 6.4. Other low-technology adaptations include screen filters, screen magnifiers positioned on a computer monitor, and Braille labels placed on folders, notebooks, and other items for identification.

Other assistive devices serve multiple purposes. For example, a closed-circuit television provides enlargement of printed text for reading, writing, and other hand tasks. Closed-circuit televisions are used in libraries to access resource materials and in a laboratory setting to enlarge specimens or data.

Assistive devices for students with visual impairments also include reading machines that allow printed text to be scanned and then spoken. Large-print books, including dictionaries and other reference materials, are available. Portable recording devices assist students in the classroom with notes and messages. Instructional materials and tests can also be enlarged on a copy machine. *Raised-line drawings,* shown in Figure 6.5, provide access to graphics such as diagrams, charts, or maps.

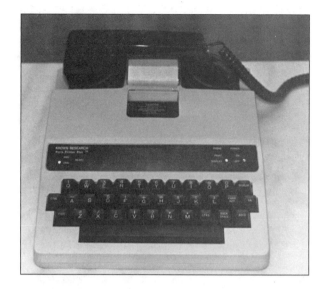

Figure 6.3. TTY device.

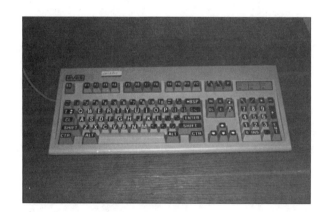

Figure 6.4. White-on-black keyboard.

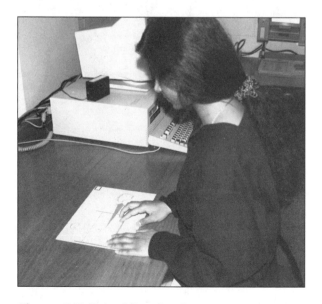

Figure 6.5. Raised-line drawing.

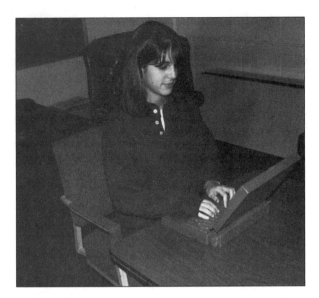

Figure 6.6. Notebook computer.

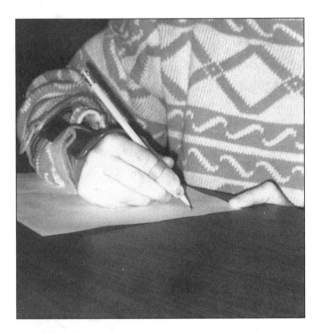

Figure 6.7. Writing splint.

Major adaptations include the use of computer technology with voice synthesizers and screen readers that explain what is displayed on the computer screen. The information read includes books on disk, reference materials on disk or CD-ROM, or typed text that is scanned into the computer. Other computer adaptations include refreshable Braille output, character enlargement software to enlarge information displayed on the screen, and Braille embossers for access to hard copies in Braille. Refreshable Braille is a series of Braille cells placed in a row.

Each cell has six or eight pins that raise and lower electronically to reproduce Braille characters. When those devices are connected to a computer, they provide dynamic tactile access to information displayed on the computer screen.

Technology for Mobility Impairments

Students with mobility impairments are affected by a number of disabilities. These range from changes in the musculoskeletal system that affect muscle use and joint function to other ailments that affect mobility and endurance, such as a respiratory illness. Students with mobility impairments have difficulty getting around campus. Limitations often include access to certain classrooms, narrow doorways, restrooms and facilities, or to sidewalks and building entrances.

Students who are unable to work or experience difficulty with walking due to an impairment use mobility devices such as wheelchairs, canes, crutches, or other devices to increase mobility. They also use transportation vehicles for mobility across campus. Easy access must be considered for these students. Environmental modifications such as ramps, electronic doors, and level thresholds improve accessibility. Other issues such as weather conditions or problems with transportation affect mobility and access.

Mobility impairments limit the amount of travel at any one time or day. This factor often requires other accommodations related to completing necessary school tasks. This includes devices to transport books and supplies and portable devices such as *laptop (notebook) computers*. A notebook computer is shown in Figure 6.6. Additional devices include adjustable-height workstations and wheelchairs.

Technology for Neurological Impairments

Neurological impairments result in a decrease of physical function, strength, sensation, or coordination due to impairments in the nervous system. Impairments in use of the extremities present problems with performance in class and in managing assignments. This frequently results in difficulty with book, paper, and pen manipulation and with tasks that relate to class assignments, homework, and writing papers. Hand movements that are impaired or painful require alternative writing tools or adaptations to other tools. Students may experience an inability to carry books and other items due to impaired ability to use their extremities or due to a loss of extremities. Speed in performing tasks is often decreased due to such a disability. Overall, these impairments may affect several areas of student performance.

Assistive technology devices include the use of tape recorders where important points can be noted for quick reference on playback of the tape, or the use of carbon paper for class lectures. Alternative typing methods or adaptations to writing tools, laboratory equipment, and machinery that provide alternative grip options or that substitute for decreased hand function are useful. For example, grip size is often increased for better hand control. A writing splint is shown in Figure 6.7. Environmental adaptations include devices such as modified doorknobs, elevator controls, and faucet handles for easier access. An example of a doorknob adaptor is shown in Figure 6.8.

Adaptive computer technology includes the use of alternative input devices for computer access. Alternative keyboards include enlarged or reduced-size keyboards, customizable keyboards, and keyboard emulators. If a student is unable to access a keyboard, alternative methods for typing into the computer are available. These include the use of voice recognition, where words are spoken into the computer, use of scanning techniques with switch activation, and the use of Morse code. Alternative pointing devices such as trackballs or head pointers allow students with only minimal movements to access graphical user interfaces. For example, a device that consists of a small dot placed on an person's forehead together with a receiver placed on top of a computer monitor that uses infrared signals provides for control of a mouse pointer and enables access to a wide variety of application programs and menu systems. The head-mouse is shown in Figure 6.9.

Assistive software is used to provide better access to the computer, including utility programs that allow for customizing the keyboard response to the user's needs. For example, software can be used to allow a student who uses one finger, or one hand, to input commands and keystrokes that require simultaneous compression in sequence instead. Word-prediction and abbreviation-expansion programs decrease the amount of keystrokes necessary to type full words. Students can preprogram words that are frequently used for assignments or papers. Word processing software provides autocorrection for typing errors, spelling and grammar checkers, and macro capability. On-screen keyboards provide alternative keyboard access by using pointing devices or switches.

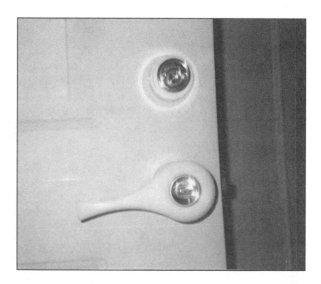

Figure 6.8. Doorknob adaptor.

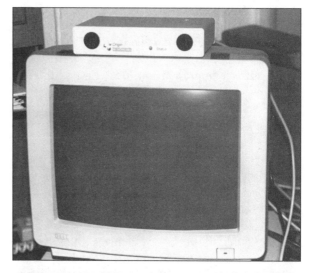

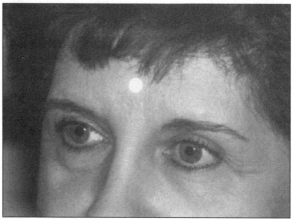

Figure 6.9. The head-mouse uses an infrared receiver placed on top of a computer monitor and a small dot placed on the user's forehead.

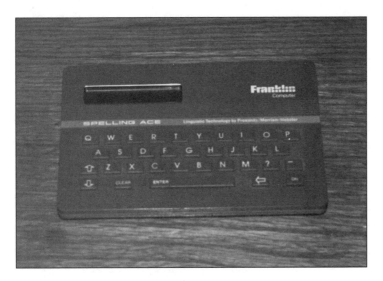

Figure 6.10. Electronic dictionary.

Technology for Learning Disabilities

Students with learning disabilities experience difficulty with oral and written expression, listening and reading comprehension, decoding skills, and performance in mathematical tasks. These difficulties affect their ability to understand lectures, take notes, perform assignments, perform writing tasks, and participate in class activities. Strategies include use of spell checkers, grammar checkers, and word processors along with instructional tutoring. Other accommodations include use of visual or auditory presentation or a combination of sensory output to obtain information for those with visual or auditory processing deficits. Other modifications include the use of tape recorders for notetaking, calculators, electronic dictionaries, and voice output. An electronic dictionary is shown in Figure 6.10. Devices also enable students with multiple disabilities to perform educational tasks that allow for a variety of alternative keyboard input methods, alternative output methods, alternative pointing devices, use of voice recognition and voice output systems, talking word processors, and assistive software.

There are many other disabilities that may require accommodations, and there are many other assistive devices and ways to adapt materials than the aforementioned devices. Many of the difficulties experienced are often compounded by other impairments, and careful planning is required to prepare students for full and active participation in college activities and work.

Computer Accessibility on College Campuses

To make college computers accessible for persons with disabilities, special equipment or devices are often added, systems are configured to incorporate an adaptive device, assistive software is loaded, and workstations are modified. Accessible computer equipment and software are procured either by the institution or by the student. Consultation between experts knowledgeable about assistive technology, the college's computer technology support, and representatives from a college's office of student disabilities frequently provides solutions for students with disabilities. Students sometimes require use of devices that are highly specialized and may require alternative funding to obtain them. It is important for students to identify campus representatives who provide the technical expertise and assistance to students. Available hardware and application programs used on campus also should be determined to establish accessibility and resolve problems related to specialized needs.

College computer laboratories offer students a wide array of computer technology. Campuses are now equipped with both Macintosh and IBM platforms. They offer a wide range of application software, networking capabilities, electronic mail, and other technology applications. Assistive technology for both platforms is now readily available.

The graphical user environment for Macintosh systems and Windows also affects the provision of technology and the way it is used. For example, character-enlargement software necessary to view menus and icons can impose challenges for the student with poor vision, especially if the student has multiple disabilities. These include orientation to the screen layout, identifying location of icons and menus and navigation through windows. Alternative ways to access this environment involve the use of keyboard commands or voice output and require additional time for learning. Adaptations and assistive devices must be configured and used to determine effectiveness. Students require options that will be available after the achievement of education goals to apply their learning to the work environment.

Many college computer laboratories have been adapted for access by students with disabilities. Lenker (1993) describes how a 2-year community college initially acquired assistive technology for use by its students with disabilities. The Coordinator of Disabled Students was proactive in pursuing assistive equipment. Funding was obtained through a federally sponsored program. Computers that were accessible needed to serve a wide student range with physical impairments, sensory impairments, and learning disabilities. A site close to offices frequently used by students with disabilities was selected. Workstations were modified with adjustable-height tables that could easily be independently adjusted by most students and had various wrist rest supports. Hardware modifications included a voice synthesizer for voice output and hardware and keyboard adaptations with high color contrast and enlarged letter and Braille symbols. Software modifications included screen-reading software, voice-output software, keyboard enhancement software, and word-prediction software. Equipment recommendation, installation, and system configuration was provided by a team of experts familiar with assistive devices. Training of college staff members on adaptive software and system troubleshooting was provided. Additional hardware and software were purchased and added to the systems as needed by students with special needs. The college assumed technical support for the system, and specific requests for assistive technology are honored on an individual basis.

Institutions have implemented campus-wide computer network systems with application programs available from a centralized network resource. This allows students to access any applications from within any networked computer laboratory. Assistive software that is networked offers students with disabilities the ability to access a variety of programs from any site connected to the centralized network server. This is advantageous in providing more flexibility for students who use assistive devices and who need to perform computer-based work. It also eliminates the need for installation of software on multiple stand-alone computer stations.

Assistive Technology Provision for Use in Higher Education

For students who are unable to use college resources, assessment for assistive technology may be required. The provision of assistive technology and modifications is a multistep process that includes:

- referral
- assessment

- procurement of equipment
- equipment setup
- training
- follow-up for continued use of devices
- maintenance and repair of devices

Referral

Referral for an assistive technology assessment may come through vocational and educational agencies, through the disabled student services department of a college, through community agencies working with the student, or through private referral or self-referral. The referral process initially defines the student's needs to participate in the educational environment and to achieve goals with use of assistive technology. Specific needs related to class requirements, necessary tasks, and other education-related activities are addressed.

Assessment

Assessment for assistive technology is provided by a team of experts who are experienced in the use of assistive devices and adaptations and who are knowledgeable about the effects of impairments on students. The assessment process frequently results in a recommendation for specific devices, hardware, software, adaptations to the computer, adaptations to the classroom and environment, or techniques to assist the student.

The technology assessment team consists of the student and various professionals knowledgeable about assistive technology devices. The team of professionals varies depending on a student's particular needs. A computer specialist is knowledgeable about computer hardware and software compatibility requirements. The occupational therapist is experienced in the use of assistive devices and addresses disability-related issues, access, and positioning. A rehabilitation engineer is knowledgeable about assistive devices and provides technical support for devices and adaptations. A seating specialist provides input into seating issues and seating posture. An architect assists with environmental modifications that facilitate independence and technology use. College representatives or education specialists are routinely included and provide valuable input as to specific educational needs, course requirements, and assistive technology available on campus. They are instrumental in helping the students to implement recommendations for assistive technology within the educational environment. Other agencies working with or providing services for the student, such as vocational rehabilitation counselors, college counselors, and trainers, are also included. Medical reports from physicians and therapists are obtained through the student or referral source.

Assessment includes evaluation of sensory and motor functions, cognition and psychosocial skills, activities of daily living (ADL), work, and play or leisure. Assessment occurs in environments deemed necessary by the assessment team. Student abilities and disabilities are studied to determine the best access method and mode of operation. Assistive software and hardware are dependent on the user's needs and abilities. In addition, the student's knowledge about assistive technology must be addressed. Based on the information collected and the expressed needs and goals of the student, various assistive devices and combinations of hardware and software are prepared for trial use during the assessment. This often requires extensive planning, research, and testing to have appropriate systems configured and devices available. These systems are then used and modified as needed according to the student's abilities, comfort, and ease of use.

Procurement of Equipment

Due to rapid changes in technology, some critical factors need consideration when recommending devices to ensure their successful and continued use. Beaver and Mann (1994) note problems in compatibility of hardware and software devices. Devices often need to be specifically configured to utilize specialized adaptive features and to allow for optimal performance. This configuration includes use of specific setups of hardware and software parameters and loading sequences. Software that uses similar commands frequently needs to be adjusted to prevent program malfunctions. For example, a student may wish to use a screen-reading program together with an electronic dictionary and a word-processing program to perform writing tasks. Each program requires consideration of specific commands that are executed to perform functions to eliminate identical commands used by one or more programs. The careful configuration of devices facilitates easy use by students and prevents conflicts in device operations that deter student performance.

Device selection that considers both current needs and future use is important in technology use. This is challenging in light of constant changes in hardware, software upgrades, and new application programs and devices. Changes in devices, along with the addition or elimination of options often occurring in software upgrades, cause variations in operation or in compatibility. Students must learn how devices operate, be aware of how changes affect current operation, and use problem-solving to ensure future use. Device selection is also affected by a student's experience with technology devices and by changing the student's knowledge and educational needs (Church & Glennen, 1992). Students who are unfamiliar with assistive technology need full orientation and training in use of individual devices.

Environments where the technology will be used and the cost of devices also affect provision of devices. Funding for devices has historically been supported through vocational agencies assisting persons with disabilities or through the educational institution. Funding sources also include other third-party payers, such as insurance companies and private payers.

After trial use of various devices, access methods, and software, a consensus is reached for the appropriate system. Recommendations for devices include specifications for computer hardware and software, assistive devices, environmental control, modifications, and use of equipment.

Equipment Setup

Systems are set up and configured, and assistive devices are customized to the student's needs. Equipment is modified, and devices are customized to meet individual needs. This is especially important when several devices are utilized.

Training

Training of the student is recommended to ensure awareness, knowledge, and comfort with the assistive devices. It also facilitates understanding of how to perform specific tasks with the assistive technology and learning how to take advantage of the capabilities of the systems. Training often places multiple learning demands on students. Training includes specific instruction in alternative access methods, setup of hardware devices, instruction in use and customization of assistive software, and instruction in use of application programs with devices and adaptations. For students, this training is extended to meet the educational demands of completing assignments, accessing on-line libraries and reference materials, and use for specific coursework. Training also includes technical support services, reference materials, and troubleshooting strategies.

Training in the use of assistive technology requires careful planning and time. Training requires the expertise of professionals knowledgeable in assistive technology, the student's disability, and concerns related to education. Evaluators and trainers must be aware of software advances inherent in each new release to take advantage of these features for students with disabilities. In addition, students receiving computer training often require training in application programs necessary to produce college-level products such as term paper formats, spreadsheet analyses, and database structures.

Follow-Up

Follow-up and monitoring is necessary as part of the assessment process. This includes technical support, especially as students become more familiar with the devices used. Modifications are often necessary due to changes in student capabilities and needs. This also helps to ensure proper equipment function, especially if many students are using the same devices. In addition, reevaluation for device use may be necessary.

Maintenance and Repair of Devices

Equipment must be maintained to be used successfully. Students need information on whom to contact when maintenance or repair is necessary. A means to address this issue is necessary for students who use assistive devices but may be unable to problem-solve or repair devices independently. The cost of maintenance and repair also needs to be considered when recommending devices.

In addition to client ability, new technology devices, cost, and the eventual goal of employment all affect the provision and use of devices. Changes in student educational choices and demands also affect technology needs and requirements and most often require intervention or assistance for optimal use. Likewise, it is difficult to predict what specific technology will meet future educational and work needs or if additional or structured instruction is required to improve choices and flexibility for the student.

Case Studies

Three case studies identify the process of selecting and using assistive technology for higher education. The students in these case studies either were unable to fully utilize the assistive technology available at their colleges or required individualized assistive technology devices to complete their educational requirements. Although it is impossible to represent all dimensions of student disabilities, these three case studies explain the basic process of assessment and device provision common to most interventions.

The clients in each of the case studies were referred to service programs at the Center for Assistive Technology (CAT). Referral forms are requested by CAT to provide information on the person's current status, specific needs, experience with assistive technology, and education. This provides a base for further assessment. Referrals for assistive technology are routed to the CAT staff who provide evaluation services. One staff member performs the preliminary task of gathering background information prior to the assessment. Once additional information is collected, staff members meet and decide who will participate in the assessment. The assistive technology team is drawn from service providers employed at CAT and from CAT projects that involve assistive technology research and education.

Each case study presents the problems of a unique person, so each case covers issues that extend beyond technology or computer access. The case studies are organized into five sections: background, assessment, intervention, outcomes, and conclusions. The background information provides preliminary information that is the basis for team selection, helps define the problem, and guides further assessment. The assessment section includes the capabilities, limitations, and educational needs of the student. The intervention section contains the recommendations or solutions for the problem and why devices are chosen. The outcomes section describes how the interventions were obtained, their effectiveness, or problems that occurred. The conclusions section briefly summarizes what insight was gained from the case study.

The first case study describes Rachel, a high school student who has juvenile rheumatoid arthritis. She is in the transition process and is planning to move from secondary education to college. The second case study, Bob, is a college student with a neurological impairment. In addition to computer needs, mobility and access are important issues related to his education. Bill, the third case study, has high-level quadriplegia and is enrolled in a specialized college program that involves independent work. His technology needs involve access to information and performance within a graphical user interface by using alternative input methods and devices

Case Study 1

Background

Rachel is a senior in high school who plans on attending a 4-year college to study biology. She has juvenile rheumatoid arthritis. As a result, Rachel experiences joint pain and fatigue most days. She usually requires a rest period after classes when she returns home. She explains that on good days, when pain and fatigue are lessened, she can participate in additional school activities.

Rachel's arthritis has caused extensive joint damage in her feet. This has affected her mobility, and she walks for only short distances. She has noticeable joint changes in her hands with her fingers drifting laterally. She also experiences pain in her arms and legs that limits activity and highly strenuous tasks. She has difficulty in rising to stand from a seated position due to the stress on her feet.

Rachel's routine is similar to those of other students her age. She attends school daily, completes daily homework assignments, and participates in extracurricular activities when her pain levels permit. She has a driver's license and uses the family car to run errands.

Rachel currently uses assistive devices to aid in her daily activities. She uses a powered wheelchair to assist with mobility in school. The powered wheelchair is left at school because it is not portable in the family car. The family car is adapted with a wheel spinner so Rachel can control the steering wheel with her decreased arm movements. Writing is difficult, and Rachel utilizes a built-up handled pen to assist with grip for writing. Because she is unable to write for long periods, she uses a word processor for typing assignments. This is also problematic, however, because she fatigues easily due to poor positioning of her arms while typing.

Rachel currently lives at home with her parents; however, she will reside in a dormitory on campus when school begins. Rachel receives assistance from her mother for self-care activities such as dressing and bathing on days when her arthritis is more active. There is concern as to how Rachel will perform ADL independently in preparation for classes when living away.

Rachel became a client of a state vocational agency through transition planning at the secondary level. This transition planning assists with needs related to her disability in preparation for postsecondary education. Rachel, her school team, her parents, and her vocational rehabilitation counselor identified a need for a computer to help Rachel complete college course requirements. She was referred to the CAT for an assistive technology evaluation to determine specific equipment that would assist her. This process provides a more comprehensive team approach to assessment, interventions, and appropri-

ate use of assistive technology. Rachel's primary need for college was the capability to write papers, complete written laboratory reports and statistical problems, and conduct library research.

Prior to her assessment at the CAT, Rachel contacted the college's center for computing and disability to determine accessibility issues on campus related to her education. Her dormitory was accessible for her powered wheelchair. The campus' computer resources included laboratories with IBM-compatible computers with word-processing software operating under the DOS system. The computer workstations within the laboratories were not equipped with assistive technology for use by students with disabilities.

Assessment

With this background information, the evaluation staff at CAT determined Rachel's assistive technology team. The team included a rehabilitation engineer, an occupational therapist, a computer specialist, Rachel, Rachel's mother, and her vocational counselor. The team had expertise in computer use, adaptive devices, and workstation modifications. A representative from the college's center for computing and disability also provided input on request.

The assistive technology team reviewed background information prior to the assessment. The background helped to identify devices most likely to be useful for school. The vocational counselor provided information to the other team members on Rachel's current status, educational goals, and her likely technology needs at college. Rachel had previous experience with Apple computers through her high school classes. She enjoyed using computers but she experienced shoulder and hand pain after short periods of use.

Rachel expressed concerns over the difficulty she had in performing computer and other functional tasks requiring stressful hand movements such as self-care activities and mobility on campus. The team made Rachel's vocational rehabilitation counselor aware of these needs, and they made recommendations for devices that could assist Rachel with these tasks. In addition, Rachel's mother confirmed her needs related to ADL and computer access.

The devices used for Rachel's assessment included alternative keyboards, alternate pointing devices, assistive typing aids, and assistive software. These devices provide alternative ways to access the computer that require less movements or control. In addition, devices to assist with positioning, such as various types of wrist supports, chairs, and foot supports, were identified. Combinations of these devices are used for evaluation to determine the best devices for computer access.

An IBM-compatible computer was used for the assessment. Rachel was familiar with the QWERTY keyboard layout and had previously developed her own typing method. The team conducted timed typing trials to compare Rachel's prowess with the standard and alternative keyboards. The evaluation team also observed Rachel's performance and listened to her comments. The results were then used to select the keyboard that was most comfortable and the least fatiguing. In addition, the team considered performance issues such as keyboard position and body position.

Rachel's disability affected her range of motion and strength. She had full active movement at the shoulders and elbows. The joint deformities in her hands decreased her ability to fully extend her fingers. Rachel used her right index finger and her left ring finger for typing due to her limitations in hand movement and joint deformity. She typed 16 words per minute (wpm) with the standard computer keyboard.

Rachel and the assistive technology team evaluated three other alternative keyboards in addition to other assistive devices.

- *Compact Keyboard.* As shown in Figure 6.11, this is a reduced-size keyboard with a smaller key surface area and with decreased space between keys that includes all standard keyboard keys. Number, cursor, and function keys are grouped together and located above the main keys. Rachel was able to reach all keys on the compact keyboard with minimal effort. Typing speed was 13 wpm. Rachel, however, thought that the key size was too small, the key press was too resistive, and that it caused hand pain during typing.
- *Miniature Keyboard.* This is a miniature keyboard that measures approximately 7 in. by 6 in. wide. It has a standard layout that is activated through contact between a stylus and the keyboard. Rachel accessed the entire keyboard with two styli with both of her arms resting on a table for support. Typing speed using this keyboard was 13 wpm. Use of this keyboard required minimal effort for typing; however, Rachel was concerned about the static positioning of her hands during continuous typing.

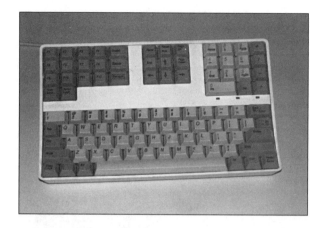

Figure 6.11. Compact keyboard.

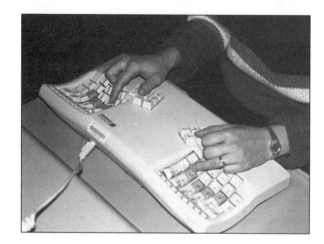

Figure 6.12. Ergonomic keyboard.

- *Ergonomic Keyboard.* This keyboard is designed to provide a more ergonomic hand position that supports the wrists and allow for more aligned finger positions. The keyboard was divided for more comfortable arm positioning. Rachel felt this position to be awkward at her wrists and palms. An example of an ergonomic keyboard is shown in Figure 6.12.
- *Typing Aid.* This is a device that is applied to the palmar surface of the hand and that tapers to a pencil-like projection. This provides an alternative to using the hands to type and eliminating pressure on the finger joints during typing. Rachel was accurate in her typing with these aids. She felt relief of shoulder and finger tension when using the aids.
- *Trackball.* Gripping the mouse was difficult and caused hand pain for Rachel. Two different trackballs, one with a 1.5 in. diameter ball

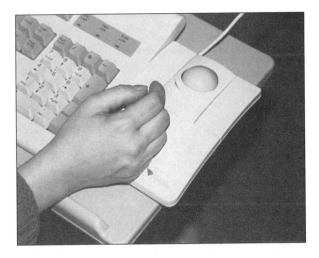

Figure 6.13. Trackball.

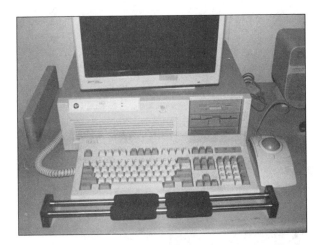

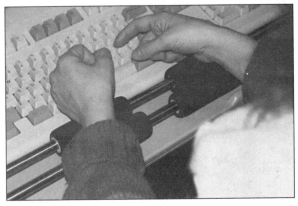

Figure 6.14. Sliding wrist rest.

with a drag button located above the ball and one with a 1 in. diameter with a drag button located below the balls were tested. Both trackballs had large surface areas for the right and left button click along with the central drag button. Figure 6.13 shows one type of

trackball. Rachel used the heel of her hand to rotate the ball and was more comfortable than when she used the mouse.

- *Wrist Rest.* Several wrist rests were used with the various keyboards to provide more comfortable positioning. These included a 2 in., vinyl-coated wrist rest positioned in front of the keyboard, an inclined keyboard support with a 3 in. plastic wrist rest attached, a foam wrist rest, and a sliding wrist rest with two cylindrical foam pieces that moved from side to side. Rachel was uncomfortable with the sliding wrist rest, which is shown in Figure 6.14.
- *Keyboard Table.* Keyboard position was determined to provide Rachel with a relaxed and stable arm position to prevent fatigue and to prevent further deterioration of the arm and hand joints. Rachel preferred an adjustable-height keyboard table to the standard desk.
- *Graphical User Environment.* Rachel worked in both a DOS and graphical user environment to determine preferences and ease of use. Rachel preferred use of the icon and pull-down menu system over DOS-based programs.
- *Keyboard-Enhancement Software.* This software is used with other software programs and provides accommodations to the keyboard. Rachel used this with word-processing software to type multiple keystrokes in sequence and found it required less effort.

To summarize, the standard keyboard was the most desirable interface for Rachel. It was familiar, and she was most comfortable using it. The assistive technology team recommended a computer system for use in Rachel's dorm room. The computer met her need to produce written assignments and perform other computer tasks. Having her own system provided Rachel with flexibility for structuring of time and pacing of activities and allowed for periods to rest especially when fatigued. It also decreased the demand on Rachel's mobility and travel to the college computer laboratories at specific times.

Intervention

The recommended computer system for Rachel was an IBM-compatible 486 DX2 at 66 MHz with 8 MB RAM, 420 MB hard drive, a SVGA monitor with .28 dot pitch, a fax/modem, and an inkjet printer. This provides a strong technical base to run the recommended software and provides for growth and flexibility as her computer needs change.

Rachel preferred using Windows, an icon-based, graphic user interface, to the DOS environment. She was more comfortable using the pull-down menu system to execute commands than she was entering keystrokes. Rachel was confident that she could learn and be more flexible with this interface even though the college computer environment was currently using software for DOS. The following software programs were recommended.

- *Microsoft Word for Windows.* Macros and word-processing features provide keystroke-saving capability in this program and eliminate the need to recommend additional assistive software to decrease the number of keystrokes. This is a powerful program that will meet Rachel's word-processing needs to produce written assignments and papers.
- *Dictionary.* A dictionary in electronic format was recommended for quick reference. This is available both on disk and on CD-ROM. This eliminates the need to manipulate a large book, which is difficult for Rachel due to hand pain and deformity.
- *Communication Software.* Communication software is necessary to use a modem and the telephone lines to communicate from one computer to another. This software was recommended so that Rachel could use her modem to perform on-line assignments and access the college library from her dorm room.

The team also recommended the following adaptive devices.

- *Trackball.* A three-button ergonomic trackball with a 1.5 in. ball was recommend as an alternative pointing device to the mouse. Rachel found this device, shown in Figure 6.15, provided a comfortable resting hand position when working in Windows. A drag button eliminated stress to the fingers. She was also able to alter hand position as needed when using the trackball.
- *Adjustable-Height Keyboard Table.* Rachel is able to raise and lower keyboard height and tilt with this table, and it enables her to assume a resting position for the shoulders during typing. It assists Rachel with flexible options for sitting aside from her standard desk chair. An adjustable-height keyboard table is shown in Figure 6.16.
- *Typing Aid.* This device, shown in Figure 6.17, provides an alternative way to type on the keyboard, eliminating finger use.

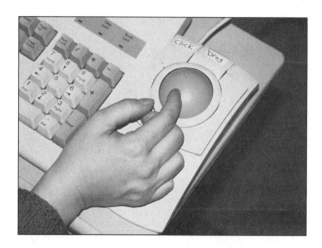

Figure 6.15. Three-button ergonomic trackball.

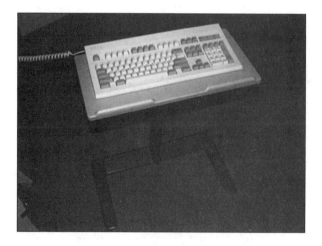

Figure 6.16. Adjustable-height keyboard table.

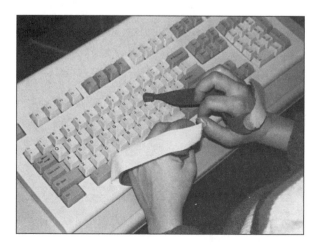

Figure 6.17. Typing aid.

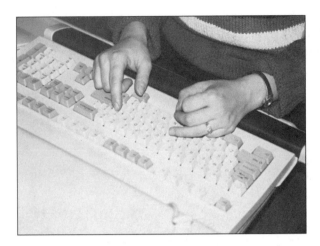

Figure 6.18. Wrist rest.

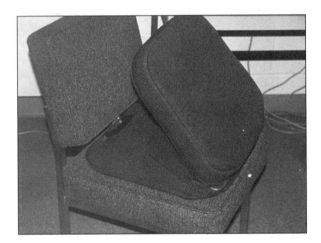

Figure 6.19. Portable cushion.

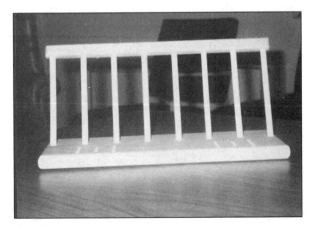

Figure 6.20. Book holder.

- *Wrist Rest.* Rachel preferred the stationary vinyl-covered rest. This provides a support surface for resting during typing. The wrist rest is shown in Figure 6.18.
- *Portable Cushion.* This device, shown in Figure 6.19, will elevate Rachel in her sitting position and assist her in rising to stand from a sitting position. Rachel has difficulty with this when sitting in standard chairs, especially for long periods. This device is portable and will be used during classes when Rachel is not using her wheelchair.
- *Electric Stapler and Pencil Sharpener.* These devices decrease stress to the wrists and hands when performing paper tasks.
- *Book Holder.* This device, shown in Figure 6.20, decreases the need to hold heavy books, which eliminates the stress on the hand and finger joints and will assist with head position during reading.

Rachel was often unable to perform independent self-care when experiencing pain. Several assistive devices were recommended to assist with daily care.

- *Bath Bench.* This would provide a sitting surface for Rachel when bathing to decrease stress on her feet.
- *Long-Handled Bath Sponge.* This would assist with reaching all body parts during bathing.
- *Stocking Aid.* This would assist Rachel when she was unable to reach her feet for dressing.
- *Reacher.* This would assist with reaching items to decrease stress on shoulders.
- *Battery-Operated Scissors.* These eliminate stress to the hands during cutting.
- *Luggage Cart.* This would eliminate the need to carry large objects or packages.
- *Cylindrical Padding.* This would allow Rachel to build up grip surfaces to decrease stress on hand joints.
- *Key Holder.* This provides a larger surface area to grab and manipulate keys.

Outcome

The vocational rehabilitation service agency funded the recommended computer system and assistive devices. In addition, the vocational rehabilitation agency funded 25 hours of training in the use of these devices. Rachel quickly learned about her system and how to use the recommended software. She was able to use the computer for completion of papers and assignments when college classes began. Rachel's computer system is shown in Figure 6.21.

The need for independence in self-care activities, class-related tasks that involved hand manipulation, and written assignments was also addressed. Rachel was independent in self-care with adaptive equipment. She was able to perform other hand-manipulation tasks without relying on others for assistance.

Conclusion

Although assistive technology was beneficial to Rachel in performing college coursework, she continued to experience pain in her joints that decreased the length of time available for school-related tasks. The devices allowed her more flexibility to perform computer work when she felt best.

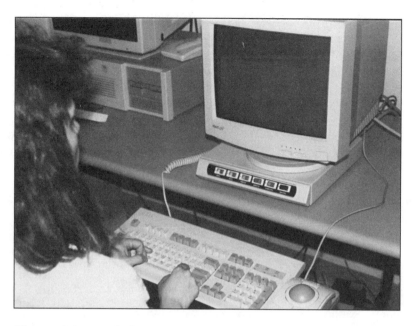

Figure 6.21. Rachel's computer system.

Rachel used a variety of devices to assist her with tasks that were not computer-related but still affected her overall performance. These tasks require consideration to enable not only computer access but also independent performance of other daily activities, especially for self-preparation for daily school activities.

Rachel was concerned about the effects of using devices as the disease progressed in her bone and tissue structures. It is important to consider the course of a disease or illness when providing assistive devices. Alternate devices may be required to offer different access options.

Rachel was not experiencing any acute inflammatory processes at the time of assessment. However, she reported that her work time was decreased to approximately 5 to 10 min. when she was experiencing pain. Rachel could benefit from an alternative computer-access method if her disability reduced her ability to use direct access for typing. Alternative methods to keyboard typing include use of voice recognition. This technology has improved and provides access without physical effort, decreasing the amount of hand use for typing papers and reserving energy for other tasks. The team made Rachel aware of this option for future consideration.

In addition, Rachel was sensitive about the outward appearance of her disability. The noticeable joint changes and use of devices affected her physical appearance. The lack of privacy in the college dorm eventually caused Rachel to transfer from the college to a local university. Rachel now resides at home. Rachel is still assessing options for assistive devices to address her mobility limitations that impede her movement around the university grounds.

Case Study 2

Background

Bob is a 19-year-old student studying engineering technology at a 4-year college. He has C8 quadriplegia secondary to transverse myelitis and a resultant mobility impairment. He has paralysis of his lower extremities and partial use of his upper extremities. Bob's hand and finger dexterity is impaired.

Bob lives at home with his mother. He has no siblings. His mother provides assistance with daily care for dressing. He requires assistance for other ADL such as meal preparation, homemaking, and managing finances. He is independent in other self-care activities except mobility. Bob propels his manual wheelchair independently on flat surfaces; however, he is unable to access his home, which has a step at both the front and back door. His mother helps him enter and exit his home.

Bob's dependence in mobility at home presents both educational and safety dilemmas. Because Bob's mother works evenings, Bob's current routine is to return home from school before his mother leaves for work. His ability to perform course-related work or to participate in other campus activities is compromised. He is unable to depend on neighbors or friends for assistance. When left alone, safety is a concern due his inability to exit his home. During the summer months, Bob spends a great amount of time indoors due to his mother's work schedule. Also, participation in social or recreational activities is severely restricted due to Bob's mobility limitations.

Bob requires assistance for transportation and commutes to school through a wheelchair-van service. Limited transportation hours and cost limit the amount of time Bob spends at school. He is unable to utilize many of the college's resources, including the computer laboratory for educational tasks. Bob does not have a driver's license.

Bob was referred to the CAT for assessment to determine computer adaptations to assist him with course requirements in pursuing a degree. The state vocational rehabilitation office made the referral and funded the assessment. The referral contains demographic information about the client, the goal of the client, the educational program the student is enrolled in, and information about previous computer use.

Assessment

The assistive technology team included Bob, an occupational therapist, a rehabilitation engineer, and Bob's vocational rehabilitation counselor, who made the referral. The occupational therapist is knowledgeable in assistive technology, disability, and computer-access issues. The rehabilitation engineer assists with device selection and modifications of devices. An architect was later added to the team to contribute expertise on accessibility issues within the home.

Although basic information is received from the vocational rehabilitation agency's case file as part of the referral process, the team collects additional background information to help identify Bob's capabilities, educational goals, and specific needs related to computer use. The vocational rehabilitation counselor provided background information, including the reason for the referral, Bob's current status, and Bob's medical history.

Bob provided details about his functional capabilities and disability, information on his vocational goal, and concerns he had related to technology and his education. He had prior computer experience in high school but had not used a computer for 2 years. He reports a limited knowledge about computers and is uncertain as to whether he could use a computer. He wants to earn an engineering degree.

A representative from the engineering department contributed information related to Bob's education and course requirements on the types of software currently used for course assignments and the projected computer needs for the near future. The college's Disabled Student Services Coordinator contributed information about accommodations and modifications available for Bob to participate in the education process and expressed a concern about accessibility needs in the classroom. Bob was enrolled in a drafting class and needed to access the drafting tables to perform class assignments.

Bob needed a computer system that would enable him to independently perform course assignments required within the engineering program and to write papers for other courses. He also needed access to the college VAX machine, the college's mainframe computer. Bob enjoys drawing and has developed a method to hold and use a pencil by using residual movements on his right side. This works well for Bob, and he wants to extend his drawing abilities with the computer. In addition, Bob needs improved accessibility especially within the home, to allow for a more flexible college schedule and to allow Bob to take advantage of college resources and activities.

Computer-access devices were identified by the assistive technology team that would assist with hand function when using the computer. The team used these devices for the evaluation. Other devices can be substituted or added depending on the student's needs. These devices include alternative keyboards, pointing devices, and positioning devices.

Bob's physical impairment limited his access to the computer. He has full active bilateral range of motion at the shoulder and elbows. He demonstrated only partial wrist extension to neutral, a straightened position on the right, and was unable to perform full finger flexion and extension or isolated finger movements. Bob's hand motion on the left was impaired, and Bob demonstrated minimal functional use. His sensation at the hands was impaired for light touch.

The assessment process used both an IBM-compatible computer system in DOS and Windows environments and a Macintosh computer. Due to impaired hand function, Bob's typing method was two-finger typing with the right thumb and middle finger on the standard keyboard. Seven devices were used to determine the most efficient and comfortable access mode for Bob. The team used direct observation and timed typing trials to evaluate Bob's capabilities. The following devices were selected.

- *Miniature Keyboard With Stylus.* This is a miniature keyboard that measures approximately 8 in. by 6 in. wide. It has a standard layout that is activated through contact between a stylus and the keyboard. This device is shown in Figure 6.22. Bob developed a comfortable method for pencil manipulation for handwriting and drawing. He was able to use this hand position to type with the stylus on the miniature keyboard with minimal arm movements. Speed differentials to the standard keyboard were minimal.

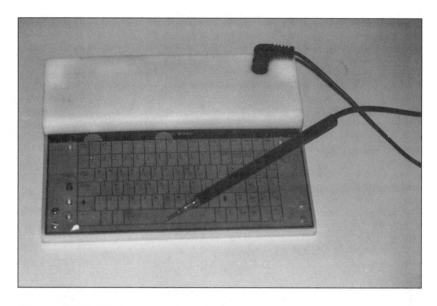

Figure 6.22. Miniature keyboard with stylus.

- *Compact Keyboard.* Because Bob accessed the computer keyboard with one hand, a smaller keyboard was evaluated that required less distance to travel to access all keys. The compact keyboard is a reduced-size keyboard with a smaller key surface area and decreased space between keys. It includes all standard keyboard keys. Number, cursor, and function keys are grouped together and are located above the main keys. Typing speeds were slightly higher with this keyboard. Bob liked the shorter distance between letter keys and the overall layout for one-handed use.

- *One-Handed DVORAK Keyboard Layout.* This key layout is ergonomically designed to allow a one-handed user more advantageous access to the most frequently used keys. A DVORAK keyboard layout designed for use with one hand is shown in Figure 6.23. Use of this keyboard requires learning the new layout and training. Although Bob uses one hand to type, he found this layout confusing and he did not want to learn a new key layout.

- *Three-Button Trackball.* Bob was unable to grip a mouse for pointing due to limited movement and coordination. He requires use of a pointing device to perform class assignments for computer-aided design. This device provided a means for Bob to use gross hand movements without a static grip to operate the mouse pointer.

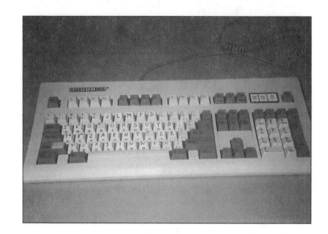

Figure 6.23. DVORAK keyboard layout.

- *Keyboard-Enhancement Software.* Bob had difficulty with typing commands or letters that required two or more keys to be pressed simultaneously. This is a program that allows for customization of keyboard function. He uses a feature that enables multiple keystrokes to be typed in sequence.

- *Crank Adjustable-Height Table.* This device is height adjustable and was used to determine an accessible yet comfortable table height to access the computer with a wheelchair.

As a result of the assessment, Bob preferred use of the compact keyboard as an alternative to the standard keyboard, with a shorter travel distance between keys for one-handed use.

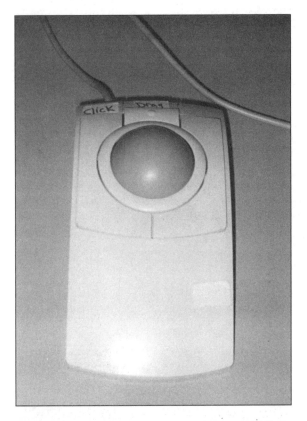

Figure 6.24. Ergonomic, three-button trackball.

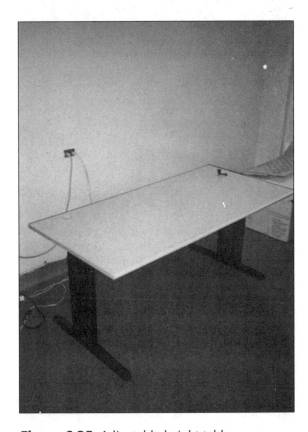

Figure 6.25. Adjustable-height table.

Intervention

The team recommended a home computer system for Bob due to his limited mobility, transportation issues, and remote access to the campus computer laboratories. They selected an IBM-compatible computer that was compatible with Bob's home system and the computers used both in the computer laboratories and in the engineering department at school. The team also obtained specific hardware that would run programs used by the engineering department. The recommended system included a 486 processor at 66 MHz, 8 MB RAM, SVGA monitor with .28 dot pitch, a 340 MB hard drive, a fax/modem, and an inkjet color printer.

The following software programs were selected.

- *Keyboard-Enhancement Software.* This enabled Bob to type multiple keystrokes in sequence to eliminate awkward finger positioning and prevent unnecessary typing errors.
- *Computer-Aided Design.* Bob's instructor recommended a student version of the computer-aided design program used at the college.
- *Word Processing.* This software is necessary to produce written reports and papers. The word-processing program selected is the same as the software used in the college computer laboratories. Bob can use the college's technical support service if he requires assistance.
- *Telecommunication Software.* This will allow Bob to use a modem to log on to the computer and perform computer tasks on the VAX from home. It will also provide on-line access to the library.

The following devices were also selected.

- *Trackball.* An ergonomic, three-button trackball, as shown in Figure 6.24, was recommended as an alternative to a mouse pointer. The ball is approximately 1.5 in. in size, and the select and drag buttons have a large surface area. Bob can easily activate these without exact finger pointing. It provides a resting hand position for Bob and allows movement of the mouse pointer without using a hand grip. The drag function will automatically hold while dragging eliminating the need for Bob to hold and drag, an especially useful function for use with his computer aided design software.
- *Adjustable-Height table.* This was recommended so that Bob could position his work-

station for wheelchair accessibility at home. An adjustable-height table is shown in Figure 6.25. This table has a crank adjustment located in front that Bob was able to manipulate with gross shoulder and elbow movements. It allows for flexibility in positioning of devices and access, especially if Bob changes wheelchairs.

Adaptations on Campus. Bob is unable to use the college's drafting table located in the engineering department with his wheelchair. Access was necessary to participate in required class laboratories. A request was made to CAT by the coordinator of disability services at Bob's college for an adaptation.

A standard drafting table currently used in the laboratory was adapted by the rehabilitation engineer. Although a product search for adjustable-height drafting tables was performed, the college opted to have table elevators constructed. Wooden blocks were constructed and applied to the legs of the table. These elevated the table approximately 2.5 in. to accommodate Bob's wheelchair. This adaptation was implemented through the CAT assistive technology team and was funded through the vocational rehabilitation agency.

Home Assessment. Bob needs independent access to his home. A home visit was necessary to assess Bob's accessibility to enter and exit the home, the entrances of the housing structure, and other related mobility needs. This assessment was performed by an architect. The evaluation process included observation, specific measurements, and a low-scale drawing.

Bob was independent in propelling his wheelchair up and down a ramp. Because Bob resided in a rented home, portable ramps were researched. Issues related to tenant rights, owner responsibility, and cost estimates for purchase and installation were investigated. Fair housing amendments mandate that a landlord cannot prevent a tenant from making adaptations to a home; however, the tenant is responsible for costs. The tenant is also responsible to remove the adaptation or change the structure to its previous state before moving.

A recommendation for a portable, aluminum ramp was made by the architect. After consultation with the property owner, Bob and his mother decided to move to another residence that was wheelchair accessible. As a result of the assistive technology evaluation and due to Bob's continual need for transportation to complete his education, the assistive technology team recommended a driving assessment

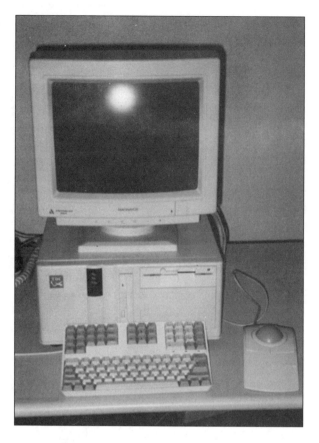

Figure 6.26. Bob's computer system.

to Bob's vocational rehabilitation counselor. Bob is reliant on van service; however, he is interested in driving. A driving assessment would determine his ability to drive and contribute toward independent transportation. This evaluation is a specialized service and is frequently performed at rehabilitation facilities.

In addition, Bob's wheelchair has a broken support in the back rest. This resulted in a poor and uncomfortable sitting posture for Bob. The technology team recommended that the chair be repaired to prevent impairments due to poor seating or orthopedic changes.

Outcome

Bob received all the recommendations made for a computer system and assistive technology. Vocational rehabilitation services provided funding for the assessment, equipment, and training. An assistive technology trainer at CAT set up and configured Bob's computer system and devices and installed the software. Bob's computer system is shown in Figure 6.26.

Bob received training in setup of his system, in use of his assistive devices with application programs, and in problem-solving techniques concerning his system. The assistive technology trainer provided reference materials as well as ongoing technical telephone support.

Bob demonstrated basic competence in the use of his equipment on completion of training. He was able to use his system for college work and assignments. However, he required major technical support that required reconfiguration of his computer system after he deleted part of his computer operating software.

Conclusion

Often students experience other needs in addition to the need for assistive technology for computer use. For Bob, his mobility impairment greatly impeded his participation in his educational endeavors.

With the recommendation of minimal adaptation, Bob was able to participate in all of his classes and meet course requirements. Also, even though students are trained in use of equipment, technical support is frequently necessary to assist them with ongoing problems and equipment failures.

Case Study 3

Background

Bill, a 40-year-old man, was traumatically injured in a car accident that resulted in a spinal cord injury when he was 30 years of age. Before the accident, he was employed as an auto mechanic. He lost his job soon after his injury because he was no longer able to perform his job duties. After receiving traditional rehabilitation services such as occupational and physical therapy, Bill returned home. He is dependent in his ADL. He is unable to participate in the many familiar daily tasks and activities he was used to that involved physical exertion.

Bill lives in a ranch home that he had previously built with his wife, daughter, and son. He has one married son and a granddaughter. Family members are a main support system and assist with daily needs. He lives in a rural, hilly area that is approximately 2 hours from the nearest major city. He is unemployed and on a fixed income. His wife is his only caregiver and is also a homemaker. His house was previously equipped with a hospital bed; however, he does not independently control the bed functions. He uses a speaker phone for telephone conversations. He uses a powered wheelchair for mobility. He acquired a van that was adapted with a

wheelchair lift for transportation. Bill has a difficult time with travel due to his medical limitations, such as dizziness from sitting upright for long periods, and can only travel short distances.

Bill was eligible for services under a state vocational services agency. He explored options for higher education and employment under this service. He decided to enroll in a college program. His vocational rehabilitation counselor referred Bill to CAT for an assistive technology evaluation by his vocational rehabilitation counselor. The evaluation was to determine how technology could assist with his needs to accomplish his educational plan. The vocational agency funded his assistive technology referral.

The occupational therapist who performs technology assessments at CAT collected background information prior to the technology assessment. Bill's previous spinal cord injury resulted in C5 quadriplegia with severe physical impairments. Past medical reports were provided by Bill and his counselor. He was spending a great amount of time in his home because he is limited functionally due to his disability. He was interested in enrolling in school to study business management. His goal was to become self-employed within the home. Bill graduated from high school but had no additional postsecondary education. He needed a computer system that would allow him to work on completing college courses and prepare for employment within the home. Bill wanted to become active and believed that he had potential to be productive. He was aware of the enormous changes and advances in computer technology. He was unaware of what would assist him to achieve his goals.

The college program that Bill enrolled in was designed to assist students who were unable to take traditional courses on a college campus. Coursework is structured so students perform much of their work independently. Meetings with instructors and counselors facilitate this process.

Bill needed a computer system to help complete college assignments in a timely manner as course requirements demanded, provide a way to communicate with instructors, and access the library. He required an access method that would capitalize on his abilities and would accommodate his disability.

After background information was collected, a plan by the assistive technology team was devised to prepare for the assessment. The evaluation team included Bill, an occupational therapist, and a computer specialist. These team members would evaluate computer access and computer-related needs. Other professionals such as a seating specialist, a rehabilitation engineer, or technician are often included on the team to address any specialized seating needs, or special adaptations related to computer needs; however, their particular expertise was not required for Bill's assessment.

Assessment

Bill had complete paralysis of his lower extremities, so he used a powered wheelchair for mobility. Bill had intact head and neck movements. He had minimal active movement of his left forearm and utilized a weak tenodesis movement (wrist motion) for a limited amount of activities (such as hitting an accessible wall switch). He used residual right arm movements at the shoulder for body support and stabilization. Bill had no active finger movements or grasp function. His balance was impaired, and he required stabilization of his upper body to use his left arm for any activity. His cognitive skills were intact, and his verbal communication skills were good.

Loss of upper-extremity movements limits Bill's access to and ability to use a computer. The computer assessment included evaluation of access to the computer with a variety of assistive devices and assistive software. Bill labored to hit keys on a standard keyboard. He was unable to reach all keys with his residual movement. He was unable to manipulate any assistive hand devices. He had never used a mouthstick and preferred not to utilize this device for computer access. Bill needed an alternative access method to the keyboard.

The following devices:

- *Keyboard Emulation Using a Proportional Chin Controller.* Bill had intact head and neck movements that he could use to manipulate devices. He found using this device, which is controlled through chin movements, too tiresome for repetitive typing needs. He did not believe he currently needed the integrated system that this device offered. An example of this device is shown in Figure 6.27.
- *Voice Recognition.* Bill had good verbal communication skills and was able to train a vocabulary with consistent vocal performance. In training a vocabulary, the person vocalizes words as prompted by the computer program. The computer then recognizes these commands. He found this not to be physical-

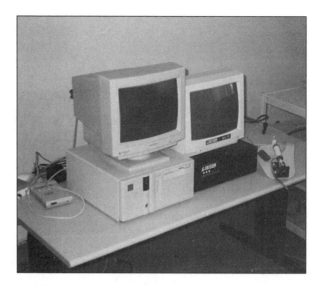

Figure 6.27. Proportional chin controller.

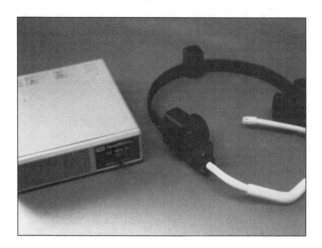

Figure 6.28. Head-pointing device.

ly demanding and was able to work for longer periods without fatigue.
- *Head-Pointing Device for Alternate Mouse Pointing.* Bill was able to use head movements for operation of this pointing device through use of a headset with an ultrasonic signal and switch activation for mouse clicks. This device is shown in Figure 6.28. He found use of head movement somewhat fatiguing.

He wanted more independent access and was unable to position the headset independently.

- *Digital Joystick.* This device, along with a hardware interface, is attached to the computer and provides alternative mouse pointing access. The joystick is controlled with chin

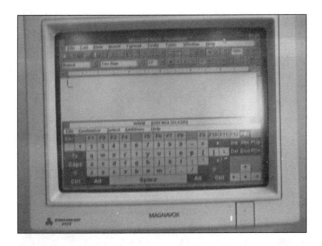

Figure 6.29. On-screen keyboard.

movements. This device does not allow for diagonal mouse pointing. Bill found this more difficult to operate.

- *Three-Button Trackball.* This trackball had a 1.5 in. ball with large select button surfaces and with a drag mode. Bill was able to operate this ball with residual gross arm movements. Movements were slow; however, Bill was comfortable using his arm to operate this device.

- *On-Screen Keyboard.* This software provided keyboard access when using an alternative pointing device. An on-screen keyboard is shown in Figure 6.29. This allowed Bill to type letters by centering the mouse pointer over the letter on the screen to type keystrokes. Bill was able to use this keyboard to type keystrokes.

- *Word Prediction.* The word-prediction list provides possible word choices that the computer could then type automatically if selected. This feature is used to reduce the amount of keystrokes that the user must type and thus decrease the amount of effort and fatigue required. Bill was most successful when using this with the onscreen keyboard.

To summarize, Bill favored voice recognition as his main access method. Voice recognition software allows for speaking words and letters instead of typing keystrokes. This method was faster, less fatiguing, and less physically demanding to input words and characters than the other methods. Bill demonstrated poor motor control and fatigued easily from the various devices that required arm or head movements. He also fatigued from the physical demands needed to maintain his balance when necessary.

Intervention

The recommended system is an IBM-compatible 486 DX2 tower at 66 MHz with 32 MB RAM, 420 MB hard drive, a SVGA monitor with .28 dot pitch, a tape backup, dual-speed CD ROM, a fax/modem, and an inkjet printer. This high-powered system was necessary to run the voice recognition software along with other application programs within a graphical user interface. The hard drive will also decrease the need to manipulate diskettes when accessing his application programs and saving his work. It will provide Bill with flexibility to use a variety of software programs while using the adaptive devices and other assistive software. The tape backup will be used to back up his voice and work files to eliminate unnecessary retraining. The CD-ROM is needed for access to reference materials as Bill is unable to manipulate books due to his disability.

- *Voice-Recognition Software.* Together with hardware, this will provide use of voice recognition as an access method. It allows voice commands to be used for navigation within Windows and for activating mouse movements.

When first evaluated, Bill used voice recognition within a DOS environment. This access became available for use within a graphical user interface. Bill favored Windows and opted to use this as his main computer environment.

- *Word for Windows.* This is a powerful word-processing program that Bill will need to produce written reports within a Windows environment. Macros and word-processing features provide keystroke-saving capability in this program and eliminate the need to recommend additional assistive software to decrease the number of keystrokes. Bill was able to use the trackball to operate the program menus within the graphic environment.

- *FAX/Modem Software.* This provides Bill with the ability to send faxes from his computer. This was necessary to send messages and assignments from home to his instructors.

- *On-Screen Keyboard.* This software will provide Bill with an alternative access method if he is unable to use voice recognition.

- *Communication Software.* This software will allow Bill to use his modem to access on-line reference and library material through the phone lines. It will provide access to the Internet and other on-line services. This is important for Bill due to his mobility impairments and his limitations in travel.

- *Reference Materials on CD-ROM.* This software provides electronic access to reference materials. Bill is unable to manipulate books, and these will assist with college work.
- *Encyclopedia on CD-ROM.* This is another program that Bill needs for quick reference.

Bill also required the following devices.

- *Adjustable-Height Table.* This table allows for wheelchair access, along with proper positioning of devices for comfortable use.
- *Trackball.* Bill was able to control this device with residual arm movement. He preferred using these movements even though they were initially slow. Other options for pointing devices could include head-pointing devices that do not require placement of a headset for more independent access.
- *Stand-Alone Microphone.* This device will allow Bill to use voice recognition without a headset for more independent access.

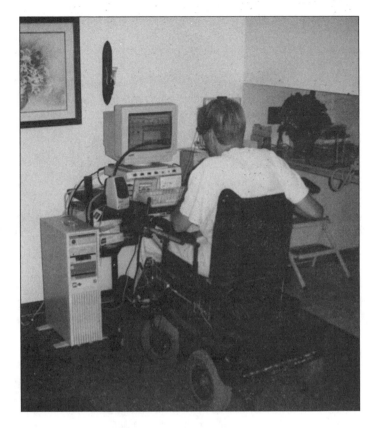

Figure 6.30. Bill's computer system.

Outcome

Bill is receiving training in the use of his system though funding by the vocational rehabilitation agency. This system is shown in Figure 6.30. Due to the presence of multiple complex components, training in use of voice recognition, Windows access, and word processing are the highest priorities to assist Bill with his course assignments. Bill has shown great interest in learning about the computer and its uses. He has developed skill at using his on-screen keyboard as an alternative input method to voice recognition and continues to independently explore the system programs and options.

Conclusion

Bill was informed during his assessment of other possible options for computer use in occupations (i.e., computer-aided design). These work and education areas can be further explored at Bill's request. Although a highly sophisticated system was recommended, most users of assistive technology face the issue of equipment obsolescence. Continued advances make technology outdated and require updating by the client.

There are new learning issues for Bill as he returns to school. For example, Bill needs to learn how to perform school tasks such as writing papers, doing library research, and developing studying techniques. Bill's learning demands are compounded because he has no computer knowledge. In addition to schoolwork, he must also learn about basic computer function, correct use of his access methods, and software operation. The multiple components to Bill's system require additional learning for full operation of his system. Extended training periods must be considered to allow time for both college work and computer operation. Continued support is necessary to ensure optimal and successful usage.

Bill's ultimate goal was for self-employment within his home. Bill will need to integrate his education and acquired skills into competitive work. This may necessitate changes or additions to the assistive devices that Bill is using. Reassessment and additional technical support may be required to help Bill accomplish his goals.

Summary

Assistive technology can help students realize educational and life goals. There is a wide range of assistive devices that are successfully used to accomplish these goals. Improving and new technologies continue to provide options for access to information. It is important to provide education about assistive technology to students, educators, and agencies working with students with disabilities to provide optimal educational opportunities.

The transition process is an effective means for facilitating the provision of assistive devices for students at the secondary level with postsecondary goals for higher education. This allows for a more comprehensive preparation process and can provide students with the necessary skills to use technology before entering college. Students need to learn how to use their devices to be competitive and productive.

The successful transition from postsecondary education to employment can be facilitated with assistive technology. This requires careful planning and integration into the workplace. In addition to learning new jobs skills, students' technology needs may change. Issues related to device compatibility, workstation design, and accessibility must be addressed. Employers need to be more aware of how assistive devices can make students eligible for competitive employment and how use of technology can assist them in performing jobs.

Several issues are related to the successful choice and use of assistive technology for education. Student abilities and disabilities are examined to determine the best access method and mode of operation. Assistive software and hardware are dependent on the user's needs and abilities. Educational requirements, device compatibility, student experience and expertise, and future needs all affect the provision and use of devices. In addition, ongoing technical support and maintenance often is required for continued use. When recommending assistive technology, it is important to make provisions for the installation of devices, compatibility with other devices and the environment, upgrading, and follow-up.

Successful assistive technology interventions often require an interdisciplinary team approach and coordination and collaboration among schools, agencies, and students. It is important to remember that high- and low-technology solutions are available, and college resources often provide the necessary adaptations. A thorough assessment of the student is to determine what type of intervention will best meet that person's needs. It is also necessary to consider psychosocial factors and learning when recommending assistive technology.

Training in the use of assistive technology is also an important issue for students. Training includes instruction on how to use devices and also requires integration of the technology for completion of educational tasks. For example, students may need to use assistive computer devices to access and perform on-line assignments.

Students with disabilities often require other services or additional assistive technology to assist with self-care, preparation for school, or mobility, as noted in the case studies. These needs can affect overall college performance and must be addressed.

Students with disabilities may require assistance in exploring options for use of assistive technology for education and work areas. Many students are unaware of what educational or employment tasks can be achieved with assistive technology.

Chapter 6 References

Arnold, E., & Czamanske, J. (1991, April). *Can I make it? A transition program for college bound learning disabled students and their parents.* Paper presented at the Annual Conference of the Council for Exceptional Children, Atlanta, GA.

Beaver, K., & Mann, W. (1994). Provider skills for delivering computer access services: An assistive technology team approach. *Technology and Disability, 3*(2), 109–116.

Brown, C. (1987). *Computer access in higher education for students with disabilities.* San Francisco, CA: George Lithograph.

Castorina, C. (1994, March-April). Project ease: Spreading the word about adaptive technology. *Change,* pp. 45–47.

Church, G., & Glennen, S. (1992). *The handbook of assistive technology.* San Diego, CA: Singular.

College Consortium of Disability Advocates. (1993). *Effective college planning.* Western New York Transition Resource Center, Buffalo, NY. *Individuals With Disabilities Education Act, (1990), 20*(33). Pub. L. 101–476.

Coombs N., & Cartwright, G.P. (1994, March-April). Project ease: Equal access to software and information. *Change,* pp. 42–44.

Deykes R., & Anthony, K. (1994). *Career planning and employment strategies for postsecondary students with disabilities.* Heath Resource Center (Higher Education and Adult Training for People with

Handicaps). Washington, DC: National Clearinghouse on Postsecondary Education for Individuals with Handicaps.

Hasazi, S.B., Hock, M.L., & Cravedi-Cheng, L. (1992). *Vermont's post-school indicators: Using satisfaction and postschool outcome data for program improvement.* In F.R. Rusch, L. DeStefano, J. Chadsey-Rusch, L.A. Phelps, & E. Szymanski (Eds.), *Transition from school to adult life* (pp. 485–506). Sycamore, IL: Sycamore.

Health Resource Center (Higher Education and Adult Training for People with Handicaps). (1994). *Make the most of your opportunities—A guide to postsecondary education for adults with disabilities.* Washington, DC: National Clearinghouse on Postsecondary Education for Individuals with Handicaps.

Lau, C., & O'Leary, S. (1993). Comparison of computer interface devices of persons with severe physical disabilities. *American Journal of Occupational Therapy, 47,* 1022–1030.

Lazzaro, J.L. (1993). *Adaptive technologies for learning and work environments.* Chicago, IL: American Library Association.

Lenker, J. (1993). *Final report: Assistive technology on campus.* Unpublished manuscript. State University of New York at Buffalo.

Mann, W.C., & Lane, J.P. (1991). *Assistive technology for persons with disabilities.* Bethesda, MD: American Occupational Therapy Association.

Murphy, H. (1991). *The impact of exemplary technology-support programs on students with disabilities.* Washington, DC: National Council on Disability.

Nochajski, S. (1993). *The transition process.* Unpublished manuscript.

RESNA Technical Assistance Project. (1992). *Assistive Technology and the Individualized Education Program.* Washington, DC: RESNA Press.

Rubenstein, L.S., & Milestein, B. (1993). Redefining equality through the ADA. In P. Wehman (ed.). *The ADA mandate for social change* (p. 318). Baltimore, MD: Brookes.

Spiers, E. (1992). *Students who are blind or visually impaired in postsecondary education.* American Council on Education, Heath Resource Center (Higher Education and Adult Training for People with Handicaps). Washington, DC: National Clearinghouse on Postsecondary Education for Individuals with Handicaps.

Wagner M., Blackorby, J., Cameto, R., & Newman, L. (1993). What makes a difference? Influences on postschool outcomes of youth with disabilities. In *The Third Comprehensive Report from the National Longitudinal Transition Study of Special Education Students.* Menlo Park, CA: SRI International. ED 365 G85.

Yuditsky, I. (1991). *Effective empowerment.* Toronto, Ontario, Canada: Canadian Rehabilitation Council for the Disabled.

Chapter 6 Study Questions

1. Describe two major federal Acts that have had an impact on students with disabilities.

2. Describe the use of assistive technology for students with each of the following types of impairments:
   a. hearing impairments
   b. vision impairments
   c. mobility impairments
   d. neurological impairments
   e. learning disabilities

3. Contact your campus office that provides services for students with disabilities. Ask about the services available for each of the impairments listed in question 2. Ask specifically about issues of assistive technology services. If you have already graduated from college, call your alma mater.

4. How accessible is your campus, both in terms of mobility impairment and electronic accessibility? Do your computer centers have any special equipment to assist persons with disabilities? Are your libraries computerized, and if so, do they have special equipment for access by students with disabilities?

5. Interview a student with a disability on your campus. Discuss his or her use of assistive technology and issues of accessibility. Be prepared to refer the student to an appropriate agency should there be assistive technology needs that have not been met.

Chapter 7:
Technology in the Workplace

I. Introduction

II. Legislation
- A. The Rehabilitation Act
- B. Rehabilitation Act Amendments
- C. Education for All Handicapped Children Act
- D. Individuals With Disabilities Education Act
- E. Technology-Related Assistance for Individuals With Disabilities Act
- F. Americans with Disabilities Act

III. Assistive Technology in the Workplace
- A. Cumulative Trauma Disorders
- B. Sensory Impairments
- C. Neurological and Physical Impairments

IV. The Process of Providing Assistive Technology for the Workplace
- A. Referral
- B. Assessment
  - 1. Home Environment
  - 2. Work Environment
- C. Procurement of Equipment
- D. Equipment Setup
- E. Training
- F. Monitoring for Continued Use of Devices
- G. Maintenance and Repair of Devices

V. Assistive Technology Issues

VI. Case Studies
- A. Case Study 1
  - 1. Background
  - 2. Assessment
  - 3. Evaluation
  - 4. Intervention
  - 5. Outcomes
  - 6. Conclusions
- B. Case Study 2
  - 1. Background
  - 2. Assessment
  - 3. Computer

196

7.

Technology in the Workplace

Susan M. Nochajski, MS, OTR/L, and Christine R. Oddo, MS, OTR/L

Introduction

Assistive technology has made it possible for many persons with disabilities to seek and achieve successful employment. Through the use of a variety of assistive technology devices, persons with disabilities have the potential to be successful in employment opportunities not previously afforded them. The number of persons using assistive technology to perform jobs has increased considerably over the past several years. Assistive technology has enabled these persons to advance through the employment process, obtain competitive employment, and achieve life goals.

For many persons with disabilities, computer technology enables them to participate in workplace skills and engage in meaningful employment. The computer serves as a tool for them to perform reading and writing tasks and to control the environment. For example, within the work environment, computers may be used to prepare reports, enter data, perform designing tasks, work on spreadsheets, compose music, and perform a variety of other jobs.

Legislation

Transition to the workplace can be viewed as two distinct yet interrelated processes: the initial transition from school to work, and transitions within the work environment from sheltered to supportive to competitive employment or to greater functional independence in the present work situation. The use of assistive technology facilitates transitions both to and within the workplace. Legislation has influenced the work potential of persons with disabilities. Six key pieces of legislation influencing transition and employment will be discussed briefly:

1. The Rehabilitation Act of 1973
2. Rehabilitation Act Amendments of 1986
3. The Education for All Handicapped Children Act of 1975 (EHA)
4. The Individuals With Disabilities Education Act of 1990 (IDEA)
5. Technology-Related Assistance for Individuals With Disabilities Act of 1988 (TRAID)
6. The Americans With Disabilities Act of 1990 (ADA)

The Rehabilitation Act

The Rehabilitation Act of 1973 was a milestone for persons with disabilities seeking employment. Section 504 of the Act prohibited discrimination against a person based solely on that person's disability in any program receiving federal assistance. This legislation had widespread implications because employers were prohibited from discriminating against an otherwise qualified person in a wide range of employment activities such as job application procedures, compensation, and advancement.

This legislation established a priority for the Rehabilitation Services Administration to serve persons with severe disabilities and to establish and regulate sheltered workshops as alternative places of employment for those persons unable to work in competitive employment (Reed, 1991).

Rehabilitation Act Amendments

The Rehabilitation Act Amendments of 1986 defined rehabilitation technology services as "the systematic application of technology, engineering methodologies, or scientific principles to meet needs of individuals with handicaps in areas which include education, rehabilitation, employment, transportation, independent living, and recreation" (p. 35). By defining rehabilitation technology, this legislation acknowledged the value of assistive technology in the workplace and encouraged rehabilitation technology services.

The Rehabilitation Act Amendments also enabled state employment programs to purchase services such as assessment, job placement, and training that are necessary for persons with disabilities to obtain and productively apply assistive devices (Rusch, Chadsey-Rusch, & Johnson, 1991).

Education for All Handicapped Children Act

The EHA was enacted in 1975 to ensure that students with disabilities receive a free appropriate public education. This legislation, although not affecting employment directly, provided a basis for education and skills related to employment through special education and related services. A major component of the EHA mandates several items including an individualized education program (IEP). The IEP is defined as a written statement designed by the teacher, parent, and a school representative that must include:

- the child's present education level,
- annual goals, including short-term educational objectives,
- the specific education services to be provided and the extent to which the child will participate in regular educational programs,
- initiation date and length of services, and
- evaluation procedures.

Individuals With Disabilities Education Act

The IDEA (an amendment to the EHA), enacted in 1990, has two new mandates pertaining to the IEP that will have a substantial effect for students with disabilities. The new IEP components are related to transition services and the use of assistive technology.

The IDEA legislation requires that, by the time a student with a disability reaches 16 years of age, a statement of the transition services that he or she needs must be included in the IEP. Transition services are defined in the legislation as:

> a coordinated set of activities for a student, designed within an outcome-oriented process, which promotes movement from school to post-school activities, including post-secondary education, vocational training, integrated employment (including supported employment), continuing and adult education, adult services, independent living and/or community participation. (20 U.S.C. Chapter 33, 1401 [a] [19])

In addition, the individual student's needs, taking into account his or her preferences and interests, must be the basis for the coordinated set of activities. These activities should include instruction, community experiences, the development of employment, and other postschool adult living objectives. When appropriate, ADL and functional vocational evaluation should also be included (NICHY, 1993).

The IDEA also requires that "all children with disabilities have available to them...a free appropriate public education which emphasizes special education and related services designed to meet their unique individual needs..." (20 U.S.C. Chapter 33, 601[c]). Assistive technology is subsumed under the category of related services and "can be a form of supplementary aid or service utilized to facilitate a child's education..." (RESNA Technical Assistance Project, 1992, p. 15).

With a broad interpretation consistent with other federal legislation, the IDEA defined assistive technology as both a device and a service. An assistive technology device is defined as "any item, piece of equipment or product system, whether acquired commercially off the shelf, or customized, that is used to increase, maintain, or improve functional capabilities of individuals with disabilities" (20 U.S.C. Chapter 33, 1401 [25]). Assistive technology service is "any service that directly assists an individual with a disability in the selection, acquisition, or use of an assistive technology device" (20 U.S.C. Chapter 33, 1401, [26]). Assistive technology services may include evaluation; purchasing, leasing, or providing devices; selecting, designing, fitting, customizing, adapting, applying, maintaining, repairing, or replacing devices; coordinating and using other therapies, intervention, or services; and providing training and technical assistance for a person with a disability or for professionals who provide services for persons with disabilities.

Technology-Related Assistance for Individuals With Disabilities Act

The development of assistive technology continues at a rapid pace. For consumers to be aware of devices and their availability, the TRAID was enacted in 1988 and reauthorized in 1994. This federal legislation provides funding for states to develop and implement statewide programs to provide information on assistive technology and technology-related assistance to persons with disabilities of all ages.

Americans With Disabilities Act

Title I of the ADA prohibits an employer from discriminating against any qualified person with a disability. The legislation defines a "qualified individual with a disability" as one who, with or without reasonable accommodation, can perform the essential functions of the job, that is, those listed in the job description. A reasonable accommodation is one that does not impose an undue hardship on an employer, such as bankruptcy or laying off another employee to pay for the accommodation.

Reasonable accommodations generally fall into one of three categories: environmental modifications, equipment modifications, and procedural modifications. Examples of environmental modifications include the removal of architectural barriers, for example, making the job site accessible by installing a ramp or opening doors.

The provision of assistive devices and special tools is categorized as an equipment modification. Environmental control units, voice-activated telephones, enlarged key-caps, and adjustable chairs are all examples of equipment modifications. Procedural modifications include such things as restructuring tasks, altering work methods, and changing work schedules.

Assistive Technology in the Workplace

Assistive technology can include specific devices or modifications to equipment that assist or enable a person to perform work tasks; it can also include modifications to the environment. By using technological or environmental interventions to overcome the effects of a particular disability, a worker with a disability is able to become engaged in meaningful employment or continue in his or her current work roles. For example, a worker with a disability resulting in paralysis of the extremities is able to input information and commands into the computer with voice recognition instead of the traditional keyboard. Work options may include competitive employment either within or outside the home, work in sheltered or supported employment, volunteer work, or homemaking.

Competitive employment is "work that produces valued goods or services at minimum wage or above, offers opportunities for advancement, and is in an integrated setting" (Clees, 1992, p. 235). It is the traditional work for pay by persons who are able to obtain and maintain work independently. Frequently, this option has not been viable for persons with severe disabilities who require assistance and ongoing support. Consequently, alternative work placements have been developed that aid persons with disabilities in employment. These alternatives include sheltered and supported employment.

Sheltered employment is work in a structured, supervised setting in which workers are paid a percentage of the minimum wage based on their productivity. Sheltered workshops usually receive contracts for work from a variety of businesses.

Supported employment has become an increasingly popular alternative to sheltered employment and a stepping stone to competitive employment for many persons with severe disabilities. Supported employment is "paid work in a variety of settings, particularly regular work sites, especially designed for handicapped individuals: (i) for whom competitive employment has not traditionally occurred; and (ii) who, because of their disability, need intensive ongoing support to perform in a work setting" (Hughes & Wehman, 1992, p. 184). For supported employment to be as effective as possible, it is essential for the trainer or job coach to be aware of how a specific task may be modified and assistive devices that are available. With this information, the trainer and worker can problem-solve to ensure that the worker becomes as productive as possible. Other options for work include volunteer work, nonpaid employment, and homemaking.

Persons with disabilities frequently require the use of devices or modifications to the environment for them to engage in work. An interdisciplinary team determines the necessary devices, or modifications, and procures, and integrates these items into the work setting. The team includes the person with the disability, the employer, other employees, various service agencies, funding sources, medical practitioners, and professionals knowledgeable about assistive devices. The integration of devices and

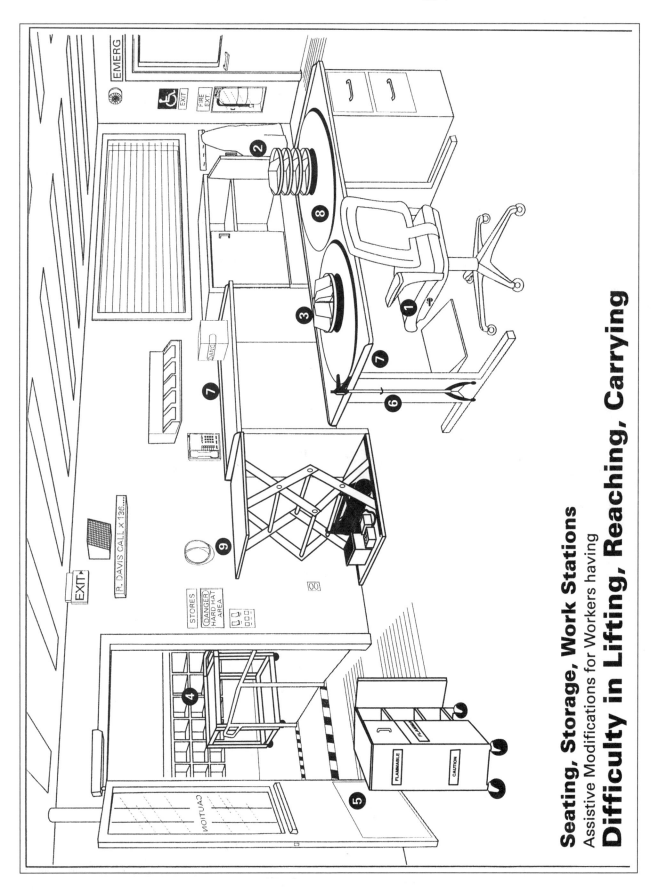

Seating, Storage, Work Stations
Assistive Modifications for Workers having
Difficulty in Lifting, Reaching, Carrying

Figure 7.1. Example of a workstation design.

Difficulty in Lifting, Reaching, Carrying

(Impaired mobility, range of motion, and/or strength in trunk or upper extremities)

Approximately 4.6 million U.S. workers (ages 18-69) report difficulty in lifting, reaching, carrying as a result of a chronic disabling condition. (Other workers may also experience this limitation due to minor or temporary conditions).

Following are modifications to Seating, Storage and Work Stations which should be considered with the input of these workers.

Seating

1. Locate adjustment controls as close as possible.

Storage

2. Store items within 18" reach from body (or use pull-out shelves or "lazy suzan" carousels); if space is cramped, use suspended storage.

3. Provide desk-top files/organizers.

4. Facilitate sliding rather than lifting of containers heavier than 2 lbs., or provide wheeled cart or other aid for carrying materials.

5. Use securely-enclosed carts, other equipment for messy/ hazardous materials.

6. Minimize need for reaching up, reaching behind, or bending down; provide mechanical "reachers" and keep in convenient location.

Work Stations

6. Provide mechanical "reachers", other materials handling equipment.

Work Stations (Continued)

7. Provide raised edge to keep materials from falling.

8. Provide "lazy suzan" work surface.

9. Install powered "lift tables" for positioning heavy work.

Attach cords to tools to keep within reach.

Cluster materials, tools within 18" reach radius from body.

41

Figure 7.2. Example of a workstation design.

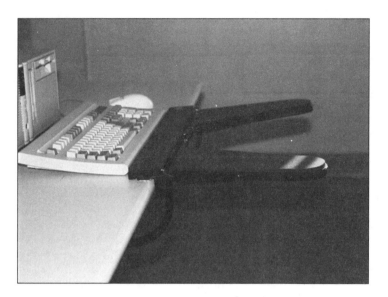

Figure 7.3. Wrist support.

accommodations into the workplace can be a complex process because the needs of many persons must be addressed.

Steinfeld and Angelo (1992) proposed the adaptive work placement model to address the integration of assistive technology into the workplace. This model stresses the importance of professional services across disciplines as well as employer education and support to facilitate technology acquisition, modifications, and use. In addition, the model places emphasis on the entire work environment, including accessibility to the building, workstation design, and setup and the work tasks.

The ACHIEVE project developed a process to assist persons using assistive technology in the workplace (Angelo, Hurlburt, & Oddo, 1992). In addition to assessment of work tasks and workstation and building accessibility, this project included assessment of current technology use, the home environment, and transportation issues. After assessment, the client was matched with the appropriate technology to facilitate employment or expand employment opportunities.

Mueller (1990) provided useful information on how to modify and incorporate assistive technology into the workplace. Suggestions for seating, storage, computers, and workstation design were provided. The information is especially useful because it shows both major and minor modifications. The specific modifications depend on the person's impairment and the particular equipment that must be accommodated within a workspace. Figures 7.1 and 7.2 provide an example of a workstation design.

Posture and positioning that is comfortable for the worker and makes optimal use of body mechanics is important to prevent the occurrence of fatigue and injuries. The worker's functional capabilities and the need to change position during a work period are considered when recommending assistive devices or modifications (Angelo, Hurlburt, & Oddo, 1991). Many devices are available to improve positioning. Adjustable-height tables provide a flexible work height that will benefit most employees. The table surface can be raised or lowered to provide a comfortable arm and hand position during work. This eliminates the tendency of the worker to use poor body mechanics to reach the work surface. Adjustable-height tables also make it easier for persons with wheelchairs to access the work surface.

Workstation designs are often altered to meet the needs of the worker with a disability. When arranging the workstation, it is important to consider the organization of the space needed to perform work tasks, the efficient use of additional work space, and the availability of space for other work needs. The shape of the workstation must be considered in the design or modification process. A variety of workstation designs offer different options for access and more efficient use of space. These shapes include the kidney-bean, L, U, and E designs. Selection of a specific shape is determined by the tasks to be performed, the worker's functional abilities and limitations, and the organization of work equipment and assistive devices.

To provide accessibility and prevent the need for excessive arm reach and twisting movements, table surfaces are available that can be tilted to various angles, recessed, or extended. Rearrangement or mounting of devices or tools within the reach of the worker, are also considered adaptations. Work tools and assistive devices used most often are positioned close to the worker for easy access.

A variety of arm- and wrist-positioning devices provide the worker with arm and hand support. This is especially useful during performance of repetitive tasks.

Figure 7.3 shows one example of a wrist support. Ergonomically designed chairs that allow for adjusting seat height, width, depth, and tilt facilitate a comfortable and aligned sitting position. Footstools provide additional support to stabilize the lower body, hips, and feet.

Other adaptations that enable a worker with a disability to access the work site include lowered or enlarged switches, environmental control devices, voice-activated telephones, and automatic page turners. Automated equipment, such as electric pencil sharpeners and staplers, make work tasks easier for all workers.

The assistive technology described above is useful for persons with a wide range of disabilities; devices for more specific disabilities are now discussed briefly herein. Although these devices and adaptations are useful, the list is by no means exhaustive.

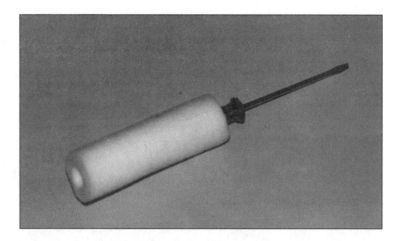

Figure 7.4. Tool modified with cylindrical padding.

Cumulative Trauma Disorders

Cumulative trauma disorders (CTDs) is a term used to describe a variety of disorders or impairments of the upper extremities, including carpal tunnel syndrome and repetitive strain disorder. These disorders primarily affect the hands and wrists, and occur from excessive or repetitive use of the joints and soft-tissue structures. Hand and arm tasks that involve continuous, awkward, or static positions (such as grasping a tool or sustained reaching), or tasks that involve repetition of movement without recovery time (such as keyboarding) put workers at risk for developing or worsening these disorders (Williams & Westmorland, 1994).

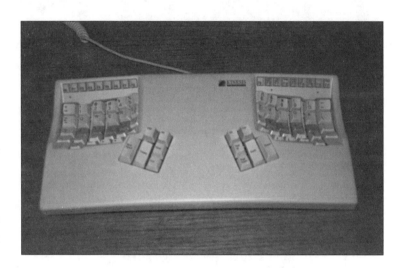

Figure 7.5. Kinesis keyboard.

Assistive technology is used in the workplace to help prevent or to decrease the effects of CTDs. Analysis of the job (including positioning, workstation design and setup, task demands, necessary tools, and time requirements) is required. Adaptations are made to decrease stress on the hand and joints and to fit the user. These include enlarged handles, padded surfaces, and contoured grips. Tool positions are modified to facilitate aligned wrist movements and prevent awkward wrist positions (Beaton-Starr, 1992). A tool modified with cylindrical padding is shown in Figure 7.4.

For example, alternatives to the standard keyboard include the use of specially designed ergonomic keyboards. These keyboards are designed to facilitate a more natural hand position through the rearrangement of frequently used keys and through alternative positioning of keyboard sections. Other

features of various ergonomic keyboards include support for the wrist and minimization of hand and finger movements. The Kinesis keyboard is shown in Figure 7.5. In addition, software is available that alerts the user, through an auditory signal or visual message, to change body positions. For example, this software is used as an adjunct to worker education programs. A message may appear on the screen prompting the worker to remove hands from the keyboard and to perform preinstructed hand and wrist exercises.

Sensory Impairments

Persons with sensory impairments and primarily vision and hearing impairments comprise a large segment of the workforce who have disabilities. Although other chapters in this book address vision and hearing impairments, this chapter discusses cer-

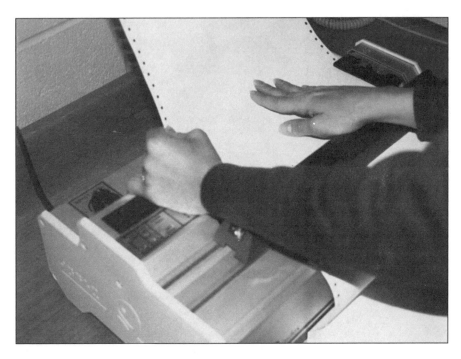

Figure 7.6. Braille output from Braille embosser.

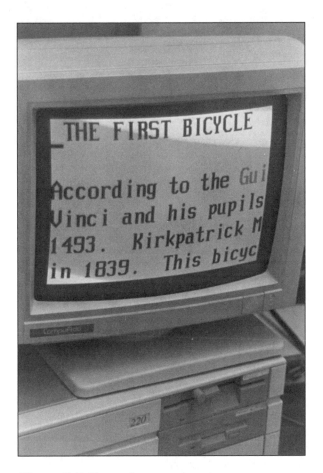

Figure 7.7. Text-enlargement system.

tain technology useful in the workplace. Often a place of employment has an existing computer environment where individual workstations are networked together and use software stored on a mainframe computer in another location. Networked computers allow coworkers to send and receive electronic mail and share reports and documents stored on disk.

For persons with hearing impairments, the use of electronic messages facilitates communication in the workplace. Software that provides a visual cue to alert a user is used to replace auditory feedback from computers. For persons with visual impairments, computer technology is adapted with screen readers, used in conjunction with voice synthesizers, to provide auditory presentation of the screen display. For example, a person using a word-processing application program to write a report is able to hear the letter, word, sentence, or paragraph being typed. In addition, information displayed on the screen, such as pop-up screens and electronic mail messages, is heard to enable the worker to communicate with and to share documents with coworkers. Printed text that is scanned into the computer provides access to other written information needed to complete a job task. Other useful workplace adaptations include Braille or tactile labels displays and hard-copy Braille output produced by Braille embossers, as shown in Figure 7.6.

Text enlargement helps persons with poor vision read information displayed on a computer screen. Figure 7.7 illustrates a text-enlargement system. A portable talking notetaker with headphones is used to perform writing tasks at meetings or in other work situations when a desktop computer is not practical.

Neurological and Physical Impairments

Neurological and physical impairments include a wide range of disabilities and often include involvement of the nervous system, muscles, and joints. These disabilities frequently result in impairments in mobility, motor control, strength, coordination, dexterity, and overall function. These impairments often result in an inability to perform routine work tasks such as writing, typing, or using traditional tools.

Numerous devices assist persons with these types of disabilities. A wide variety of alternative input devices help with access to the computer. Alternatives to the standard keyboard include expanded or customizable keyboards and compact, miniature, and ergonomic keyboards. A customizable keyboard can be used to program functions that require multiple commands into macros. The worker can then select one key to perform a multistep task. This is beneficial in reducing the number of keystrokes for workers who fatigue easily. Examples of these keyboards are shown in Figure 7.8.

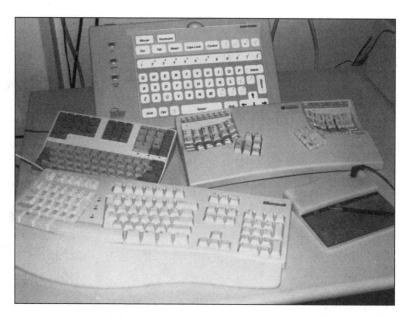

Figure 7.8. Alternative keyboards.

Numerous alternative pointing devices assist persons who are unable to use a mouse to control the mouse pointer on the screen. For example, a worker with limited hand movement and poor coordination can use a trackball instead. This device is attached to the computer in the same manner as a mouse. It enables the worker to use gross hand movements to move the trackball to perform mouse functions of selecting and using menus. This device also eliminates the need to hold and drag when moving items on the screen. Figure 7.9 shows one type of trackball.

In addition to hardware adaptations, specialized software also improves computer access and use. These programs, in conjunction with hardware, provide options for use of scanning, Morse code, and voice recognition as input methods. In addition, word prediction, voice output, on-screen keyboards, and keyboard adjustment utilities assist with more efficient computer work.

The Process of Providing Assistive Technology for the Workplace

Assistive devices are recommended to make persons with disabilities more independent at work. The provision of assistive technology and environmental modifications in the workplace is a multistep process that includes:

- referral,

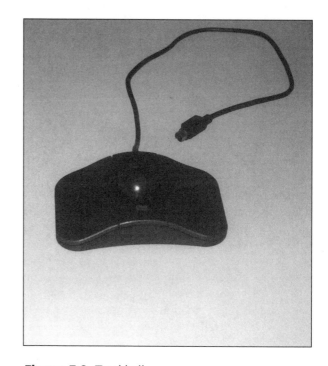

Figure 7.9. Trackball.

- assessment,
- procurement of equipment,
- equipment setup,
- training,
- monitoring for continued use of devices, and
- maintenance and repair of devices.

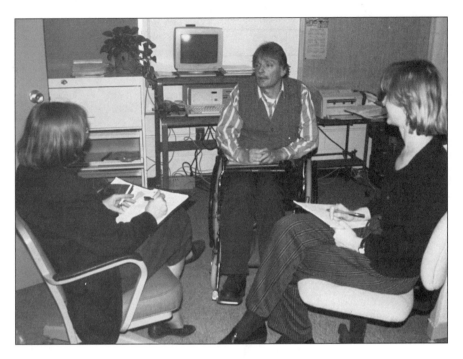

Figure 7.10. A meeting of the assessment team.

Referral

Referrals for assistive technology in the workplace come from a variety of sources. Many vocational or service agencies refer clients to assist with job accommodations and to assist with increasing competency necessary for competitive employment and advancement. Employers who realize the necessity for accommodations in order to enhance or sustain work skills and contributions of employees with disabilities will make referrals. This assists with the transition from being a worker without a disability to one with a disability or to assist with beginning work. Referrals enable the worker with a disability to maintain productivity and the ability to continue working. Self-referral from clients is also a common source of referral. Referral sources can also include other professionals and third-party payers.

Assessment

Assessment is an extremely important issue in workplace accommodation, adaptation, and modification. The evaluation process, or problem analysis, is initiated by defining the person's need for assistance to work. Assessment is used to determine appropriate assistive technology and environmental modifications needed to become employed or to improve employment. A thorough assessment of the problem is an essential first step in providing assistive technology. Not only the person but also the environment and the person–device fit must be assessed. Environmental assessment includes not only the workplace itself, but also the home environment as it relates to the person's ability to prepare for work. Assessment of transportation issues is also included, depending on individual needs. In view of the diverse nature of assessment, a team approach is essential.

The technology assessment team should always include the person with the disability and the employer. The team of professionals knowledgeable about assistive technology devices will vary depending on the worker's particular needs. Professionals from the fields of occupational therapy, rehabilitation engineering, and architecture are often core members of the team. The occupational therapist is experienced in the use of assistive devices and addresses disability-related issues, positioning, and the worker's functional capabilities and limitations. A rehabilitation engineer is knowledgeable about assistive devices and provides technical support for devices and adaptations. An architect assists with the design of the adapted environment and makes recommendations for environmental modifications that facilitate independence and foster assistive technology use. Figure 7.10 portrays a meeting of the assessment team.

Depending on the needs of the worker, additional persons on the team include professionals with expertise on computers, augmentative communication, and seating. A computer specialist is knowledgeable about computer hardware and software requirements and can contribute information about device compatibility and networks. The augmentative communication specialist shares knowledge about alternative communication systems and assists in integrating communication devices into the workplace. A seating specialist provides input into seating and positioning systems to ensure that they are functional in the workplace.

Other agencies working or providing services for the worker are also team members. Vocational rehabilitation counselors, college counselors, trainers, physicians, nurses, and therapists are also included.

Many factors affect a person's ability to become employed or maintain employment. Assessment includes evaluation of sensory and motor functions, cognition, and psychosocial skills as well as the person's performance on activities of daily living (ADL), work, play, and leisure. Worker needs related to job requirements, necessary tasks, and other work-related activities are also assessed. The assessment also includes evaluation of the work environment and other areas determined necessary. Additional work issues that should be assessed include communication, socialization, and education of other employees about assistive technology.

Worker abilities include what the person can do, current work skills and qualifications, education, and special needs. For example, if a worker needs to substitute use of another body part for impaired hand function, it is necessary to assess the worker's ability and endurance to perform the job and what modifications are involved.

Assessment is an ongoing process. Based on the information collected and the expressed needs and goals of the worker, various assistive devices are prepared for trial use during the assessment. For workers using computers, combinations of hardware and software are also prepared. This requires extensive planning, research, and testing to have devices available and appropriate systems configured. These devices and systems are then used and modified as needed according to the worker's abilities, comfort and ease of use.

Home Environment

Assessment of the home is important if the home is a factor in determining whether someone can be employed. For example, if the worker uses a wheelchair, the home should be evaluated for accessibility to ensure that the worker is able to prepare and depart for work with relative ease in a timely manner. The use of assistive devices to increase independence in preparing for work can assist with successful employment. Some workers are employed within the home. In addition to accessibility, workstation needs and equipment for work are evaluated.

Work Environment

In addition to the provision of assistive technology, many persons require or could benefit from modifications to the worksite to facilitate job performance. A worker with a disability must be able to access the work area to perform job tasks. Assessment of the work area will enhance the capabilities of the person.

It is important to identify the work locations or spaces where the person will work. This can include where a specific workstation is located, and other locations such as restrooms, lounges, cafeteria, parking areas, or other rooms that the employee uses to perform the job. It is important to identify the workstation and equipment being used. In addition, it is equally important to determine the job tasks and responsibilities and any other mechanism in place to accomplish the job. For example, if a person is going to use a computer for work, it is important to determine equipment type, application programs used, what the person must learn, if the computers are networked, if electronic mail is used, and any other pertinent questions that relate to the job and employee performance.

At the work site, assessment includes analysis of job tasks and functions, and other work-related needs including mobility, ADL such as eating and hygiene, workstation design, equipment compatibility, and modifications to current assistive technology.

Procurement of Equipment

After trial use of various access methods, assistive devices, or software, a consensus is reached by the team as to the most appropriate intervention. This includes specific recommendations for computer hardware and software, assistive devices, environmental control, modifications, and use of equipment.

Equipment can be used "off the shelf," but it is often necessary to customize and configure devices to meet individual needs. This is especially important when several devices are required and utilized. Device procurement includes not only adaptations to existing work equipment but also the fabrication of new devices to facilitate work performance.

Careful selection of assistive devices is important so that there is a high level of acceptance by the worker (Thiers, 1994). Workers should demonstrate a willingness to learn to use devices that facilitate work skills. Durability, reliability, portability, and ease of maintenance and service are desirable device features (Smith, 1991). Devices are often procured through the employer, vocational organizations, third-party payers, and private acquisition.

Funding of assistive technology is a concern for both employees and employers. Vocational rehabilitation agencies have traditionally helped persons with disabilities prepare for work. This has included the acquisition of assistive technology for work purposes. Work incentive programs, available through the federal government, serve to encourage both

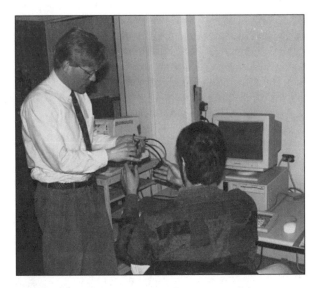

Figure 7.11. An assistive device being set up.

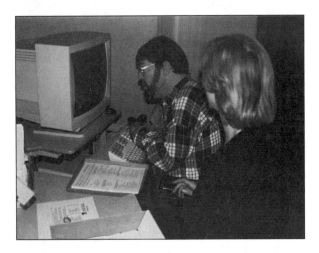

Figure 7.12. Training being provided.

part-time and full-time employment. They assist workers with issues related to the initiating employment, maintenance of benefits, and tax incentives (Woodward, 1993). Persons with disabilities may rely on these programs to purchase devices or equipment, to receive personal care and transportation, and to encourage the hiring of persons with disabilities.

Equipment Setup

Assistive devices will require special setup and adaptations. The team member most knowledgeable about a specific device or piece of equipment is responsible for accomplishing this task. Devices frequently need to be fitted to the worker. In addition, use of assistive technology must be integrated within the work setting for optimal worker performance. Figure 7.11 shows an assistive device being set up.

Training

Training is an extremely important component in the provision of assistive technology in the workplace. A worker requires specialized training in device use; training provides a way to ensure knowledge about and comfort with the device. Training also gives the worker an understanding of how to perform specific tasks with the assistive technology and how to take full advantage of the capabilities of the assistive technology. Users must be familiar with their devices and how the device can be used for increased proficiency in job performance and independence in work. In addition, user readiness and knowledge of the job requirements can facilitate easier transition to the workplace (Chamot, 1989). Figure 7.12 shows training being provided.

Training places many learning demands on workers. For workers with computers, instruction includes training on alternative access methods, orientation and setup of hardware devices, use and customization of assistive software, and use of application programs. These skills are then integrated into the workplace. Training also includes technical support services, reference materials, and troubleshooting strategies.

Training within the work environment involves on-the-job training with assistive technology. This is important to facilitate performance and completion of job requirements, to ensure compatibility with the job, and to promote worker and employer satisfaction with devices.

Issues in training include the timing of training, who will train, and payment for training. Initial training in the use of assistive technology should be done by a professional knowledgeable about the device. However, in order to integrate the technology into the workplace, on-the-job training includes input from the employer or others involved in the work environment.

Another area concerning the use of assistive technology in the workplace involves training of job tasks with the assistive devices. Workers may require new skills to perform the job with the assistive technology. Problems in work compatibility, performance demands, and the technology must be corrected to ensure maximum performance. This can be especially challenging for persons who are new to using assistive devices for performing work tasks. Mann and Svorai (1994) describe a training program for persons with cognitive impairments (COMPETE) who use computers for training in keyboarding and data entry. Their findings, in addition to the use of assistive technology for access to computers and the workstation, support the need for an interdisciplinary approach, education of employers, and follow-up support after job placement.

Monitoring for Continued Use of Devices

To facilitate continued use of assistive devices, workers and their employers are provided with training on problem-solving and troubleshooting, and information on the availability of technical support. Monitoring is necessary to provide modifications or adjustments as the worker gains expertise in job performance or experiences changes in level of impairment.

Maintenance and Repair of Devices

Equipment must be maintained to be used successfully. This issue should be addressed for the worker using assistive devices who may be unable to problem-solve or repair devices independently. Workers and employers require information on whom to contact when maintenance or repair is necessary. The cost of maintenance and repair also needs to be considered when recommending or procuring devices.

Assistive Technology Issues

Several issues are related to the successful choice and use of assistive technology for work. In addition to worker ability and expertise and equipment compatibility, devices using new technology, cost, and future needs of the worker all affect the provision and use of devices. In addition, ongoing support, maintenance, and flexibility of the device also effect use.

The level of involvement is an important consideration in the provision of services to persons with severe disabilities. Additional time is often needed for evaluation of devices, resolution of compatibility issues, training in the use of equipment, and developing on-the-job performance and competence. Often persons with severe, lifelong disabilities have not had the opportunity to experience activities that enable them to develop work habits. Assistive technology provides solutions for problems arising from skill limitations, but one also needs to consider other limitations. For example, consider a person with a traumatic brain injury. Although his work skills were adequate, he had trouble remembering to take his medications, which led to performance problems on the job. A device called the NeuroPage was used as an intervention. The device consists of a computer

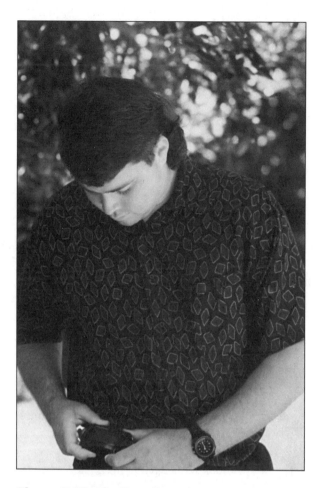

Figure 7.13. The NeuroPage.

with preprogrammed messages and times that remind him to take medications, and a beeper that signals the message. The beeper is carried by the person at work. It beeps and gives the reminder to take medication at the appropriate time. This device enables him to remain gainfully employed. The NeuroPage is shown in Figure 7.13.

Bushrow and Turner (1994) describe barriers to technology use in special education. These concerns are also manifested when assistive technology is used in the workplace. Assuming responsibility for implementing the technology into the workplace, learning about devices, and problem-solving with the technology is a concern for many employees. A person using technology may affect the employer. The employer often shares responsibility for equipment, training, and maintenance. The employer may need to provide equipment to make the necessary accommodations so the employee can perform the job. This can be costly. Also, equipment maintenance, updating, and training become concerns.

Environmental adaptations and assistive devices for the worker with a disability also have an effect on other workers. For example, work space and equipment are used by all employees. Modifications to the work area will have an effect on not only the worker using the assistive technology but also other employees. The attitudes and acceptance of other employees will assist in making the use of technology and devices successful in employment.

Other issues that are important to successful employment with assistive technology include coordination of services between agencies, addressing transportation needs, the choice of part-time or full-time employment, long-term commitment to the employment process, disability benefits, and the economic climate.

Case Studies

Through the use of three case studies, this chapter provides an in-depth look at the process of providing assistive technology in the workplace. The case studies include persons with rheumatoid arthritis, quadriplegia, and cerebral palsy with mild mental retardation. The cases consider both high- and low-technology solutions to problems.

The persons in each of the case studies were referred to various service programs at the Center for Assistive Technology (CAT). Referral forms are requested by CAT to provide information on the person's current status, specific needs, experience with assistive technology, and information about the job site. This information provides a basis for further assessment. Work-related referrals for assistive technology are routed to the CAT staff who provide evaluation services. One staff member performs the preliminary task of gathering background information prior to the assessment. Once additional information is collected, staff members meet and decide who will participate in the assessment. The assistive technology team is drawn from service providers employed at CAT and from CAT projects that involve assistive technology research and education.

Each of the case studies are organized into five major sections: background, assessment, intervention, outcomes, and conclusions. The background information provides preliminary information that is the basis for team selection, helps define the problem, and guides further assessment. The assessment section also includes not only the capabilities, limitations, and interests of the person, but also the home and work environments. The intervention section contains the recommendations or solutions for the

problem. The outcomes section describes how the interventions were obtained, their effectiveness, or problems that occurred. Finally, the conclusions section briefly summarizes what insight was gained from the case study.

Case Study 1

Background

Mary is a 55-year-old woman who is employed as a machine operator for a small manufacturing company. Mary has a longstanding history of rheumatoid arthritis that affects all of her extremities. She experiences intermittent joint pain throughout the day. She has decreased ability to move both upper extremities. She has multiple joint deformities of the hands. She experiences ankle and foot pain after brief periods of movement.

Mary lives alone and owns her home. She does not have any relatives living in the area. She has a small circle of friends that she socializes with on a weekly basis. She is independent in ADL; however, daily self-care and chores are difficult on days when pain and fatigue are more severe, especially on workdays. She works approximately 30 hours a week.

Mary's main work duties are those of a seamstress. Her job entails assembly of fabrics and patterns, cutting materials, and sewing pieces together on an industrial sewing machine. Mary experiences difficulties in performing all job tasks due to her limited movements, pain, and fatigue when working.

Mary is a client of a state vocational services agency. Under this service, options to assist her with work tasks were explored. Mary was referred to CAT for an assistive technology evaluation by her vocational rehabilitation counselor. This was to determine how technology could assist with Mary's needs to accomplish work tasks and continue employment. The vocational agency funded this assistive technology referral.

Assessment

The occupational therapist at CAT assumed the responsibility for gathering preliminary information about Mary, her job, and what needed to be addressed through the assessment. The occupational therapist's experience with a variety of disabilities and assistive devices facilitated this process. Initial intake forms developed through the EXTEND project at CAT are used to collect information related to a person's current function and abilities, work experience and needs, and home activities. An example of the intake form is shown in Figure 7.14.

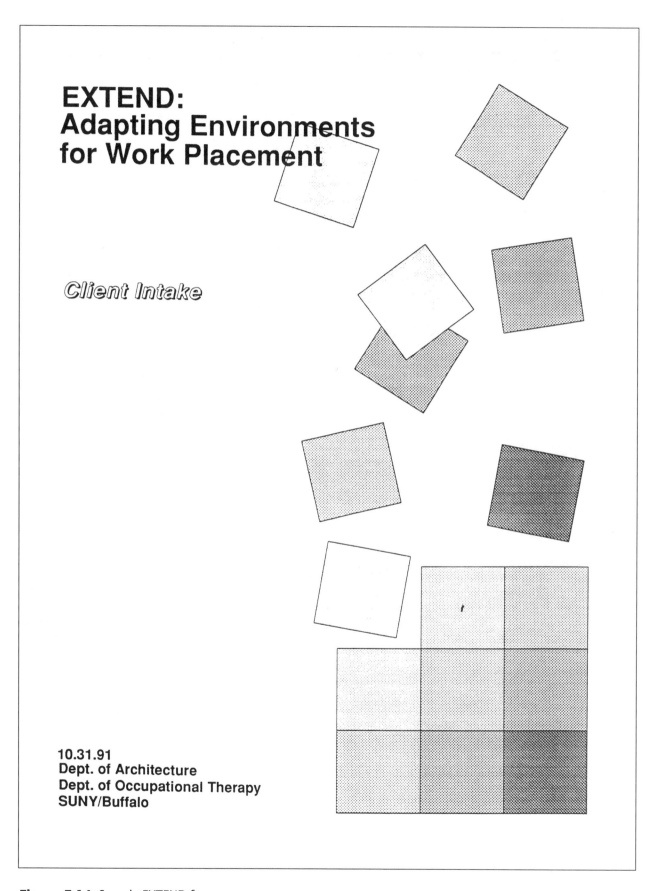

Figure 7.14. Sample EXTEND form.

```
EXTEND                                                          Client  Intake
═══════════════════════════════════════════════════════════════════════════════


    Interviewer:_____


    1. Personal Data:

    Name          _____
    Address       _____   Phone    _____
    City          _____   Soc Sec # _____
    Zip code      _____


    Date of enrollment in RDP project:  ____/____/____

    This is:

              1 _____ An original enrollment
              2 _____ A reenrollment (after withdrawal or unsuccessful job
                      placement)

    Disability program:

              1 _____ SSI
              2 _____ SSDI
              3 _____ SSI & SSDI
              4 _____ Application pending

    Length of time on disability prior to enrollment: ___ yr

    Date of birth:  ____/____/____

    Sex:

              1 _____ M
              2 _____ F

    Race:

              1 _____ Black
              2 _____ White
              3 _____ Hispanic
              4 _____ Other



                                   CI - 1
```

Figure 7.14. Sample EXTEND form (continued).

EXTEND   **Client Intake**

2. Referral Source:

Agency _____

Name and Position _____

Phone _____

3. Home Environment:

Lives: alone   1_____   with family   2_____   other   3_____

_____

_____

Please indicate present type of residence:

family home	1_____		apartment	4_____
group home	2_____		institution	5_____
hospital	3_____		other	6_____

4. Transportation Used Most Often

w/c van service	1_____
bus/lift	2_____
subway	3_____
other	4_____
personal car or van	5_____
who drives	_____

_____

Is transportation: Public   1_____   Private   2_____

Problems with transportation   _____

5. Ambulation:

Independent:	yes 1_____	no 2_____
with device:	yes 1_____	no 2_____
device used:	_____

CI - 2

Figure 7.14. Sample EXTEND form (continued).

EXTEND   **Client Intake**

6. Communication:

Verbal: yes 1_____   no 2_____

Is speech fully understandable to:

    familiar others   yes 1_____   no 2_____

    'unfamiliar others   yes 1_____   no 2_____

If communication system is used, please check types:

Voice synthesizer	_____	Writing	_____
Signing	_____	Gestures	_____
Symbols	_____	Pictures	_____
Line drawings	_____	Objects	_____
Other	_____		

If other, please specify type:

_____

7. Assistive Devices:

Please check if presently using one or more of the following devices:

Crutches	_____	Cane	_____
Walker	_____	Glasses	_____
Hearing Aid	_____	Prosthesis	_____
Artificial limb	_____	Braces	_____
Splints	_____	Communication system	_____
Power W/C	_____	Manual W/C	_____
Other	_____		

If other, please specify:

_____

8. Current W/C:

Size   _____

Age   _____

Armstyle   _____

Wheels/Tires _____

Frontrigging _____

Figure 7.14. Sample EXTEND form (continued).

EXTEND   **Client Intake**

Laptray   _____

Seatbelt   _____

Positioning devices used _____

If power, what is the control box and where is it located:

                          _____

Vendor where purchased   _____

Vendor used for repairs   _____

9. Education:

Less than high school graduate   1_____

High school graduate   2_____

Some college   3_____

College graduate or more   4_____

Are you presently taking classes: yes _____   no_____

If yes, where: _____

Education Level   _____

10. Work History:

Last place of employment _____

How long at this site   _____

Type of job   _____

Job duties   _____

Full Time _____   Part Time _____   If Part time, #hrs/wk._____

Former places of employment:

    Name and reason for termination:

    1. _____

        _____

    2. _____

        _____

Figure 7.14. Sample EXTEND form (continued).

EXTEND   **Client Intake**

Career Goals:

_____

_____

_____

11. *Medical Information:*

Diagnosis   _____

Onset of diagnosis   _____

Other medical concerns (other medical problems, seizures, swallowing problems, diabetes, etc.)

_____

_____

Medications   _____

Precautions   _____

Recent medical, surgical or dental procedures   yes   1____   no   2____

Planned medical, surgical or dental procedures   yes   1____   no   2____

Do you have a hearing impairment?   yes   1_____   no   2_____

     If yes, please specify   _____

Do you have a visual impairment?   yes   1_____   no   2_____

     If yes, please specify   _____

Are you currently receiving therapy?   yes   1_____   no   2_____

     If yes, please specify type and frequency

12. *Skin Care*

Sensation impairment or absent in any part of body:

          yes   1_____   no   2_____

Do you have a history of pressure sores?

          yes   1_____   no   2_____

CI - 5

Figure 7.14. Sample EXTEND form (continued).

EXTEND   Client Intake

If yes, specify type and frequency:

_____

_____

Please specify if have active pressure sores:

     yes   1_____   no   2_____

Are you receiving treatment for your pressure sores?

     yes   1_____   no   2_____

What kind of pressure relieving device do you use or in what way do you relieve pressure?

_____

What is your schedule to shift weight?

_____

13. Bladder/Bowel:

Do you have voluntary control over your bladder and bowel?

     yes   1_____   no   2_____

If no:

Are you on a bladder/bowel program?

     yes   1_____   no   2_____

In what way has your bowel or bladder problems interfered with work or socializing?

_____

Do you need assistance from others:

    getting to and from bathroom: yes 1_____   no 2_____

    with transfers in bathroom: yes 1_____   no 2_____

    Positioning in bathroom: yes 1_____   no 2_____

    Managing toileting or clothes: yes 1_____   no 2_____

CI - 6

Figure 7.14. Sample EXTEND form (continued).

EXTEND   **Client Intake**

14. Self Care Skills:

Indicate level of functioning (Independent, Dependent or Assistance) in column 1

List devices used to accomplish task in column 2

Specify number of years device used in column 3

I=Independent
D=Dependent
A=Assistance   Devices   Years

feeding	_____	_____	_____
dressing	_____	_____	_____
toileting	_____	_____	_____
grooming	_____	_____	_____
writing	_____	_____	_____
talking	_____	_____	_____
opening doors	_____	_____	_____
telephoning	_____	_____	_____
walking	_____	_____	_____
other	_____	_____	_____

Are you experiencing difficulty with any of the above tasks, the individuals assisting you or the devices you use?

_____

_____

General tolerance/endurance _____

_____

Number of hours spent engaged in activities daily (ie. self care, longest amount of time in wheel chair) _____

_____

If assistance is required for any of the tasks above, who provides it?

_____

_____

_____

CI - 7

Figure 7.14. Sample EXTEND form (continued).

EXTEND — **Client Intake**

15. Medical Emergency:

Notify _____
Relationship _____
Phone _____
Address _____

Name of person completing questionnaire (if not client)

_____

Relationship to client _____
Telephone _____

Adapted from :
Hugh McMillian
Adaptive Device Center

CI - 8

Figure 7.14. Sample EXTEND form (continued).

ACHIEVE
ASSESSMENT FOR EMPLOYED PERSONS

Date _____

Name _____

Address _____ Phone _____

City _____ State _____ Zip _____

Disability _____

Date of Occurrence _____ Date of Birth _____

Referral Source:

    Agency _____

    Name and Position

    _____

EMPLOYMENT

Work History

I will ask you several questions about jobs you have had and also the one you have now.

  (1)
1. Current Employer _____

2. Address _____

3. Do you work at this address or another?

   If you work at another, where?

Figure 7.15. ACHIEVE form.

4. Title ______________________________

5. Date employment started ______

6. Name of Supervisor ______________________

7. Phone Number __________________________

8. Hours per Week ________________________

9. Provide one:
   a. Annual Salary ______________
   b. Bi-Weekly ______________
   c. Weekly ______________
   d. Hourly ______________

10. Job Description ___________________________

(2)
11. Place of employment ________________________

12. Dates of employment Starting ______ Ending __

13. Title ___________________________________

14. Reason for terminating _____________________

15. Hours per Week ___________________________

16. Salary Per Hour, Week or Year ______________

17. Job Description ___________________________

(3)
18. Place of employment ______________________

19. Dates of employment Starting ______ Ending ______

20. Title _______________________________

21. Reason for terminating _____________________

22. Hours per Week ___________________________

Achieve Assessment for Employed Persons 2

Figure 7.15. ACHIEVE form (continued).

23. Salary Per Hour, Week or Year _____

24. Job Description _____

Now let's go back and talk about your current job.

25. How did you become aware of this job?

26. How did you obtain this job?

27. What are the specific tasks that you perform?

28. Were any tasks changed because you could not perform them?

29. What tasks do you need others to assist you to complete?

30. How quickly do you complete your job tasks compared to your co-workers?
    much faster ____
    faster   _____
    the same   ____
    slower   _____
    much slower   ___

31. Are you satisfied with your current job?
    Yes __   No __

32. What are your present career goals?

Achieve Assessment for Employed Persons   3

Figure 7.15. ACHIEVE form (continued).

33. Did the employer make modifications to the work tasks for you?

Figure 7.15. ACHIEVE form (continued).

WORKSITE EVALUATION

Work Task Performance Capabilities

1. List the five most important work tasks that you complete.   These are the tasks that are most important in getting the job done.

Five most important work tasks Ranking

1.

2.

3.

4.

5.

2. Rank them, one being the most important and the highest number being the least important.

3. Indicate frequency that you do each task, Daily, Weekly, Monthly and number of hours spent in completing the task. List devices used if applicable.

Task	D, W, M	# of hrs ,	Device
1.			
2.			
3.			
4.			
5.			

Achieve Assessment for Employed Persons   5

Figure 7.15. ACHIEVE form (continued).

4. List any work tasks you cannot perform but you feel would be important to your job or career if you could perform them.

Work Tasks	Reason you are not performing task
1.	
2.	
3.	
4.	
5.	

Achieve Assessment for Employed Persons 6

Figure 7.15. ACHIEVE form (continued).

ASSESSMENT OF ASSISTIVE DEVICES USED AT WORK

Now I want you to ask you about the assistive devices you use at work.

1. List all the assistive devices that you use at work. Rank them. One being the device that you think is most important to you at work and the highest number being the least important device at work.

	Assistive Devices	Rank
1.		
2.		
3.		
4.		
5.		

2. What do you like best about the device you ranked as number one?

3. What do you like least about this device?

Achieve Assessment for Employed Persons   7

Figure 7.15. ACHIEVE form (continued).

ASSESSMENT OF ASSISTIVE DEVICES USED AT WORK

I will be asking you some questions about the devices you use at work. Answer the questions with:

<u>S</u>trongly <u>D</u>isagree, <u>D</u>isagree, <u>N</u>eutral, <u>A</u>gree, or <u>S</u>trongly <u>A</u>gree.

	Device 1	Device 2	Device 3	Device 4	Device 5
Name of Device					
1. It is easy to operate					
2. It was easy to learn how to use					
3. I needed special training to learn how to use it					
3a. If yes, who gave special training					
3b. how long was training					
4. The controls and displays are accessible					
4b. where are they located?					
5. It responds accurately to my commands					

Figure 7.15. ACHIEVE form (continued).

	Device 1	Device 2	Device 3	Device 4	Device 5
6. I am comfortable when using this device					
7. It does what it is suppose to do					
8. I am happy with this device					
9. I am completely independent in setup and operation of this device					
9a. if not, who helps set up					
9b. how often is help required?					
10. I use it daily					
11. It is low maintenance					
12. It is not too difficult to get it repaired					
13. It is convenient to use					
14. It makes my life easier					
15. I am proud to use it					

Figure 7.15. ACHIEVE form (continued).

16. It is easy to keep it working					
17. It increases my speed					
18. It works well with other devices (list devices)					
19. It makes me more independent					
20. I can use it for a variety of tasks					
21. It looks good					
22. It helps me interact with others					
23. Other people like this device					
24. I would like a different device					

Figure 7.15. ACHIEVE form (continued).

Open Ended Questions

	Device 1	Device 2	Device 3	Device 4	Device 5
Name of Device					
1. What functions does the device performed?					
2. What position are you in while using device? (seated, standing)					
3. What movement is needed to operate device?					
4. How much time do you use this device each day?					
5. When did you purchase this device?					
6. What did you pay for it?					

Achieve Assessment for Employed Persons   11

Figure 7.15. ACHIEVE form (continued).

Now I would like to ask you some general questions about the devices you use at work.

1. What specific reason made you choose this item?

Device 1

Device 2

Device 3

Device 4

Device 5

2. What is your back up system for this device?

Device 1

Device 2

Device 3

Device 4

Device 5

3. What improvements would you like to see made to this device?

Device 1

Achieve Assessment for Employed Persons 12

Figure 7.15. ACHIEVE form (continued).

Device 2

Device 3

Device 4

Device 5

4. What problems are you experiencing with the present device?

Device 1

Device 2

Device 3

Device 4

Device 5

5. What would you like to tell the assistive device developers
about the devices made for people with disabilities?

6. What are the major qualities you look for in the device you
use for work activity?

7. Do your feelings about the devices change the longer you use
them?   How?

Achieve Assessment for Employed Persons   13

Figure 7.15. ACHIEVE form (continued).

8. Please finish this sentence
    Using assistive devices at work is comfortable because...

9. Please finish this sentence
    My employer encourages me to use assistive devices because...

10. What other assistive devices have you used and discarded?
    1.
    2.
    3.
    4.
    5.

11. Why were they discarded?
    1.
    2.
    3.
    4.
    5.

Figure 7.15. ACHIEVE form (continued).

USE OF ADAPTIVE DEVICES TO ACCESS OFFICE EQUIPMENT

Please list other equipment you use in the office and, where needed, the adaptive device that assists you in using the office equipment.

Equipment   Device Used To Improve Access

1. Typewriter

2. Stapler

3. Fax

4. Copy Machine

5. File Cabinets

6. Book Shelves

7. Postage Meter

8. Binders

9. Hole Punchers

10. Telephone

11. Thermostat

12. Light switch

13. Elevator

14. Office door

15. Windows

16. Other

Figure 7.15. ACHIEVE form (continued).

BUILDING AND WORK SPACE DESIGN CONFIGURATION

                        Yes   No
1. Access to building
    a. Ramp   __   __
    b. Surface   __   __
    c. Evenly paved, no cracks__   __
    d. Slope less than 1:20__   __
    e. Curbcuts   __   __
    f. Hand rails   __   __
    g. Doors
                    width min. 32"__   __
                    Threshold bevelled__   __
                    Door operable with closed fist   __   __

2. Describe work space/area

3. Describe Work Station
    a. Present seat height:_____

    b. Present table height:_____

    c. Present monitor height:____

4. What other rooms do you use in the building? List all rooms used and how they are accessible.

    a. Bathroom
    b. Break Room
    c. Cafeteria
    d. Library
    e. Lounge
    f. Mail Room
    g. Smoking Area
    h. Supply Room
    i. Other

5. What modifications would make them more accessible?

Figure 7.15. ACHIEVE form (continued).

6. What is the emergency evacuation plan (i.e. fire)?

Figure 7.15. ACHIEVE form (continued).

TRANSPORTATION

1. What form of transportation do you use daily to get to work?

   car _____ van/lift ___ bus ___
   bus/lift _____ subway _____
   other _____

   Are you satisfied with it?

   Transportation is: Public _____ Private _____

   Is transportation easily obtained?

2. How far from your home do you travel to get to work?
   ____ miles

   How much time does it take?

   Does the weather affect your travel?

   If yes, how?

3. Please tell me which of these mobility aids you presently use:
   Crutches _____ Cane ___ Walker ___
   Power W/C _____ Manual W/C _____
   Other _____

   If other, please specify:

   _____

4. Do you need to travel much within your building?
   yes   no

   If yes, how many rooms do you need to use?

   Are there obstacles that prevent you from moving into these others rooms?

Figure 7.15. ACHIEVE form (continued).

EDUCATION

1. Highest degree obtained

    __ college
    Degree in ______________________________

    __ junior college
    Degree in ______________________________

    __ high school diploma

    Do you have any college credits?

2. Are you presently taking classes? yes ______ no ______

    If yes, where: ____

    What classes are you taking? ____________________

COMMUNICATION

1. Verbal: yes ________ no ________

2. Speech is fully understandable to:

    familiar others yes ________ no ________

    unfamiliar others yes ________ no ________

3. Communication system is used:
    All the time?, Once a day?, or oCcasionally?

    Electronic Device _______ Writing _______
    Signing _______ Gestures _______

Achieve Assessment for Employed Persons 19

Figure 7.15. ACHIEVE form (continued).

Symbols	______	Pictures	______
Line drawings	______	Objects	______
Voice Output		Other	______

If other, pleases specify type:

____

Achieve Assessment for Employed Persons 20

Figure 7.15. ACHIEVE form (continued).

LIVING SITUATION

1. What type of home do you live in?

    Family home ___ Apartment ___ Group home ____
    Iinstitution ___ Hospital ____ Other   ____

2. Does anyone live with you?   Yes ___ No ___
    If yes, who?
    Parents ____   Spouse   ___
    Children ____   Live in Atendent ___
    Other   ____

3. How long have you been living in this type of residence?

4. Type of setting:

    urban ___ suburban ____ rural ____

    sidewalks: yes ____ no ____

5. How much time does it take you to get ready for work?
        ___ time

    Do you get ready independently for with assistance of others?

        independently __
        with assistance __
          who is the assistant? __

6. When do you retire in the evening?

Home Activities

    Please tell me if you are Independent (**I**), Independent with a Device (**ID**), or Dependant (**D**). If you use a device, please tell me the name and how many years you have been using it.

	I, ID, D	Device	Years in Use

Achieve Assessment for Employed Persons   21

Figure 7.15. ACHIEVE form (continued).

Feeding			
Dressing			
Toileting			
Hygiene			
Writing			
	I, ID, D	**Device**	**Years**
Mobility			
Other			

What are your comments or problems regarding use of these devices?

Device	**Comments**
1.	
2.	
3.	
4.	
5.	
6.	
7.	

Figure 7.15. ACHIEVE form (continued).

MEDICAL INFORMATION

1. Do you have any other medical conditions such as seizures, diabetes, loss of vision, swallowing problems?

____

____

____

2. Do you take any medications regularly?
   If yes, what do you take?

Medication	Dosage	Times/Day
1.		
2.		
3.		

3. Are you currently receiving therapy?
   yes ______ no _______

   If yes, please specify type and frequency

   ____

SKIN CARE

1. Do you have a history of pressure sores?
   yes ______ no _______

   If yes specify, type and frequency.

   ____

   ____

   Are you receiving treatment for your pressure sores?

   ____

Achieve Assessment for Employed Persons 23

Figure 7.15. ACHIEVE form (continued).

2. Do you have a schedule to shift weight?

____

BLADDER/BOWEL:

1. How do you take care of your bowel and bladder needs at work?

2. Do you need assistance from others?

   a. Getting to and from bathroom_____
   b. With transfers _____
   c. Positioning in bathroom _____
   d. Hygiene

3. Has your bowel or bladder problems interfered with work or socializing?____

____

Achieve Assessment for Employed Persons 24

Figure 7.15. ACHIEVE form (continued).

BENEFITS

Do you currently receive government benefits?

1. If so, what type?

2. If you do not receive benefits, how did you get off of them and still retain attendant care?

Achieve Assessment for Employed Persons 25

Figure 7.15. ACHIEVE form (continued).

Through telephone conversations with Mary, her counselor, and her employer, background information was collected prior to the technology assessment. Information gathered about the work environment included work locations, jobs or activities performed in these locations, necessary work skills, productivity levels required to maintain employment, and problems Mary experiences in performing her job.

Once background information was compiled by the occupational therapist, the assistive technology team was determined by the CAT evaluation staff. The assessment team included Mary, her work supervisor, two occupational therapists, a rehabilitation technician, and an architect. This team had expertise in the use of assistive devices and modifications to existing devices, workplace accessibility, and issues related to Mary's disability. Mary's work supervisor provided necessary information related to the overall job process, work requirements, and equipment used through a tour of Mary's work site.

Home Evaluation. The assessment included a home visit to determine Mary's capabilities and needs related to activities performed at home that affect her employment. This was to ensure that needs related to preparation for or transportation to work did not interfere with the ability to maintain employment. Information was collected with an interview format. This tool was developed through the ACHIEVE project at CAT and is shown in Figure 7.15.

Mary experiences difficulty with self-care activities such as bathing and grooming. However, she uses several assistive devices, such as a bath seat, grab bars, and a long-handled sponge and comb.

She has difficulty with hand grasp and manipulation of small items, including the use of her house and car keys and opening her car door. This affects her ability to prepare for work and to independently transport herself to and from work. On days when her arthritis was more painful, Mary lost work time due to these difficulties.

Workplace Evaluation. The main machinery room and the bathroom were the work locations assessed, because they presented problems for Mary. The building entrance had a flat threshold with an electric door and was accessible to Mary. Her work department was on the same level. She used the elevator within the building when necessary. The cafeteria was also accessible to Mary; however, she did not use this area because she remained in her department for breaks.

Within the work environment, specific job tasks were explained and demonstrated by the work supervisor to the assessment team. Mary's overall job was to sew a variety of clothing items. This task included several steps such as laying out and cutting the fabric and sewing the pieces of material together. Mary cuts the needed fabric once or twice a day, and the majority of her work time is spent at the sewing machine. Mary's workstation setup and performance on the job were observed by the assessment team to facilitate a better understanding of the way Mary operated work equipment and performed work tasks. She experienced the following difficulties.

- The first step of the job is to assemble and manipulate long yardage of a heavy fabric to prepare for cutting. The fabric is positioned on a table 5 ft. long, 30 in. wide, and 45 in. high. This workstation setup was too high for Mary and required her to continuously reach up with her arms to perform the task. Continual positioning of the fabric with an uncomfortable reach caused repetitive stress on her arm joints and was extremely painful for Mary. She was unable to perform this task without adjusting her posture and stretching her arms. Due to decreased arm strength, additional force was required to push and manipulate the fabric. After a day's work, Mary experienced extreme pain in her arms and fatigue.
- Mary experienced difficulty utilizing standard dressmaker scissors to cut the fabric due to decreased hand strength and joint deformities. The cutting motion causes stress and pain on her finger joints. She attempted to compensate for this problem by cutting the fabric with both hands on the scissors.
- Mary experienced pain in her feet when operating the treadle bar on the sewing machine. This bar requires continuous ankle movement during sewing. Figure 7.16 shows the treadle adaptation.
- Mary sat on a small stool when sewing at the machine. She had difficulty rising to stand after sitting. As a result, she refrained from taking her work break away from her machine. She had similar difficulty when using the restroom; it was difficult for her to rise from the toilet.

The equipment Mary used for her work tasks was functional for the small size and number of products produced. The employer preferred to con-

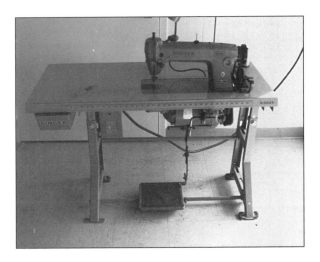

Figure 7.16. Treadle adaptation.

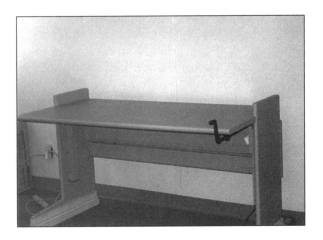

Figure 7.17. Adjustable-height table.

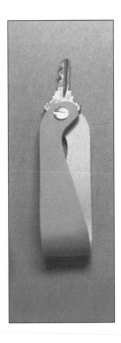

Figure 7.18. Key holder.

tinue using this equipment and she expressed an interest in adapting the work environment and in using other equipment within the building to assist Mary rather than automating the tasks. The employer was concerned about Mary's limited work tolerance and stressed the need for Mary to maintain work quality and productivity.

Mary's coworkers were concerned about the difficulty Mary was experiencing in performing her duties. Their concerns involved both support and opposition. Some workers thought it was unfair that Mary did not have to meet daily work quotas. Other workers thought that adjustments to existing equipment would benefit all of the workers.

Mary took pride in her work and enjoyed the sewing tasks she performed. Mary did not want to be treated differently from other workers. However, she felt compelled to perform limited work or less strenuous jobs due to daily pain. She expressed concern over her ability to continue working.

Evaluation

The occupational therapist on the team evaluated Mary's sensorimotor function to determine Mary's abilities and specific limitations in range of motion, coordination, strength, and endurance. This is necessary to determine how her impairments limit job performance and to make adaptations and recommendations that she is capable of using.

Mary had deficits in active movements throughout her upper extremities. She had joint deformities at the hands and was unable to perform full finger flexion or extension. She had a lateral drift of the fingers on both hands. Range of motion of the shoulders is limited as well. Strength of the upper extremities and hands was decreased, and Mary fatigued easily. She ambulated without assistive devices; however, her gait was slowed due to pain. Arthritic changes were noted at the feet.

Mary had difficulty grasping objects and used arm and partial finger movements to grasp and position work items. She was able to hold items and manipulate objects with a larger grip size. She was also able to perform knee movements without pain that could replace use of ankle and foot motions for work tasks.

Intervention

The assistive technology team explored possible assistive devices and modifications. They recommended a total of 12 devices and modifications as possible interventions. These included both provision

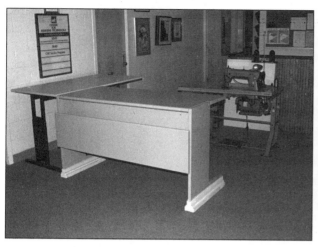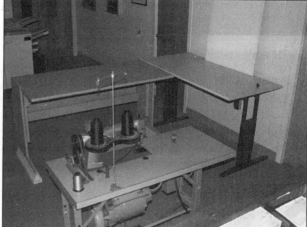

Figure 7.19. Final modification plans.

of new devices and modifications to existing equipment as described below.

- *Adjustable-Height Table.* This table was adjusted to a work height that is comfortable for Mary to reach and work on without straining her upper extremities. It also provided flexibility in workstation height for other employees. This table is shown in Figure 7.17.
- *Surface Area Width Increase.* Mary needed a longer work surface area, such as a longer straight workstation or an L-shaped work station to support large yardage of fabric. This provided a support area where the fabric could be moved without lifting to position it for cutting.
- *Electric Scissors.* This device provided a way to perform the necessary cutting tasks without a resistive force on the hands and fingers.
- *Adjustable-Height Stool.* This device affected sitting height to provide elevation to assist Mary with rising to stand. This provided increased ease in changing position during work.
- *Footstool.* This device was recommended to provide a support surface for Mary's legs when sitting on the elevated stool. This helped to eliminate stress on the lower extremities and allows for resting the feet during work.
- *Elevated Toilet Seat for Bathroom.* This device was recommended to assist Mary with rising to standing from a sitting position to meet personal needs during the workday.
- *Knee Pedal Adjustment.* An adaptation was made to the sewing machine with an existing knee pedal. The pedal was padded for more comfortable use and attached so that Mary could use her knee to operate the sewing machine instead of operating the treadle with her foot.
- *Enlarged Knobs on Sewing Machine.* The sewing machine was also adapted by enlarging the existing knobs with padding to make it easier for Mary to make machine adjustments while sewing.
- *Lever Faucet Handles.* Lever handles were recommended for restroom faucets to allow for easier operation through pushing motions and to decrease stress on hand joints.
- *Key Holder.* A key holder was recommended to provide a larger and longer surface area to grasp when using keys. An example of this device is shown in Figure 7.18.
- *Car Door Opener.* This device provides a longer lever arm and decreases the force needed to open the door handle. This also reduced the amount of stress on the hands.
- *Cylindrical Padding.* This was tubing with a padded large surface area that was used to enlarge grip sizes of tools used. This was used to build up handles on home items such as a toothbrush and writing tools that Mary uses for daily activities.

Pictures of the final modification plans are shown in Figure 7.19.

Outcomes

The CAT team provided specific information on the recommended devices, including possible vendors, to

Mary's employer and vocational rehabilitation counselor. The employer purchased and set up the adjustable-height table, adjustable-height stool, and footstool and adapted the sewing machine with the knee pedal. The vocational rehabilitation agency made money available for the sewing machine adaptations and for additional assistive devices. Modifications to the restroom were not implemented because Mary did not feel a need for them at the time. She thought the above modifications were sufficient and did not want her disability to draw more attention to herself from the other employees.

Mary continued with her same work tasks; however, she reduced her number of work hours to accommodate her periods of pain and fatigue. She eventually eliminated the job tasks that required manipulation and cutting of fabrics and assumed more tasks that required sewing.

Conclusions

Mary was able to continue her current job with assistive technology and modifications provided jointly by her employer and the vocational rehabilitation agency. However, these modifications were not sufficient to prevent the effects of her disability from reducing her ability to work in certain areas over time.

Monitoring of progress and reassessment provide assistance once devices are implemented. Mary may require other devices if the disability progresses. For example, electric door locks are currently available for both car doors and standard doors that replace the need to manipulate keys.

Case Study 2

Background

Paul is a 50-year-old teacher who sustained a spinal cord injury at the C4 level. He has quadriplegia with paralysis of his upper and lower extremities. Paul has taught high school English for over 25 years. He previously coached football and maintains an interest in sports. He owns a home and lives with his only sister.

Paul's injury resulted in severe physical impairments that limit his functional abilities. As a result, he spends a great amount of time in his home. He requires assistance for all of his ADL and receives caregiver assistance 4 hours per day. His sister attends to his needs at all other times. Due to his disability, Paul requires a powered wheelchair for mobility. He uses a collar with a chin controller for wheelchair operation. Paul is unable to control his living environment, including activities such as oper-

ating lights, the radio, and television or using the telephone due to his physical limitations.

Although Paul is unable to use his hands, he is able to use head and partial neck movements to operate a mouthstick. He has two mouthsticks that he is able to use proficiently. He uses these primarily for a minimal amount of writing that consists of signing his name or writing short notes.

Paul became acquainted with assistive technology during his rehabilitation process. He received only a few devices on discharge due to an unstable medical course and his need for acute care. Paul found his health improving and was proactive in seeking information and services that would enable him to obtain assistive devices to control his environment and to work again. He became a client of a vocational rehabilitation agency and requested assistance in planning work options and a means to acquire assistive technology.

Through this service, options for continued employment were explored. Paul decided not to return to daily teaching in the classroom but opted to teach evening classes and to provide individual tutoring. He identified job tasks that needed to be addressed with assistive technology. His major need is a writing system to perform work tasks. He is unable to use his mouthstick for writing for long periods. In addition to writing, he needs to have access to printed material, perform routine planning functions, and use the telephone.

Paul was referred for an assistive technology evaluation to address both environmental control and computer access by his vocational rehabilitation counselor. The referral was to determine how and what technology could help him attain his vocational goals. The state vocational agency funded his assistive technology referral.

After background information was collected by the rehabilitation engineer, a plan was devised to prepare for the assessment by the assistive technology team. The evaluation team included Paul, an occupational therapist, and a rehabilitation engineer. These team members would evaluate control of the environment, computer access, and computer-related needs. A seating specialist, a computer specialist, and a technician were involved to address any specialized needs or adaptations related to Paul's assistive technology needs.

Assessment

Environmental Control. Paul was initially assessed within his home. He identified several items within his home environment that he needs to control. Most of these items were located within his bedroom, where he currently spends most of his time. Items to be controlled included his lights (both an overhead light and a bedside lamp), a fan, a radio, a television, his telephone, and an electric door opener. Additionally, he considered control for his drapes and electric bed, but thought control of these items was unnecessary at the time.

Paul's work plan includes a work office located within his home. He needed devices that would be flexible and that could be used in various locations within his home. He needed a computer system that would allow him to work within the home. Paul wanted to become active and believed that he had potential to be productive.

Evaluation of motor function identified areas for control of devices. Paul has minimal movement of his left forearm. He has active head and partial neck movements; his speech is fluent. Paul chose to explore the use of all of these movements as activation sites for control of assistive devices to be evaluated.

Paul and the team evaluated five devices for use in environmental control.

1. *Scanning-Based Hand-Held Remote.* This is a compact device that operates through infrared transmission and uses an attached switch for activation. It allows for control of the television and radio. With additional attachments, it can be used to control lights and other appliances. The remote is shown in Figure 7.20. Paul was able to operate this device independently with a chin-controlled switch when the remote was mounted on his bedrail. He found the LED display difficult to see from various positions in bed.

2. *Scanning-Based Dedicated Environmental Control Unit.* This device allows for control of lights and appliances, telephone, television and radio, and other electronic devices by using scanning as a selection method. Paul found this device easy to operate with a chin-controlled switch, and he was able to clearly see the LED display. However, this device is large and must be positioned on a separate table.

3. *X-10 Based Controller.* This device uses house wiring to send signals. Four different X-10 controllers were evaluated with a direct selection method. Each featured a different type of activation switch with a characteristic

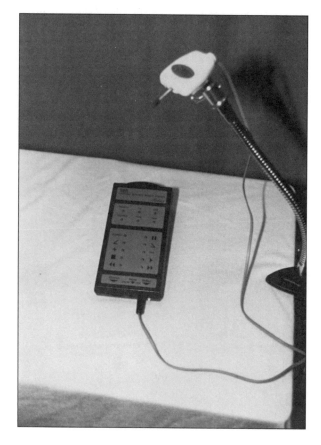

Figure 7.20. Scanning-based hand-held remote.

button size and activation force. All required specific positioning within Paul's range of motion. Paul was able to use his mouthstick to operate the switches. Figure 7.21 shows Paul using the X-10 controller.

4. *Switch-Controlled Telephone.* This device uses a speakerphone and specialized hardware to assist with making and receiving telephone calls. Paul is able to operate this device independently.

5. *Electric Door Opener.* Paul is able to use this device independently to operate his outside door. Consultation with a construction company for installation was provided.

Computer

Loss of upper-extremity movement limits Paul's access to and ability to use a computer. The computer assessment included evaluation of an access method to the computer with a variety of assistive devices and assistive software. Due to Paul's inexperience with computers and the various access methods evaluated, observation and feedback from Paul were the primary methods of assessment.

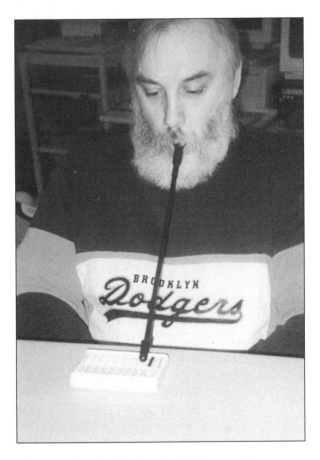

Figure 7.21. Paul using the X-10 controller.

The computer used for assessment is an IBM-compatible computer. Devices evaluated included:

- *Standard Keyboard With Mouthstick.* Paul was unable to reach all keys on the standard keyboard due to incomplete neck movements.
- *Compact Keyboard With Mouthstick.* This is a reduced-size, space-saver keyboard that includes all standard keys. Number, cursor, and function keys are grouped together and located above the main keys. Paul was able to reach all keys; however, he thought it was strenuous to type for long periods.
- *Miniature Keyboard.* This is a miniature keyboard that measures approximately 8 in. by 6 in. with a standard layout that is activated through contact between a metal wire connected wand or mouthstick and the keyboard. Paul accessed the entire keyboard with a mouthstick; however, he had difficulty seeing the keys on this keyboard.

- *Keyboard Emulator With Chin Controller.* This is a computer workstation that replaces the keyboard without hardware or software modifications. It is accessed through use of head and chin movements. This device provides control for an integrated system of computer use, phone access, and environmental control with the same controller. Paul preferred a different access method for computer use. Because he had other methods of access to environmental control, he did not have a need for an integrated system at this time.
- *Voice Recognition.* A combination of hardware and software allows for computer access with voice input. Paul had good oral communication skills with consistent vocal performance. He was able to train the computer to recognize his spoken words and commands. He found this to be not physically demanding and was able to work for longer periods without fatigue.
- *Head-Pointing Device for Alternate Mouse Pointing.* This is an optical pointing device that uses infrared signals to control movements. A small target was attached to Paul's forehead, and he was able to use head movements for operation of the mouse pointer. Mouse click was performed with a switch attached to the optical sensor. Paul demonstrated good control of the pointer and was comfortable with this device. The head mouse is shown in Figure 7.22.
- *On-Screen Keyboard With Word Prediction.* This is software that provides a keyboard on the computer screen and is accessed with an alternative pointing device. Paul was able to type letters by centering the mouse pointer over the letter on the screen to type keystrokes. Paul was able to visualize and comprehend use of this keyboard to type keystrokes. The word-prediction list provides word choices that the computer types automatically if selected. This feature reduces the number of keystrokes that the user types and thus decreases the amount of effort required for input.

To summarize the assessment results, Paul preferred voice recognition as his main access method. This method allows for speaking words, letters, and commands instead of typing keystrokes. This method was faster, less fatiguing, and less physically demanding for input than the other methods tested.

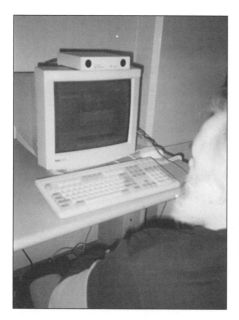 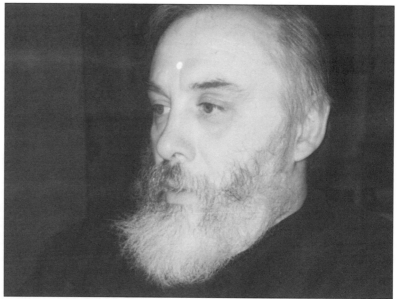

Figure 7.22. Head-pointing device for alternate mouse pointing.

Paul demonstrated poor motor control and fatigued easily from the various methods that required head movements to operate devices.

Intervention

Environmental Control. Paul's ability to use a mouthstick for reliable selections helped rule out the options that use scanning or a switch. Although these systems were more comprehensive, Paul preferred the more direct control he had with the mouthstick. Paul was also able to use his mouthstick to operate his television remote control when it was mounted in front of him on his over-the-bed table. The following devices were recommended for Paul.

- *X-10 Wireless Remote Control and Light Dimmer System.* This device provides on/off control for up to 16 items. It includes both light and appliance modules and allows for dimmer control of the overhead light.
- *14 In. Mouthstick and Docking Station.* Paul required a third, shorter mouthstick to operate the switches for environmental control. The docking station holds the mouthstick when it is not being used and is necessary for independent access to his mouthsticks.

Computer. The recommended computer system is an IBM-compatible 486 DX2 tower at 66 MHz with 32 MB RAM, 420 MB hard drive, a SVGA monitor with .28 dot pitch, a tape backup, dual-speed CD-ROM, a fax/modem, and a laser printer. This high-powered system is necessary to run the voice-recog-

nition software along with other application programs within a graphical user interface. Because Paul is unable to manipulate diskettes, the large hard drive allows for additional storage for software and files. It will provide Paul with flexibility to work with a variety of software programs while using the adaptive devices and other assistive software. The tape backup is used to back up his voice and work files to eliminate unnecessary retraining. CD-ROM is needed for access to reference materials because Paul is unable to manipulate books.

Software.

- *Voice-Recognition Software.* Together with hardware, this would provide use of voice recognition as an access method. It would allow voice commands to be used for navigation within Windows and for activating mouse movements.
- *Windows.* When first evaluated, Paul used voice recognition within a DOS environment. This access became available for use within a graphical user interface. Paul favored Windows and opted to use this as his main computer environment.
- *Word for Windows.* Paul required a powerful word-processing program to perform his work tasks and writing. This program provides built-in shortcut features such as macros and autocorrection along with preprogrammed templates for a variety of writing functions.

- *Fax/Modem and Communication Software.* This would provide Paul with the ability to send and receive faxes from his computer and a way to access on-line information and databases, along with reference materials. This was important for Paul due to his mobility impairments and travel limitations.

- *On-Screen Keyboard.* This software would provide Paul with an alternative access method when he was unable to use voice recognition (see Figure 7.23).

- *Reference Materials on CD-ROM.* This software would provide electronic access to reference materials. Paul is unable to manipulate books, and this would assist with his work.

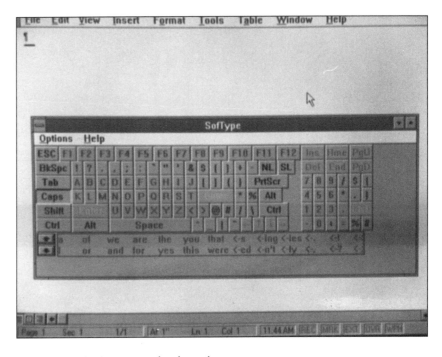

Figure 7.23. On-screen keyboard.

Other Recommended Assistive Devices. The following devices were also recommended for Paul.

- *Adjustable-Height Table.* This table allows for wheelchair access along with proper positioning of devices for comfortable use.

- *Stand-Alone Microphone.* This device would allow Paul to use voice recognition without a headset for more independent access.

- *Alternative Pointing Device.* Paul was unable to use a mouse due to his physical limitations. He was able to control the screen pointer with an alternative pointing device that included a dot placed on his forehead and an infrared signal.

Outcomes

The state vocational rehabilitation agency provided funding for the assistive devices recommended for environmental control. The CAT rehabilitation engineer set up the devices and trained Paul in their use. It took approximately 3 hours to set up the equipment, and Paul required 2 hours of training to use the unit to control bedroom lights, radio, and television. The rehabilitation engineer demonstrated how to use the control device. Paul then had the opportunity to practice using the mouthstick to operate the environmental control unit and to ask any questions that he had.

Training for environmental control within his work area will need to be addressed when Paul becomes employed.

The CAT team recommended purchase of a computer system and training on its use for Paul. This recommendation was made to the state vocational rehabilitation agency, and approval for funding was being processed by the agency according to their policy.

Training for the computer system requires instruction in basic hardware components and function, including CD-ROM operation and use of tape backup. The team will also provide instruction in the use of voice-recognition software and integration with other programs, use of the head pointer for mouse navigation, use of the on-screen keyboard for alternative access, use of application programs to perform work tasks, and use of on-line information retrieval. The team expects initial training to take approximately 25 to 50 hours. Additional training or consultation is often required.

Conclusions

Provision of assistive technology is a long process for persons with severe disabilities. Persons with severe or multiple disabilities require more time for evaluation of devices, have more compatibility issues to be resolved because they use more devices, and require more intensive training in the use of devices. Training in the use of multiple devices is also necessary to integrate devices and skill for work purposes.

Case Study 3

Background

The previous case studies, particularly Paul's, illustrated the use of relatively high-technology interventions to workplace accommodations. This case study demonstrates an effective low-technology solution to workplace modification. The person in this case study was referred to the Applied Studies program at the CAT. Applied Studies is an interdisciplinary, interagency program that focuses on providing graduate students an opportunity to solve actual problems experienced by person with developmental disabilities. Funded by the New York State Office of Mental Retardation and Developmental Disabilities (OMRDD), Applied Studies participants include students and faculty from the disciplines of occupational therapy, physical therapy, speech and language pathology, architecture, engineering, rehabilitation counseling, and nursing, as well as clinicians and staff members from various developmental disability service organizations (DDSOs).

A DDSO is an administrative unit within the New York state OMRDD system. Based on the concept of a catchment area, or geographic area, DDSOs were developed to meet the needs of persons with developmental disabilities by providing and coordinating residential and program services in one or more counties. Most states have similar organizations, although different names such as "regional centers" are often used.

DDSO personnel refer problems to the Applied Studies group. It is important that referrals are stated in the form of a problem, not a potential solution, as this often limits the possible outcomes. The Applied Studies project coordinator reviews the referral, and the problem is then assigned to a team of students. Applied Studies students and faculty work collaboratively with the referring DDSO personnel to further identify and define the problem. After the problem is objectively defined, the Applied Studies team continues to work collaboratively with DDSO personnel to further assess the problem and to develop and try out possible solutions.

Thomas is a 40-year-old man who has cerebral palsy with spasticity. Motor function in all four extremities is limited due to spasticity, muscle weakness, bilateral contractures, and limited range of motion. Thomas is also diagnosed as having mild mental retardation and a controlled seizure disorder. He is not ambulatory and independently uses a powered wheelchair, controlled by a joystick, for mobility. Because Thomas is unable to communicate verbally, he uses an alternative communication device, a Touch Talker, for communication. He operates the Touch Talker by direct selection.

Thomas has worked in a sheltered workshop under the auspices of a DDSO for several years. He enjoys going to work and wants to be productive. Sheltered workshops procure contracts for jobs from area businesses. Workshop contracts typically fall into one of three categories: packaging, light assembly, and collating. Sheltered workshop employees are paid a percentage of the minimum wage that is based on their productivity. Workshop staff perform a time sample on a job to determine how many items are produced in an hour. This is viewed as the standard, and the sheltered workshop employees' performance is compared to this standard.

Many of the jobs available in Thomas' workshop require strength, coordination, and manual dexterity. Due to his physical limitations, Thomas is able to complete few of the jobs in the sheltered workshop.

As a result of his inability to be productive in the workshop, a referral was made to the Applied Studies program. Thomas and workshop personnel asked that an attempt be made to modify some of the tasks so that he would be able to complete them. As part of the referral process, DDSO staff completed a screening form that provided the Applied Studies team with preliminary information on Thomas and the problem. This screening form is shown in Figure 7.24.

After review of the screening form, the next step in the process was to clearly define the problem, in this case, to determine which of the several workshop tasks would be modified so that Thomas would be as successful and independent as possible. The Applied Studies team and workshop personnel met to discuss the advantages and disadvantages of modifying various tasks.

A major criterion in determining which task was to be modified was how often the workshop received a contract for that particular task. The task to be modified should be one that the workshop receives a contract for on a frequent, consistent basis. Another consideration was the complexity of the task. A more complex task—that is, one with several steps (pack-

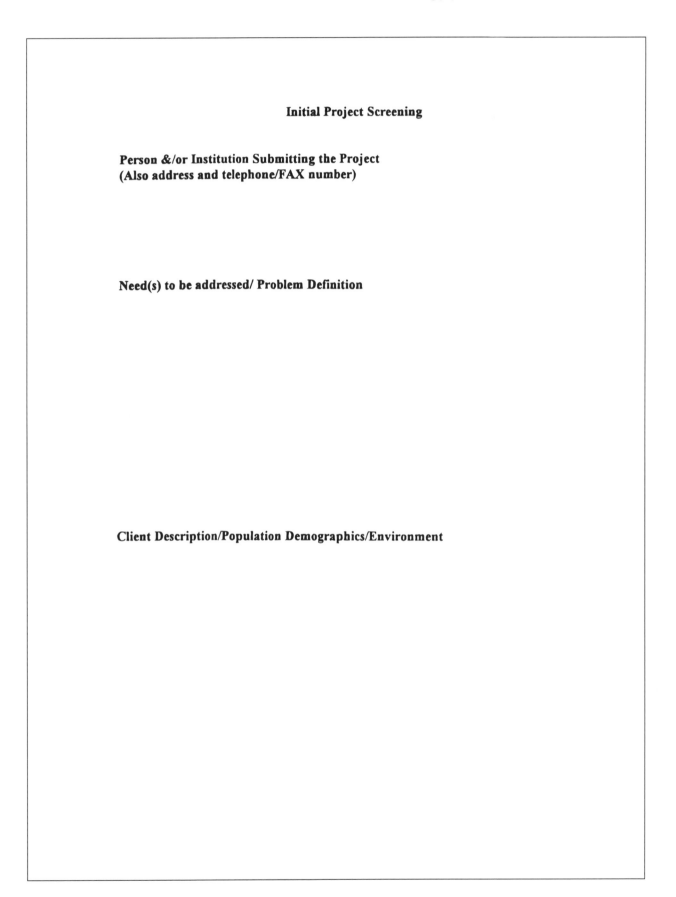

Figure 7.24. Screening form.

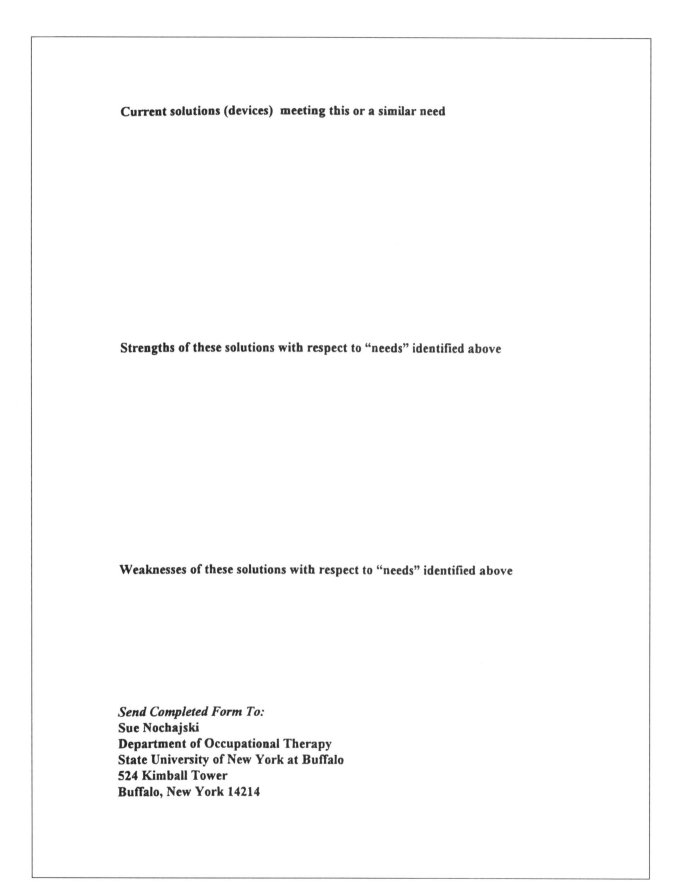

Current solutions (devices) meeting this or a similar need

Strengths of these solutions with respect to "needs" identified above

Weaknesses of these solutions with respect to "needs" identified above

Send Completed Form To:
Sue Nochajski
Department of Occupational Therapy
State University of New York at Buffalo
524 Kimball Tower
Buffalo, New York 14214

Figure 7.24. Screening form (continued).

aging seven items, for example)—is more difficult to modify. In addition, the necessary adaptations would be complex as well. The modification or adaptation should be as simple as possible to avoid breakdown of parts and complicated maintenance.

After observing the tasks available in the workshop and discussing the tasks with Thomas, workshop personnel, and the Applied Studies students and faculty, the team decided that a stamping task would be modified. This contract is received monthly and is expected to be a longstanding job. The task is relatively simple and uses little equipment, so it was anticipated that task modification would be relatively easy to accomplish.

A local business uses self-adhesive labels stamped with a quality-control number on its products and contracts with the sheltered workshop to supply these labels. This contract is received by the sheltered workshop on a monthly basis, and 5,000 labels are to be stamped each month. The task consists of stamping a quality control number on each label by using an adjustable rubber stamp, with at least eight numerals and one letter, and an ink pad. The labels to be stamped are on a sheet consisting of 10 rows and 3 columns of labels.

Assessment

In this particular situation, it was necessary to assess Thomas's functional capabilities as well as the task to be completed. The team for this project included a rehabilitation engineer and two occupational therapy graduate students from Applied Studies, as well as Thomas, his work supervisor, and his program occupational therapist. After the Applied Studies project coordinator and the workshop staff discussed the problem and background information, this team was selected by their mutual agreement. The team was appropriate because occupational therapists are most able to complete a functional assessment and task analysis, the rehabilitation engineer is able to assist in the design and fabrication of an assistive device if one is warranted, and the work supervisor is most familiar with Thomas's work performance. As always, the client is considered to be an integral member of the team.

This team is somewhat unique because many facilities do not have the services of a rehabilitation engineer. Typically, professionals such as occupational therapists are involved in workplace modifications and adaptive devices. Not all therapists have the skills and expertise to design and fabricate mechanically sound devices. Because of this, stu-

dents in the Applied Studies program are encouraged to use commercially available products and devices as much as possible. These devices are used "off the shelf" or are modified. If a new device is to be designed, commercially available parts are used as much as possible.

Assessment of Thomas. The team from Applied Studies worked together with the workshop team to assess Thomas. The Applied Studies team acts in a consultative role to the DDSO personnel, and the staff most familiar with the client plays an active role on the team. Therefore, Applied Study students rely a great deal on the staff most familiar with Thomas and the problem situation for assessment information. The students do not typically do an independent functional assessment.

Thomas's occupational therapist and workshop supervisor provided the Applied Studies team with copies of reports on his functional capabilities. Prior to their first visit to the workshop, the students telephoned the occupational therapist and workshop supervisor to discuss the information. The therapist stated that Thomas had bilateral active and passive range of motion limitations in all joints of his upper extremities. He demonstrates preference for his right hand and does not use his left hand. Both hands have finger deformities. Flexor tone dominates Thomas's upper extremities, and extensor tone dominates the lower extremities. Thomas has bilateral wrist contractures; the resting position of his hand is at approximately 85 degrees of flexion. To promote wrist extension, Thomas wears a splint on his left hand for 30 min. three times per day. He does not wear a splint on his right hand. Thomas's upper-extremity strength is also limited; it was difficult for the occupational therapist to use manual muscle testing to determine actual muscle strength. Thomas was not able to grasp a dynamometer to measure grip strength. Through estimation, it was determined that Thomas can apply a force of approximately four times the weight of the hand with his right upper extremity.

Based on workshop observation, the work supervisor reported that Thomas's work habits and behaviors are good. He understands, retains, and follows multistep directions; maintains attention to the task; and is not easily distracted. Thomas readily accepts constructive criticism and suggestions. Thomas is motivated to work and would like to be more independent and productive at the workshop. Thomas and his workshop supervisor established a goal that Thomas work at 50% of the productivity of other employees in the workshop.

On the first visit to the workshop, the Applied Studies team further discussed previous assessment results with Thomas and the occupational therapist. The students had additional questions about Thomas's seating system and the way the job was set up. The discussion provided answers to these questions.

Assessment of the Task. The Applied Studies team observed and videotaped the work environment and Thomas's work performance on the stamping task on several occasions. Videotaping enabled the team to consult and problem-solve without directly observing Thomas again. The distance between the workshop and the university is more than 50 miles, so videotaping Thomas' performance for further review is both time- and cost-effective.

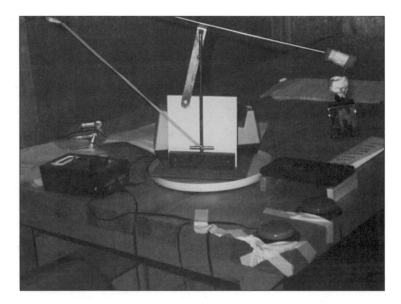

Figure 7.25. The stamp was suspended from a supporting arm that was mounted on a swivel base.

Workshop staff previously adapted the task by suspending the stamp from a supporting arm that was mounted on a swivel base, as shown in Figure 7.25. The swivel action enabled Thomas to maneuver the stamp from the ink pad to the sheet of labels. In an attempt to improve neatness and accuracy, staff also folded sheets of labels into three parts to decrease the available surface area to be stamped. Thomas would stamp one column of the labels and then the supervisor would set up the sheet again. This required much supervisor assistance, and Thomas was not able to complete the task as independently as he would have liked.

However, due to his physical limitations, he continued to have difficulty with precise placement of the stamp on the label. Workshop personnel were not completely satisfied with the device they designed and noted several limitations:

- There was difficulty with securing the base of the device to the work table. The device frequently moved and tipped over when in use.
- The swivel arm mechanism on the device moved too freely, requiring Thomas to "chase" the stamp, and decreasing the control Thomas had in positioning the stamp over the label.
- There was difficulty in proper adjustment of the tension used to connect the swivel arm with the base of the device.
- The depression point on the swivel arm of the stamp lacked adequate resistance, causing

Thomas's hand to fall off the device when he depressed the stamp. This is particularly evident when he applied greater force.
- The stamp being used has a rounded stamping surface and Thomas must roll the stamp for all the numbers to appear on the label.
- The ink pad was not securely attached to the table and moved easily when Thomas pressed the stamp on it.

Intervention

After analyzing the task and Thomas's performance, the team decided that modifying the stamp and using an adaptive jig to hold and slide the labels would be an appropriate solution. The team also decided that the solution should include two specific design features: (a) the use of continuous label sheets to solve the problem of the work supervisor folding the sheets of labels, and (b) a self-inking stamp instead of the separate ink pad and stamp. This would solve the problem of the ink pad being unstable and would also simplify the task by decreasing the number of steps in the process.

A product search was conducted using HyperAbleData, a database of numerous assistive devices. Nothing was found that could be used as is so a commercially available self-inking stamp was purchased from a local office supply store for approximately $70. This stamp was adapted and was a primary component of the task modification. Additionally, no commercially available devices were found that would position the labels under the

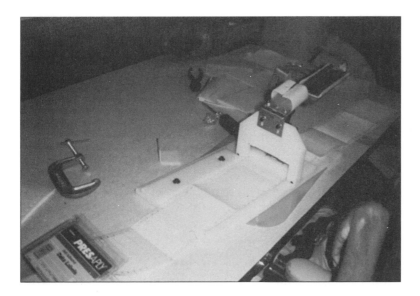

Figure 7.26. Adapted stamp.

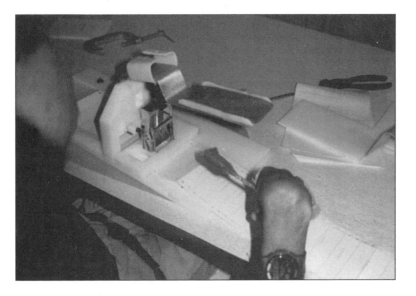

Figure 7.27. Adapted stamp with universal cuff.

The jig consisted of a base 6 in. wide, 18 in. long, and 1/2 in. thick, with a recess to hold the stamp and a bridge attached to the base to hold the stamp. The measurements for the bridge are 1 in. by 4 in. by 3 in. The jig directed the motion of the sheets of labels so that Thomas could move them himself. It also included a window for lining up each label, that allows him to stamp the number in the middle of the label each time. The bridge is mounted to the base with a hinge and a handle made from aluminum is attached to the bridge. The stamp is placed under the handle next to the bridge. Thomas presses the aluminum handle to depress the stamp. This adaptive device is shown in Figure 7.26.

Outcomes

Several trials and modifications were necessary to devise a workable solution. Due to his diminished physical strength, Thomas had difficulty pressing the stamp hard enough to leave an imprint. The length of the aluminum handle was increased to decrease the amount of force necessary to depress the stamp.

The rehabilitation technician fabricated two handles, one that reduced the force Thomas had to apply by one half and the other that reduced the force by two thirds. Thomas tried both handles and found that the handle that required less force worked better for him.

Due to his hand deformities, Thomas continued to have difficulty depressing the stamp. Thomas tried to depress the stamp with several parts of his upper extremity, such as his palm, elbow, and forearm, in addition to the pads of his fingers. The results were still not satisfactory and on the basis of discussions with Thomas, the team decided to use an adapted universal cuff with an attached stick to assist him in pressing the stamp. This design is shown in Figure 7.27. A universal cuff is similar to a splint. It is worn around the wrist and has a pocket in the palmar surface that allows attachments of articles such as a pencil or spoon. The stick was a small steel wrench. Using the wrench to depress the aluminum handle

stamp. The team decided that a jig was necessary to position the labels and would be designed.

Working with the rehabilitation engineer and rehabilitation technician, an Applied Studies student designed a jig. The rehabilitation technician fabricated the jig from high-density polyethylene. This material was chosen because it is easy to shape with a mill and other machinery. High density polyethylene also has a low coefficient of friction that decreases resistance when Thomas slides the labels along the jig, which makes the task easier for him.

caused another problem. The two metal surfaces slid on each other too easily, making it hard for Thomas to work the handle. This problem was solved by adding Dycem, a nonskid material, to both surfaces. With these modifications, he was able to perform the task. In addition, the modification permitted Thomas to use the extensor strength in his right arm. This change could eventually increase his active range of motion, as shown in Figure 7.27.

Thomas needed training and practice to familiarize himself with the device and to enable him to use it satisfactorily. The Applied Studies team initially provided on-site training, and Thomas's work supervisor continued the process.

Conclusions

This case study demonstrates that low-technology solutions often provide effective solutions to worksite modifications. Low-technology solutions do not necessarily imply low-technology expertise. Much thought and consideration were necessary to design and fabricate the assistive device. The adapted stamp enabled Thomas to work at one task accurately, neatly, and productively. This case study demonstrates that it is appropriate and often easier to use commercially available products, adapted when necessary, to provide assistive technology accommodations.

Summary

Successful workplace interventions often require an interdisciplinary team approach and coordination and collaboration among agencies and individuals. It is important to remember that high-technology solutions are not necessarily better than low-technology solutions. A thorough assessment of the client and the environment is necessary to determine what type of intervention will best meet that person's needs. It is also necessary to consider psychosocial factors and to determine whether the person is willing and motivated to use assistive technology.

Many person may not be aware of the technology that is available or how to use it. It is important to provide education to consumers, employers, and agencies working with persons with disabilities to provide optimal work opportunities. Training on the use of assistive technology is also an important issue. Training not only includes instruction in how to use devices, but also requires integration of the technology within the work environment. This includes instruction to the worker with a disability, the employer, and coworkers.

When recommending assistive technology, it is important to make provisions for the installation of devices, compatibility with other devices and the environment, upgrading, and follow-up. By following these guidelines, assistive technology can make the workplace more productive for persons with disabilities.

Persons with disabilities often require other services in addition to assistive technology to assist with preparation for work. For example, persons may have other needs for education, a job coach, and rehabilitation, and placement into work may take an extensive time period. Many persons require assistance with searching for work, filling out applications, preparing resumes, and learning about appropriate work skills and habits.

Clients may require services from a variety of agencies in addition to services that provide assistive technology. These can include agencies that serve persons with disabilities, such as vocational rehabilitation agencies. However, they also include other organizations that provide assistance with job skill developments. These services must be coordinated. In many cases, persons benefit from comprehensive services that assist the clients through the process of finding employment, implementing the assistive technology, and follow-up to ensure that work is successful or to assist with changes.

Employers and consumers need to understand the benefits of assistive technology and how it can be used to facilitate competitive employment. This improves employees' job performance, assists in the prevention of disability, and contributes to continued employment.

Chapter 7 References

Angelo, J., Hurlburt, M., & Oddo, C. (1992). *ACHIEVE: Final report.* Unpublished manuscript. State University of New York at Buffalo.

Angelo, J., Hurlburt, M., & Oddo, C. (1991). The function of the computer work station for the physically disabled worker. *WORK, 1*(4), 22–28.

Beaton-Starr, M. (1992). Carpal tunnel syndrome and the workplace. *WORK, 2*(4), 61–66.

Bushrow, K., & Turner, K. (1994). Overcoming barriers in the use of adaptive and assistive technology in special education. In D. Montgomery (Ed.) *Rural partnerships: Working together. Proceedings of the Annual National Conference of the American Council on Rural Special Education* (ACRSE).

Chamot, D. (1989). Technology and employment: An overview. In L. Perlman & C. Hansen (Eds.), *Technology and employment of persons with disabilities*. Alexandria, VA: National Rehabilitation Association.

Clees, T. (1992). Community living. In P.J. McLaughlon & P. Wehman (Eds). *Developmental disabilities* (pp. 228–267). Boston: Andover Medical.

Hughes, T., & Wehman, P. (1992). Supported employment. In P.J. McLaughlon & P. Wehman (Eds.), *Developmental disabilities* (pp. 184–205). Boston: Andover Medical.

Mann, W.C., & Svorai, S. (1994). COMPETE: A model for vocational evaluation, training, employment, and community for integration for persons with cognitive impairments. *American Journal of Occupational Therapy, 48*, 446–451.

Mueller, J. (1990). *The workplace workbook*. Washington, DC.: Dole Foundation.

National Information Center for Children and Youth With Disabilities (NICHY). (1993, March). *Transition services in the IEP; NICHY transition summary, 3*(1), p. 127.

Reed, K.L. (1991). History of federal legislation for persons with disabilities. *American Journal of Occupational Therapy, 46*, 397–408.

Rehabilitation Act Amendments, Pub. L. 99506 No. 51. *Fed. Reg.* 35592 (1986).

RESNA Technical Assistance Project. (1992). *Assistive technology and the individualized education program*. Washington, DC: RESNA Press.

Rusch, F.R., Chadsey-Rusch, J., & Johnson, J.R. (1991). Supported employment: Emerging opportunities for employment integration. In L.H. Meyer, C.A. Peck, & L. Brown (Eds.), *Critical issues in the lives of people with severe disabilities* (pp.145–169). Baltimore: Paul H. Brookes.

Smith, R.O. (1991). Technological approaches to performance enhancement. In C. Christiansen & C. Baum (Eds.), *Occupational therapy: Overcoming human performance deficits* (pp. 744–786). Thorofare, NJ: Slack.

Steinfeld, E., & Angelo, J. (1992). Adaptive work placement: A "horizontal" model. *Technology and Disability, 1*(4), 110.

Thiers, N. (1994, November 27). Abandoned! Why do people abandon or not use assistive technology? *OT Week*, pp. 22–23.

Williams, R., & Westmorland, M. (1994). Occupational cumulative trauma disorders of the upper extremity. *American Journal of Occupational Therapy, 48*, 411–420.

Woodward, J. (1993). *The ACCESS guide to federal work incentives*. Tallahassee: Center for Independent Living of North Florida, Inc.

Chapter 7 Study Questions

1. Briefly describe each of the following federal Acts, and relate how they could impact the employment of persons with disabilities.
   a. The Rehabilitation Act and Amendments to it
   b. Individuals with Disabilities Act
   c. Technology Related Assistance for Individuals with Disabilities Act
   d. Americans with Disabilities Act

2. What are cumulative trauma disorders? How might assistive technology be used for persons with this condition?

3. Describe the impact of a vision impairment on a person working in:
   a. an office (as a secretary)
   b. a restaurant (as a cook)
   c. a store (as a cashier)
   d. a factory (as a foreman)
   How might assistive technology be used by these individuals?

4. Do the same exercise as question 3, but for a person with hearing impairment.

5. Do you know a person with a disability who is employed? Interview this person on his or her use of assistive technology. Be prepared to refer this person to an appropriate agency should there be assistive technology needs that have not been met.

Chapter 8:
Older Persons and Assistive Technology

I. Introduction

II. Considerations in Assistive Device Interventions
A. Personal Factors
1. Consumer Perspective
2. Age
3. Diagnosis
B. Social Environment Factors
1. Caregivers
2. Setting
3. Role
C. Physical Environment Factors
1. Urban/Rural
2. Climate
3. Design
D. Disability

III. Areas of Assistive Technology Interventions
A. Safety
B. Independence
1. Mobility
2. Activities of Daily Living
3. Instrumental Activities of Daily Living
4. Work
5. Leisure
C. Sensory Perception
1. Hearing
2. Vision
D. Cognition
E. Expressive Communication

IV. Assessment Instruments
A. Functional Status
1. Functional Independence Measure (FIM)
2. OARS: Older Americans Resources and Services Program Multidimensional Functional Assessment Questionnaire: IADLs Section
3. OTFACT
B. Health Status
1. OARS
2. Jette Functional Pain Index (Jette)

*Case studies for this chapter were provided by Patricia Sperle, MS, OTR and Linda Fraas, OTR, who serve as research support specialists for the University at Buffalo Rehabilitation Engineering Research Center on Aging.

8

Older Persons and Assistive Technology

William C. Mann, PhD, OTR/L

Introduction

As we grow older, we experience gradual changes in hearing, vision, and mobility. Concurrently, we may begin to experience chronic diseases, such as arthritis, heart disease, cataracts, and diabetes. These age-related changes and chronic diseases can result in impairments. These impairments, in turn, reduce a person's functional performance. Factors that determine the impact of chronic disease and aging on functional performance include severity and number of chronic conditions, age, and support available. However, environmental interventions and assistive technology may be applied to reduce the impact of impairments on a person's functional performance.

The proportion of the population in the United States represented by elders has been steadily increasing, and is projected to increase well into the next century. In 1900, fewer than 1 person in 25 was over 64 years old; by 1989, more than 1 in 8 were over 64 (U.S. Senate Special Commission on Aging, 1991). Almost 22% of this population report problems in performing at least one activity of daily living, and 28% have problems with instrumental activities of daily living (IADL). For those 85 and older, the fastest growing segment of this population, 45% have difficulty with at least one activity of daily living (Prohaska, Mermelstein, Miller, & Jack, 1993).

Looking more specifically at the nature of these functional limitations, 23% of the over-64 age group have difficulty with activities of daily living (eating, bathing, dressing); 10% of the group that have difficulty require help with these activities. An even higher percentage of the over-65 age group (27%) report difficulty with home management activities (Prohaska, Mermelstein, Miller, & Jack, 1993).

The percentage of the over-65 age group living in nursing homes is relatively small—5% (Fowles, 1988). However most persons in this age group have at least one chronic disease, and many have been diagnosed with several diseases. Deinstitutionalization of special populations has increased the number of persons with disabilities living in community settings.

In addition to a very high rate of chronic conditions among elders, and a high rate of functional limitations, another important factor for the functional abilities of older persons relates to their immediate support system. While 95% of the over-64 age group live at home, nearly one-third live alone. For many, there are no immediate relatives to assist them with activities of daily living. Services are available, but many elders are not aware of their availability. Assistive devices and environmental interventions can sustain the independence of older persons, particularly those lacking a support system of people or services.

The impact of a stroke for a 65-year-old man with a supportive spouse will be very different than for a 94-year-old blind, widowed woman who has been living alone. The number and types of assistive devices and environmental interventions useful for those elders will also be different.

A recent study compared the number of assistive devices used by elders with different impairments. The results are presented in Table 8.1.

These results show that on average, elders own and use a large number of assistive devices: They own about 14 devices and use 11 of them. Elders with physical impairments, sensory impairments, or both, use the most

Table 8.1. Number and Types of Assistive Devices Owned by Elders With Different Impairments.

TYPE OF DEVICE	1 Minimally Impaired	2 Physically Impaired	3 Vision Impaired	4 Vision and Physically Impaired	5 Cognitively Impaired	6 Cognitively and Physically Impaired	7 Cognitively and Vision Impaired	TOTAL
Physical	4.8	9.3	2.3	8.3	2.1	6.6	3.9	**6.6**[a]
Hearing	0.2	0.2	0.5	0.7	0.6	0.2	0.3	**0.3**
Visual	2.5	1.2	11.9	9.1	0.5	0.8	8.1	**3.8**[b]
Cognitive	0.2	0.1	0.1	0.2	1.7	1.1	0.0	**0.4**[c]
Other	1.9	4.1	1.5	2.7	0.8	1.9	0.9	**2.6**[d]
Total Devices Owned Per Person	9.6	15.0	16.1	20.1	5.7	10.7	13.1	**13.7**[e]

a - Kruskal-Wallis one-way ANOVA x^2 = 52.90 p<.0001   d - Kruskal-Wallis one-way ANOVA x^2 = 33.39 p<.0001
b - Kruskal-Wallis one-way ANOVA x^2 = 77.24 p<.0001   e - Kruskal-Wallis one-way ANOVA x^2 = 37.57 p<.0001
c - Kruskal-Wallis one-way ANOVA x^2 = 49.71 p<.0001

assistive devices. Individuals with cognitive impairments use the fewest (Mann, Hurren, & Tomita, 1993a, 1993b).

Elders are not only lacking information on services, they also lack current information on what assistive devices are available in the marketplace. A recent study asked 110 elders with impairments, "Can you think of a device you would like to have that you haven't been able to find—a device that may not have yet been developed?" All suggestions for new devices had already been developed and were available for sale (Mann, Hurren, Tomita, Bengali, & Steinfeld, 1994).

In response to elders' needs for up-to-date information, the Rehabilitation Engineering Center on Aging at the University at Buffalo established Project Link. Project Link is a free information service to help people learn about assistive devices. Not only are elders lacking information on assistive devices, but companies that market these products have difficulty reaching the people who most need their products. This is largely due to issues of confidentiality—agencies that have lists of people with disabilities are not able to turn them over to companies selling products. Now people can call a toll free number (1-800-628-2281), answer a few questions,

and begin receiving catalogs mailed by Project Link on behalf of companies marketing assistive devices. Each person's name is kept confidential by Project Link. Service providers can share information on Project Link with elders with disabilities.

Considerations in Assistive Device Interventions

Personal Factors

Consumer Perspective

The most important factor in the eventual utility of assistive technology and interventions is the perspective of the person who will receive the interventions. Elders must be fully informed about their disability, so they can fully participate in decisions regarding the selection of appropriate devices and interventions. Service providers must consider the priorities of elders—do they really want, or feel the need for, certain devices? Have they been given options for devices and the differences between devices?

The term *resistance* is sometimes used when discussing consumer acceptance issues. Resistance is an inappropriate label, for it reflects a failure to fully consider the consumer (elder) perspective in assistive device intervention decisions. The elder may initially choose not to accept a service provider's recommendation. The service provider must take the time to understand the reasons for this choice. In discussions with the end user, alternatives are explored, more information is provided, and the most appropriate choices are eventually selected.

Service providers typically focus on self-care issues in interventions with elders; this occurs in nursing home settings and in home health care services. Devices to assist with bathing, mobility, and grooming take precedence over leisure activities. This priority may not match the elder's priority. A recent study asked 86 elders with impairments what activity they most missed doing. The missed activities were overwhelming in the area of leisure, with some IADL further down the list (such as shopping). No one surveyed mentioned a self-care activity (Mann, Karuza, Hurren, & Tomita, 1993a, 1993b). There are well over 1,000 assistive devices for leisure activities included in ABLEDATA. While service providers may have more difficulty being reimbursed for interventions in the area of leisure activities, taking some extra time to find out what is important to the elder, and making relevant recommendations, could greatly enhance the quality of life for recipients of assistive technology services.

Age

There are "young" old, "old" old, and a group that falls in between. Persons in their mid-80s and up are different, as a group, from persons in their mid-60s. The effects of aging are greater for the older group; chronic conditions affect both groups, but much more so for the older group. Economics are different, and the number of significant others available to provide support in crises or in day-to-day management is different. When we speak of providing assistive devices, or designing work or home environments for older persons, we must recognize these differences. A 65-year-old woman with arthritis may need a device to help her open a jar or to type at her job. An 85-year-old woman may need the jar opener, a walker to travel to the kitchen, a home health care aide to assist in preparing the meal, and perhaps a medical alert device in case she suffers an accident.

Diagnosis

The underlying cause of a disability will have an effect on the assistive technology selected. Medical oversight is often needed to be certain the older person is assisted, and will not actually lose function as a result of using an assistive device.

That is, the device may typically substitute for a function involving physical motion or exertion. Atrophy may result if care is not taken to supply alternative activities to maintain the level of motion or exertion. Diagnostic categories resulting in disability cover a wide range: from cognitive/psychiatric diagnoses to neuromusculoskeletal disorders such as Parkinson's disease and stroke. Persons who have had disabilities since they were young, or were diagnosed with a condition at an earlier age, face different challenges than those who first experience disease and disability at an older age. For example, a person who has been hearing-impaired since birth has learned how to adapt to this limitation. Persons in their 70s just losing their hearing have much more difficulty adapting to this condition and often isolate themselves as a result.

Stroke and arthritis are two important diagnostic categories affecting individuals in their later years. Stroke can result in weakness or paralysis on one side of the body, as well as dysphasia or aphasia (51% of all stroke cases), memory impairment or disorientation (47% of cases), and loss of, or altered, sensation (36% of cases) (Mayo, 1993). Service providers may easily recognize one-sided weakness or paralysis. Their recommendations may include devices that make it easier to complete tasks with one hand. An example of one of these devices is a one-handed denture cleaner, which consists of brushes for cleaning on top, and suction cups on the bottom to hold the device to the sink. Service providers may not as easily recognize limitations in sensation, but should be alert for this. If an elder cannot sense heat or cold, a burn could occur by bathing or cooking with water that is too hot. Devices are available to control the temperature of water at the tap. Another solution, especially for a person who cannot afford this device, is to lower the water's temperature at the water heater. Unfortunately, this latter solution may not be feasible in apartment or group home settings.

Arthritis is an important diagnostic category for two reasons: it has high prevalence and is highly disabling. Arthritis is estimated to affect 37 million people in the United States, with the greatest prevalence among the elderly (Abyad & Boyer, 1992). The Longitudinal Study on Aging indicates that 55% of elders have arthritis (Yelin, 1992). The impact of arthritis on activities is significant: 66% of persons with arthritis experience limitations in physical activities, and 25% report limitations in ADL or

IADL. This increases for elders who have arthritis and a second chronic condition, with 82% experiencing limitations in physical activity and 41% limited in ADL or IADL (Yelin & Katz, 1990).

Arthritis can affect the small joints of the body—affecting fine motor tasks; the large joints affecting mobility if in the lower extremities, and reaching and lifting, if in the upper extremities; or both. While there are many effective assistive devices to address limitations in fine motor and gross motor tasks, the service provider must also recognize that arthritis is typically associated with pain, and often with periods of exacerbation. These factors must also play a role in decisions regarding selection of assistive devices. For example, a reacher may be recommended to assist with limitations in shoulder movement, or because the elder cannot easily stand or bend. It is important to determine not only the day-of-assessment functioning of the person's hand, but whether the person also has periods when it is more difficult to grasp a device such as a reacher. There are many reachers on the market, and some require less pressure to grasp. Some reachers even offer support at the wrist and forearm for holding the device. Each feature represents a series of tradeoffs. Service providers can work closely with elders to attain the optimal match between the person and device.

Service providers must also recognize that arthritis is a progressive disease, and that the severity of impact will vary from one person to another. A study that grouped elders with arthritis into "moderate arthritis" and "severe arthritis" determined that the severe arthritis group used almost twice as many assistive devices to address their physical disabilities as the moderate arthritis group (Mann, Hurren, & Tomita, in press).

Social Environment Factors

Caregivers

For some older persons, the difference between nursing home placement and living at home comes down to the availability of someone at home to provide assistance. But often the "assistant" is the older spouse or older child (a person in their 90s may well have children in their 70s) who is also experiencing the impact of aging. Devices that can assist the caregiver—the spouse, the child, even the home health care aide—can have a major impact on eliminating the need or delaying the time for nursing home placement of a very frail elderly person. For an elder who cannot transfer independently, a lift assists both

him or her and the caregiver. For a person with a cognitive impairment who wanders, an alerting device helps the caregiver and ensures the person's safety.

Setting

The term *congregate care setting* indicates settings such as nursing homes (skilled nursing facilities), hospitals, health-related facilities, family care homes, and day programs or outpatient settings. The process of designing or adapting the environment, or introducing assistive devices, will differ in many cases with the setting. A person sharing a room in a nursing home will require different devices and different environmental interventions than a person living at home (in most cases).

Role

Employee, retiree, homemaker, or caregiver—each role an older person fills brings with it different considerations for environmental design and adaptations, and for assistive technology solutions. Someone who works and also needs an assistive device at home may require a different device than a person with similar disabilities who does not work. For example, the device may need to be portable for the person working who also needs the device at home. Older caregivers may need specific assistive devices for themselves and other devices for use with the person for whom they are providing care.

Physical Environment Factors

Urban/Rural

Two major differences between urban and rural settings are type of housing and availability of transportation. Housing units in urban areas have less flexibility for adaptation due to multistories, tenant leases, and neighbors. There are few high-rise apartments or condos in rural areas, making major adaptations less difficult. On the other hand, transportation problems faced by older persons in rural areas are typically much greater than those faced by persons in urban areas—which is not to say that urban areas do not have serious transportation problems for persons with disabilities. Personal security and safety are another important aspect of the physical environment.

Climate

Climate has an impact on how a person dresses and on the activities in which the person engages.

Transportation, shopping, and entertainment patterns vary with changing weather patterns. Elders are more sensitive to extremes of heat and cold, and need to be able to control the temperature in their homes. The products available vary by climate. For devices used outside, different materials might need to be considered in a dry climate versus a wet climate. In Buffalo, an elder might purchase an "ice grip" for the base of his or her cane, while few are sold in Miami.

Design

The characteristics of the immediate physical environment—that is, the design of rooms, spaces, landscape features, furnishings, and building elements—have a significant influence on the independence of older people. Environments also can pose significant barriers to access, safety, usability, and security. Environments also have direct impacts on a person's life satisfaction, morale, adjustment, and physical health. Poor environmental design, therefore, can confound or even counter the positive effects of assistive technology. Moreover, environmental design and building technology can often eliminate the need for expensive technological interventions, thereby providing a more cost-effective solution to specific problems.

A study of environmental problems in the homes and neighborhoods of elders recently reported that more problems were found in the kitchen than in any other room or area, with the bathroom ranking second. However, for elders with cognitive impairments, the bathroom posed the most problems. In both the bathroom and kitchen, size is a critical factor. People need room to store things, use devices, move about, and accommodate caregivers. Fixtures are also important. Can the sink be reached? How easy is it to get in and out of the bathtub? Are the cabinets too high or too low (Mann, Hurren, Tomita, Bengali, & Steinfeld, 1994)? These are all important considerations for service providers in assessing home environments.

Design also relates to devices. Some potentially useful devices may be underutilized by older persons because they are not designed with their needs in mind. The typical hand-held remote control device is a good example. For an elder with mobility limita-

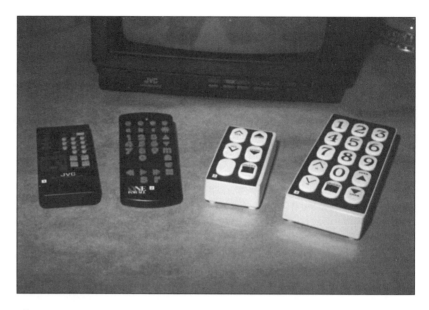

Figure 8.1. A recent study demonstrated that elders with impairments prefer TV remotes with large buttons and good color contrast.

tions, a hand-held remote may be essential for full use of a television. But if the buttons are too small and close for an elder with arthritis to operate, or too difficult for an elder with some vision impairment to see, the remote control device is not useful. A recent study demonstrated that elders with impairments preferred TV remotes with large buttons and good color contrast between button symbols and the background, as pictured in the remotes in Figure 8.1 (Mann, Ottenbacher, Tomita, & Packard, 1994). Service providers could recommend a universal remote control with large buttons, such as those manufactured by Universal Electronics Inc., manufacturer of the "One-for-All" line of remote controls (phone contact 1-800-394-3000).

Any appreciable loss of function in physical, cognitive, or sensory abilities reduces the older person's level of interactions with the environment, which in turn places his or her health and independence in jeopardy. Traditional interventions to mitigate the effects of a disability involve a caregiver substituting his or her abilities for the older person's loss in function. More recently, attention has been turned to environmental interventions and assistive device that reduce "handicapping" conditions.

Disability

Different devices and different environmental adaptations are needed for different types of disabilities. Sensory, cognitive, and motor impairments each present different challenges for structuring the environment and providing assistive devices. One of the more unique aspects of aging is the prevalence of *multiple* disabilities—presenting perhaps the greatest challenge for developing interventions.

Severity of disability is a major consideration in providing assistive technology interventions. Assistive devices appropriate for a person with minor disabilities may address a number of areas, including employment and leisure. Many older persons are employed—with changes in the labor market, changes in attitudes toward aging, and changes in available assistive technology, it is not surprising to find statements like: "The private sector and government must keep workers trained in new technology to remain productive, and retirement should be restructured to encourage older individuals to work" (Schwartz, 1989, p. 3).

A person with minor disability may benefit from a number of devices, depending on what the disability is (e.g., a button hook and jar opener for a person with some arthritis in the hands and resultant decreased strength and pain, or a magnifier and high-intensity lamp for a person having difficulty reading fine print).

Older persons who have severe disabilities will employ different assistive technology—"tools"—than a person with minor disabilities. Most assistive technology requirements will be in the areas of: (a) safety, (b) independence, (c) sensory perception, (d) cognition, and (e) expressive communication.

Areas of Assistive Technology Interventions

Safety

An older person who is disoriented and at risk for getting lost is said to exhibit "wandering" behavior. Wandering is a threat to safety. In nursing homes, staff are faced with unpleasant options: physically restrict patients, or provide more staff. Providing more staff is not often possible. At a Veterans Administration nursing home in Atlanta, Georgia, a group of investigators studied the effectiveness of using a computer-generated voice to instruct patients who "wandered" near exits to return to their living units. There was a significant decrease in the number of "exits" with the use of this device (Blasch, Saltzman, & Coombs, 1989). A recent publication provides names, address, products, and services for 11 companies that offer products for long-term-care security (U.S. Bureau of the Census, 1989).

The problem of falling is related to wandering. As we age, especially as we reach our 80s, we are more susceptible to fractures due to osteoporosis, a gradual loss of calcium from the bones. Research is underway on gait, and in particular "postural sway" —upper-body precession from the vertical axis—as postural sway is related to falling during ambulation (Farris, 1988). Assistive devices in this area have existed for centuries—from the simple cane to walkers. New devices may include microprocessor-based monitors that can track such motions as postural sway, and offer an alarm—or a voice suggestion, such as "slow down," "sit down and rest"—as a way of preventing falls.

Independence

Mobility

Mobility includes walking, with or without an assistive device, and wheeled forms of transportation, including wheelchairs and scooters. Assistive devices for walking include canes, walkers, and crutches. There are more than 4 million people in the United States who use canes for support, and more than 60% of cane users are over 65 years old (LaPlante, Hendershot, & Moss, 1992). Canes can support up to 25% of a person's weight, while walkers and crutches are usually recommended when additional support is needed, or to assist with lateral balance.

Canes are inexpensive and widely available. One result is that many elders have canes that were not provided following careful professional assessment, so there is often a poor fit between the cane and the user. A recent American Association of Retired Persons report advised its members: "A medical professional (physician, physical or occupational therapist) should recommend and fit your cane" (Norrgard, 1992, p.1). A recent study of cane use found that elders face a number of problems with canes they own, with more than half the identified problems relating to difficulty and/or risk with the use of the cane (Mann, Granger, Hurren, Tomita, & Charvat, in press). A companion study of walkers found that 61% of walker users had a problem with at least one walker they owned, and that more than half the problems were categorized as "difficult or dangerous to use" (Mann, Hurren, Tomita, & Charvat, 1995). A careful evaluation of cane or walker options should be performed in the setting where the elder will most frequently use the cane or walker.

Wheelchairs are used almost universally by nursing home patients, and many older persons living at home also use them. There are many considerations in ensuring that the wheelchair will not only provide mobility, but that that the "fit" will be both safe and comfortable. The problem of decubiti must be considered when fitting a wheelchair and when positioning the person, as well as when recommending the length of time the person should remain in the wheelchair at one time. Another aspect of wheelchairs is safety. Brakes must be in good working order. A British study determined that two-thirds of the 200,000 wheelchairs in England and Wales were used by people over retirement age, and that a significant percentage of these chairs had "inefficient brakes and flat tires" (Haworth, Powell, & Mullex, 1983).

The decision to use a wheelchair must involve the potential user, unless the person's judgment is severely impaired and he or she is not capable of participating in the decision. Many nursing home patients who are physically capable of walking choose to use a wheelchair. For some this is a result of the fear of falling; for others, multiple physical factors—pain, strength, endurance, vision, and balance—affect the decision (Pawlson, Goodwin, & Keith, 1986). Consideration of relevant physical and psychosocial factors is essential to ensure appropriate wheelchair prescription for elders.

Activities of Daily Living

There are a large number of devices available that can assist a person with eating. These devices make it easier to hold utensils or prevent food from spilling off the plate or out of the cup. Dentures are used by many older persons, and have obvious implications for eating. Getting dentures in or out of the mouth may be a problem for some, and there is even an assistive device for denture handling (Labell & Glassman, 1988). Tremors can also make eating very difficult. Broadhust and Stammers (1988) developed an assistive feeding device that includes a pivoted four-bar chain mechanism, with guidance for the hand maintained by using a spring-restrained sliding handle.

Toileting is another area of serious concern to elder persons. Incontinence is embarrassing, and can result in a person isolating himself or herself. A group of researchers is working on an electronic device that will measure the decline in electromyographic activity of the muscles of the pelvic floor prior to an involuntary contraction, and alert the patient to an impending bladder contraction that occurs with loss of urine (O'Donnel, 1989). Already available for incontinence and widely used are moisture-absorbing pads.

Transferring and lifting are very important tasks, both to the person with the disability and to any care provider involved. A number of manual and powered lift devices are available for home or institutional use.

Instrumental Activities of Daily Living

Instrumental activities of daily living include such things as food preparation, housecleaning, shopping, and money management. Elders with impairments often receive personal assistance with these tasks from family or friends, or through formal caregiving services. There are many assistive devices available that can assist an elder, either in independently doing these activities or in permitting some level of participation. Some of these devices are mainstream consumer products, such as microwave ovens, televisions from which a person can shop, and phones that can be used for banking. The service provider should consider the activities in which the elder wishes to participate and the elder's functional limitations. Together, the provider and the elder can review the wide range of traditional assistive devices, consumer products, home modifications, and adaptations of existing devices appropriate for those functional limitations.

Work

Trends in the employment of older persons suggest that higher-paid older workers are being "encouraged" to move out of the workforce. Yet as the baby boom generation grows older, the percentage of the work force represented by older persons will increase. The increased number of older workers will increase proportionately the number of older workers who have impairments. Assistive devices and environmental interventions offer the potential to accommodate the functional limitations of older workers (Mann, 1992a). Service providers can play an important role with elder workers and their employers, recognizing the combined impact of the effects of aging, such as decreased vision and hearing, and the common chronic conditions of later years, such as arthritis. Service providers should recognize the rights of older workers under the Americans With Disabilities Act (ADA). While the ADA only makes one reference to older persons, it is applicable in issues of access in public places and employment.

Leisure

Elders with impairments most miss leisure-time activities, especially crafts and other hobbies (Mann, Hurren, & Tomita, 1993). HyperAbledata lists hundreds of assistive devices for leisure activities, such as card holders for one-handed card playing, large-print cards for persons with low vision, and a variety of devices for sewing and other needlecraft. In selecting appropriate assistive devices, it is important to recognize the mix of conditions faced by elders. For example, large-print cards may make it easier for a person with low vision to play card games, but if the cards are glossy and the elder is sensitive to glare, they may not be useful—and not used.

Environmental control devices can also play a part in leisure activities. Both nursing home patients and many older persons confined to home with severe disabilities experience a loss of control over their environment. Devices can help in turning lights on and off; controlling a TV, radio, or other appliance; and operating a call switch. A recent study of nursing home patients found that providing a system that performed five functions saved nursing time, and patients gained an increased feeling of control over their environment (Symington, Lywood, Lawson, & Mclean, 1986). Another study found a higher rate of radio use by elderly nursing home residents who were given simple X-10 type remote control devices (Mann, 1992b).

Sensory Perception

Hearing

Almost one out of three persons over age 64 has a hearing impairment, and 42% of those over age 85 have at least some hearing loss (Hotchkiss, 1989). While devices are available for persons with hearing impairments, many elders accept hearing loss as a normal process of aging and do not seek assistance. Hearing loss can severely affect communication, and decreased communication can result in isolation and depression (Glass, 1986). Hearing loss can affect health and safety in other ways, for example not being able to hear fire alarms or not being able to hear instructions for taking medications.

Assistive devices available for elders with hearing impairments include hearing aids; assistive listening devices (FM, infrared, or hardwire) and telecommunication (TDD) devices; amplifiers; alternate signals (light or vibration); and closed-caption video. While elders with hearing impairments have multiple options for assistive devices, they have a very high rate of dissatisfaction with devices that address hearing impairment—especially hearing aids (Mann, Hurren, & Tomita, 1994). Very often this dissatisfaction reflects: (a) receiving the hearing aid without an audiological assessment, or (b) having

significant hearing or physical status changes that make the device no longer appropriate. Service providers must recognize problems with hearing and changes in hearing capacity over time, and make appropriate audiological referrals.

Elders with hearing impairment use many devices for other impairments they face—in fact, the majority of devices they use address physical limitations (Mann, Hurren, & Tomita, 1994). When providing training in the use of any recommended assistive devices, service providers must take steps to be sure they are being heard and understood—such as standing directly in front of the person, speaking at a normal or slower pace, or speaking louder as necessary. Demonstrating devices may overcome, to some extent, the elder's difficulty in hearing instructions during training.

Vision

Vision loss is very common among older persons. More than 20% of persons over age 64 have difficulty reading due to a visual impairment. Five percent of persons over age 64 cannot see letters or words (U.S. Bureau of the Census, 1986). Most older persons with visual impairments have some functional vision. This residual vision is called *low vision.*

Vision loss among elderly persons is associated with a decrease in outdoor mobility. A recent study determined that older individuals with normal vision for their age average about 1.5 destinations outside the home each week. Older persons with visual impairments, on the other hand, average .5 destinations per week. Only 6 out of the 35 older blind individuals in this study reported any independent travel beyond their own yard (Long, 1989).

Devices for visual impairments include image magnifiers, audio output, Braille output, synthetic voice output, tactile images, scanning, and notetaking systems.

Cognition

One of every 10 noninstitutionalized elders has Alzheimer's disease or some other organic mental disorder; for elders over 85 years of age, this increases to almost one out of every two persons (Mortimer, 1983). Alzheimer's disease and other forms of dementia can result in memory loss and impaired judgment. A low-tech solution to recollection difficulty is to write notes on paper and post them in appropriate places. An alternative, high-tech solution is to use a small electronic notebook. A number of these are available for less than $100, and most offer other features, such as a clock with an alarm. The alarm can be used to provide a reminder for taking medications. Many digital wrist watches now offer similar features.

One recent study reported the effectiveness of using of an electronic memory aid by persons with Alzheimer's disease. In this study "subjects made significantly more statements of fact and fewer ambiguous utterances." In addition, subjects showed more initiative in conversations (Bourgeoris, 1990).

Assistive devices for persons with cognitive impairment can directly address deficits in memory. However, a recent study reported that although most devices used by persons with cognitive impairment address physical or sensory limitation, fewer than 17% of assistive devices for this population address cognitive impairment (Mann, Karuza, Hurren, & Tomita, 1993a, 1993b). These elders have multiple impairments and use devices to address these noncognitive impairments. Service providers must recognize the complex interaction between cognitive, physical, and sensory impairment, and consider devices that are easy to use and safe. A person with a cognitive impairment may need more extensive training in device use. Close coordination of training in device use with care providers is essential to success.

Expressive Communication

Many elderly individuals who incur stroke, trauma, progressive neurological disorders, and cancer of the larynx (and subsequent laryngectomy) find their ability to effectively express themselves limited. Communication assistive devices range from simple pictures or word communication boards to portable or stationary computer-assisted technology with a visual display or synthesized speech production. Such devices allow the individual to interact with significant others and maintain an active social role in his or her environment.

Assessment Instruments

A number of areas must be considered when determining appropriate assistive devices and environmental interventions. The functional status of the elder is essential. In relation to this, information on health and mental status is necessary to ensure useful, safe interventions. Other factors to consider are level of social supports available, type of housing, financial resources, and experience with assistive devices.

Standardized instrument evaluations consider most of these areas. Several such instruments are described below.

Functional Status

Functional Independence Measure (FIM)

The FIM was designed to measure the level of need for assistance from another person—the "burden of care" (Ottenbacher et al., 1994). It has 18 items, each rated on a 7-point scale, with a score of 7 reflecting "complete independence" and a score of 1 reflecting "total assistance." Two major domains are measured: motor and cognitive. Both the Self-Care section and the Mobility section list specific tasks with which an individual may have difficulty, and areas that might be addressed with assistive technology and environmental interventions.

OARS: Older Americans Resources and Services Program Multidimensional Functional Assessment Questionnaire: IADLs Section

One section of the OARS focuses on IADLs, such as managing money, cooking, and going shopping (Fillenbaum, 1988). There are seven items, each scored on a 3-point scale. Like the FIM Self-Care section, the OARS-IADLs can direct the service provider to specific difficult tasks for an elder—tasks that might be addressed with assistive technology interventions.

OTFACT

OTFACT is a computerized assessment developed by an occupational therapist and marketed by the American Occupational Therapy Association. Items are organized into a hierarchy, going from role function to specific components, such as neuromuscular functions. The program prompts the therapist with questions such as, "Is the client able to put on clothing independently?" and the therapist determines if there is total, partial, or no deficit in this area. The program uses a branching decision-tree structure so only relevant questions are asked. For example, if the therapist determined "no deficit" for "self-administration of medication," the program would not ask for more detail. If the response were "partial deficit," a series of functions would be presented for evaluation: "uses correct schedule," "changes medication," "stores medication properly." While there are 985 possible questions, only a subset of relevant questions is actually asked, and most assessments are completed within 15 minutes. The program prints a report of the assessment.

Health Status

OARS

In many settings the service provider can evaluate health status through a review of the elder's medical chart. This is true in health care facilities such as nursing homes and hospitals. It may be more difficult to evaluate health status when providing home-based services, especially when services are not associated with a home health care agency. In these cases, a section of the OARS addresses health status through self-report by the elder or the elder's caregiver. The OARS Health Status instrument seeks information on the types of chronic diseases the elder has, the types of medications taken, number of physician visits in past 6 months, and number of days of hospitalization and nursing home care in the past 6 months.

Jette Functional Pain Index (Jette)

Using the Jette, the elder is asked a number of questions relating to experienced pain. A score range of 10 to 40 is possible, with 10 representing no pain and 40 representing a very high level of pain (Jette, 1980).

Mental Status

MMSE—Mini Mental State Exam

The MMSE consists of 11 items summed to create a mental status score (Folstein, 1975). Thirty is the maximum possible score. An elder who scores below 24 is likely to have some cognitive impairment. The score may suggest the need for assistive devices addressing the cognitive impairment, such as memory aids or pill dispensers. It may also suggest the need for additional training on devices to address other conditions, such as vision or mobility impairment.

CES-D—Center for Epidemiological Studies Depression Scale

Depression is common among elderly persons with disabilities. Upon recognizing depression in an elder, service providers should make a referral to a physician. Since depression should be treated medically, assistive technology interventions may be more successful following medical intervention. The CES-D can help service providers determine if an elder is depressed. The CES-D has 20 items that ask elders to describe how they have been feeling for the past week (Radloff & Locke, 1986).

Assistive Technology and Environmental Interventions

CAATU—Consumer Assessments Assistive Technology Used Instrument

Developed at the University at Buffalo as a research instrument, the CAATU provides a listing of the devices a person uses. Specific categories of devices include (a) physical disabilities, (b) hearing impairments, (c) visual impairments, (d) tactile impairments, and (e) cognitive impairments. Elders are asked what devices they own, if they use each device, and if they are satisfied with each device. If they own a device and do not use it or are not satisfied with it, they are asked to explain why. The categories of devices are presented in Table 8.2, along with questions for collecting information on device use and satisfaction.

Additional questions on the CAATU include (a) What devices do you need that you do not have? (b) Of all the devices you use, which is the most important to you? (c) Can you think of any features you would like to see added to some devices you currently use? (d) Can you think of a device you would like to have that you haven't been able to find? A device that may not have been developed? (e) Can you name one thing that you would really like to do now, that you used to do but can no longer do?

EASE—Enhancements Adapting Senior Environments

EASE is a computerized assessment designed for use by occupational therapists in home-based settings. EASE identifies potential problems in independent living by comparing the functional abilities of an elder with the functional requirements of the home. For each problem confirmed by the therapist, the program presents a variety of solutions, including products, ideas, recommendations, adaptations, suggestions for professional assistance, and services. Product solutions are accompanied by ordering information. The selected ideas and recommendations are provided in a narrative report format, and may be edited by the therapist prior to printing. Additional comments can be inserted by the therapist using the keyboard at any point in the evaluation process.

HyperHome Resource

This computerized assessment was developed at the University at Buffalo Rehabilitation Engineering Center on Aging. HyperHome Resource helps home modification service providers manage the diverse

Table 8.2. Consumer Assessments Study Interview Battery: Assistive Technology Used Instrument.

A.　Physical Disabilities:

1. Environmental Control Devices
2. Robotic Device
3. Physical Extension Device (Mouthstick, Headpointer)
4. Special Switches or Controls
5. Special Computer Keyboard
6. Balance Aid
7. Wheelchair
8. Special Seating System
9. Functional Electrical Stimulation Device
10. ADL–Bathing
11. ADL–Eating
12. ADL–Grooming
13. ADL–Dressing
14. ADL–Hygiene

B.　Hearing Impairments: General Device Type

1. Hearing Aid
2. Alerting Device
3. Assistive Listening Device
4. Telecommunication Device
5. Cochlear Implant

C.　Visual Impairments: General Device Type

1. Stand-alone Print Enlargement System
2. Character Enlargement System for Computer Screen
3. Braille Output Device
4. Audio-Tactile System
5. Scanning System
6. Laptop Computer
7. Braille 'n' Speak
8. Low-Tech Aids

D.　Tactile Impairments: General Device Type

1. Special Thermometers
2. Other

E.　Cognitive Impairments: General Device Type

1. Software Such as Spell Checker
2. Memory Aids
3. Screen-Reading Programs
4. Safety/Security Device (Alerting Device)
5. Other

F.　Other Devices Used

Code	Specific Devices	Is It Used? (Yes/No)	Satisfied? (Yes/No)	If Not, Why Not?

---

technical information on environmental design ideas and products needed for quality service. It functions more like a personal information manager than a database, allowing the user maximum individual customization. Another advantage is that the HyperHome Resource interface is simple and requires only minutes of training to master. Using HyperHome Resource, the service provider can show clients photographs and sketches of recommendations regarding home modifications. Home modifications projects vary from roof leaks to renovation of a bathroom (Steinfeld & Shea, 1993).

Summary

In determining interventions for older persons with disabilities, consider:

1. There is great diversity in the limitations, functions, and needs of each "older" person.
2. Assistive technology for older persons accommodates one or more of the following:
   - changes in cognitive abilities: dementia;
   - losses in sensory abilities: vision, hearing and tactile sensation;
   - impairments that affect communication;
   - decreasing strength, endurance, and respiration; and
   - mobility and joint impairments.
3. Some applications of assistive technology require medical oversight, while others do not.
4. The best assistive technology is often the simplest. High-tech solutions should be considered only if the person's needs require them.
5. Some assistive devices in the marketplace may not be designed to accommodate the combinations of impairments older persons present. Purchased devices may require adaptation.

Case Studies

The following case studies are based on two subjects in a research study at the University at Buffalo Rehabilitation Engineering Center on Aging. This study is testing the effectiveness of a comprehensive approach to the assessment, provision, training, and follow-up of assistive device and home modification interventions. In each of the following two case studies, subjects were provided with assistive devices through the research study when the formal third-party payer or the elder was not able to pay. Thus, for every identified need agreed upon by the elder and the assessment team, an intervention was provided.

Case 1: Mrs. Doe

General

Mrs. Doe is 70 years old and lives with her husband. She has three children; her daughter lives nearby and her other two children live in another state. She retired 9 years ago, having worked for 18 years as an administrative secretary. She was forced to retire due to symptoms of Parkinson's disease in her hands. Financially, the Does have experienced difficulty because Mrs. Doe's illness has depleted their sav-

ings. Mrs. Doe does not receive any formal, paid personal care aide assistance, but Mr. Doe provides an average of 17 hours of assistance per week.

Assessment: Environment/Housing/Resources

Mrs. Doe and her husband have lived in a ranch-style home for the past 13 years. Their home is located in a suburban area that Mrs. Doe believes is very safe. Mr. Doe made some simple home modifications to address accessibility issues. He rearranged all the kitchen cabinets so that frequently used items were within reach. He placed some of the items that were in the lower cabinets in a box with a handle, allowing Mrs. Doe to pull the box out (similar to a drawer) to locate and retrieve needed items without bending. He placed an arm chair next to the bedroom closet so Mrs. Doe can sit while dressing. He also added a hand-held shower to use with a bath transfer bench.

Assessment: Medical Status

Mrs. Doe is 5'5" tall and weighs 110 pounds. She had a total right hip replacement 1 year prior to this assessment; she had three follow-up visits to her physician within the 6 months prior to this assessment. She also has had Parkinson's disease for the past 9 years and circulatory problems in her extremities. She takes four medications. She experiences some minor pain, particularly during ambulation, with a score of 15 on the Jette.

Assessment: Physical/Sensory Status

Mrs. Doe describes her hearing and vision as very good; she wears bifocal glasses. She scored 38% physically disabled on the Sickness Impact Profile.

Activities requiring balance and coordination are very difficult for Mrs. Doe. She had three significant falls in the last year—the first resulted in the hip fracture requiring a total hip replacement (THR). She fell in her kitchen while carrying items to the kitchen table as she was assisting with meal preparation. The third fall occurred in her sewing room, where she stumbled over the carpet.

Mrs. Doe is right hand dominant, and is experiencing fine motor difficulties due to upper-extremity tremors and decreased strength; hand grasp strength measured 22 kilograms. The tremors occur primarily in the morning when she wakes up.

Assessment: Cognitive/Mental Status

Mrs. Doe demonstrates no cognitive impairment, scoring 28 (out of 30) on the MMSE, and 21 (out of 21) on the Social Cognitive section of the FIM. She scored 16 on the CESD, indicating that she may be somewhat depressed. Mrs. Doe became very tearful when describing the changes in her life as a result of declining health. She scored 34 (out of 40) on the Rosenberg Self-Esteem Scale, suggesting that self-esteem is moderately high. An aspect of Mrs. Doe's personality is that she likes to do things quickly. This is a definite factor in her falling: She is constantly testing her capabilities and thereby increasing her risk of a fall.

Assessment: Functional Status

For IADLs, Mrs. Doe scored 9 (out of 14) on the OARS. She is able to use the telephone and handle her own money independently. She is beginning to have difficulty writing legibly; this is confirmed by her husband who says he has difficulty reading her grocery lists. Mrs. Doe requires some assistance when going to places out of walking distance. Her husband drives her to all appointments, and assists with shopping for groceries and clothes, and with doing housework. Their washer and dryer are located in the basement, which Mrs. Doe cannot access safely; thus Mr. Doe does the laundry. He states that he is afraid to leave the house because his wife may attempt to do the laundry herself. Mrs. Doe does some light housework, but again, Mr. Doe would prefer to do it rather than risk Mrs. Doe falling.

Mrs. Doe requires assistance with medications; she has difficulty opening medicine bottle tops. She uses a weekly pill organizer. She also requires assistance with preparing meals. She owns a rubber jar opener and an under-the-counter jar opener but does not have the strength to use them. She uses a microwave oven. While she assists with meal preparation, she desires to be even more independent in the kitchen. Mr. Doe actually prepares most meals. He is afraid of his wife falling, so he supervises her while she sets the table.

For ADL, Mrs. Doe scored 38 out 42 on the Self-Care section of the FIM, meaning she is still fairly independent at performing self-care activities. Assistive devices clearly support this level of independence. She is independent in eating and lower-extremity dressing (she uses a sock aid). She uses assistive devices for grooming (hairdryer with brush attachment), bathing (rubber bath mat, tub transfer bench, long-handled brush, hand-held shower), upper-extremity dressing (dressing stick button, hook/zipper pull), and toileting (bedside commode). While Mrs. Doe reports that she received training in the use of the bath bench following her hip surgery,

she was observed using the device inappropriately. She simply stepped into the tub and sat down, treating the bench like a chair rather than using it to do a seated transfer. She stands for most of her shower, using the bath bench only to sit for washing her lower extremities. She grasps her sink to assist in getting out of the tub. She uses the hose of the hand-held shower as an assist in standing, and also uses a ceramic soap dish as a grab bar—there is no arm rest on the transfer bench. She drops items like soap and shampoo while standing, and finds it difficult to retrieve them.

Mrs. Doe uses panty-liners for occasional incontinence. She has difficulty getting on and off her toilet, as it is very low. She uses the side of the bathtub and the sink to assist with sitting and getting up. She performs all hygiene activities independently. She has difficulty with buttoning and other fine motor tasks such as threading needles and opening containers. Mrs. Doe also uses a reacher, cordless phone, touch-operated lamp, Gaymar seat cushion, automatic garage door opener, and TV remote control.

Mobility and locomotion are major areas of difficulty for Mrs. Doe. She requires balance aids for ambulation. She owns a folding walker and J-cane, but does not always use them in the house. She says she only needs to use them in the evening after a busy, tiring day. She was observed using the walker incorrectly, carrying it several steps before placing it on the floor, and rocking it on the back legs then forward onto the front legs. She is unable to make turns safely—her feet become entangled. She often overextends the placement of the walker, forcing her to lean forward more, thus further exacerbating her balance problem. When ambulating without a support aid, her right upper extremity is extended at the glenohumeral joint, with elbow flexion. Right lower extremity movement is delayed, and foot drop occurs with this gait pattern. Her center of gravity is anterior to her body; her head leads, forcing her to lean forward and accelerate to maintain balance.

Interventions

The following interventions were recommended:

1. *Problem:* Inappropriate use of the tub bench and hand-held shower, which could lead to a fall.
   Intervention: Mrs. Doe was retrained on transfers into and out of the tub. She was encouraged to shower seated on the transfer bench and was taught methods to bathe and rinse using the hand-held shower.

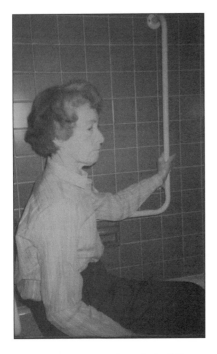

Figure 8.2. Mrs. Doe is holding the right-angled grab bar in tub area.

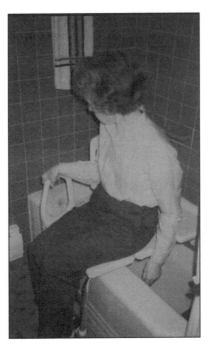

Figure 8.3. Mrs. Doe uses the portable grab bar to guide her in the seated bath transfer.

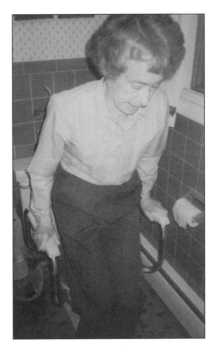

Figure 8.4. Mrs. Doe demonstrates the use of the toilet safety frame.

2. *Problem:* No grab bars are available in the tub so Mrs. Doe uses the ceramic soap dish and hand-held shower hose.

   Intervention: Although standing has been discouraged, Mrs. Doe continues to stand during part of her shower. A right-angled grab bar was installed on the wall above the tub. She is able to pull herself up to a standing position and grasp the vertical portion of the bar for balance (see Figure 8.2). A portable grab bar was placed on the outer tub rim next to the back support of the tub bench. This provides additional support for pushing up from the transfer bench and for standing once her feet are outside the tub. This portable grab bar also guides her in a seated bath transfer (see Figure 8.3).

3. *Problem:* Bathing items are dropped while in the tub.

   Intervention: A tub caddie was purchased and adapted to fit the tub. This device holds all articles necessary for bathing within reach while sitting on the transfer bench.

4. *Problem:* Mrs. Doe loses balance when standing up after toileting.

   Intervention: A safety frame was mounted over the toilet to provide stability when standing or sitting. Mrs. Doe is able to push up with

both upper extremities and hold onto the armrests until she is stabilized (see Figure 8.4).

5. *Problem:* Mrs. Doe has difficulty reaching clothing in her closet and transporting it to her bed without loosing balance.

   Intervention: Mrs. Doe has an arm chair close to the closet door, which forces her to side step between the chair and the closet door. The chair was moved away from the closet door, thus providing enough space for her to use the walker when obtaining clothes. She was trained to: (a) hold the walker with one hand while reaching for articles of clothing with the other, (b) drape the clothing over the frame of the walker, and (c) use both hands to maneuver the walker to the chair or bed where she gets dressed.

6. *Problem:* Mrs. Doe has difficulty maintaining balance while dressing her upper body.

   Intervention: Mrs. Doe was trained to dress while seated on the bed or chair and to use the walker for balance and support during dressing.

7. *Problem:* Mrs. Doe uses the walker incorrectly, and dangerously.

   Intervention: Mrs. Doe was trained in all aspects of ambulating correctly with a walker, including turning, sitting and standing, and maneuvering in the house. She requires reminders to slow down and to take smaller steps. A walker bag was purchased and attached to assist in carrying items (see Figure 8.5).

8. *Problem:* Mrs. Doe's perception of the walker making her look old has resulted in her using the walker less than she needs to.

   Intervention: Mr. and Mrs. Doe were trained on the correct use of the walker. Following discussions with this couple, they agreed that Mr. Doe would provide reminders to Mrs. Doe to use the walker correctly.

9. *Problem:* Handwriting is difficult for Mrs. Doe due to upper-extremity tremors and intrinsic muscle fatigue.

   Intervention: Mrs. Doe was trained to use an assistive writing device called the "Writing Bird" and a weighted pen. After trying both devices for 2 weeks, she decided the weighted pen worked best in reducing the tremors. She was also taught techniques to conserve her writing energy while writing (see Figures 8.6 and 8.7).

10. *Problem:* Mrs. Doe has decreased bed mobility and requires assistance getting out of bed or turning in bed. Mrs. Doe is not able to roll from her back to her stomach, or onto her side. She is also having difficulty getting into and out of bed.

    Intervention: Mrs. Doe was trained in bed mobility compensatory strategies. She was taught where to sit on the bed so that when

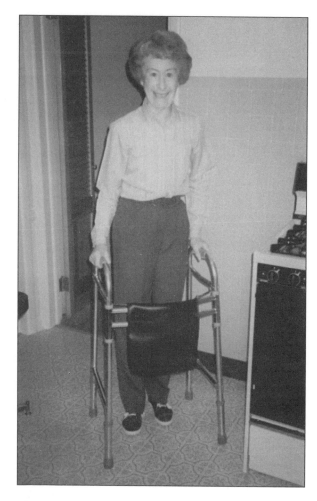

Figure 8.5. Mrs. Doe demonstrates the walker with the walker bag attached.

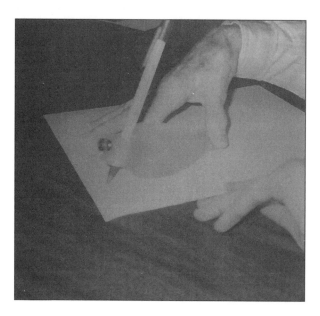

Figure 8.6. Mrs. Doe tests the Writing Bird, but finds that it does not meet her needs.

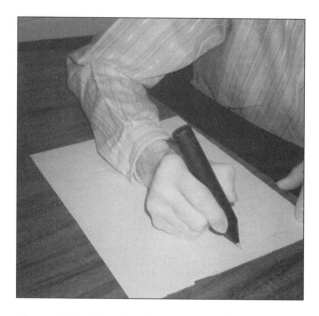

Figure 8.7. Mrs. Doe demonstrates the use of the weighted pen.

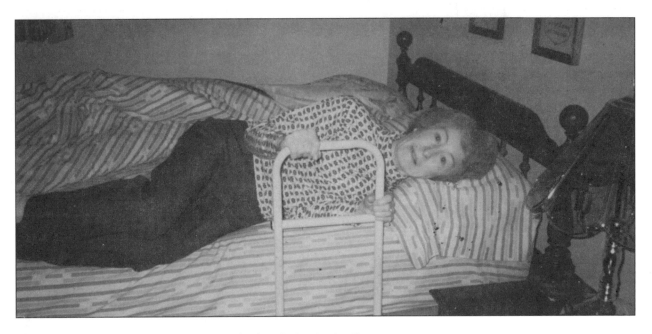

Figure 8.8. Mrs. Doe is able to turn in bed with this bed rail.

she lies down she will be in her preferred position on the bed. She was also taught to bridge her hips to shift her body over in bed, and the areas to grasp on the headboard to assist with turning to the right side. A bed rail was provided. The new bed rail permits her to turn to the left side (see Figure 8.8). She no longer can roll segmentally (initiating the turn with her head, then using her shoulder, her hip, and finally her lower extremities).

11. *Problem:* Mrs. Doe has difficulty fastening small buttons as a result of upper-extremity tremors and decreased fine motor coordination.
    Intervention: Mrs. Doe was given a button

hook/zipper pull device which, following training, she is using successfully (see Figures 8.9 and 8.10).

12. *Problem:* Mrs. Doe had difficulty drinking from glasses and cups and had been spilling hot and cold liquids.
    Intervention: Mrs. Doe was given a weighted cup with a lid, which has eliminated liquids spilling (see Figure 8.11).

13. *Problem:* Mrs. Doe's kitchen chair is a swivel-type. When going from standing to sitting, she does not always end up sitting squarely on the seat. She also has difficulty determining the seat's position.

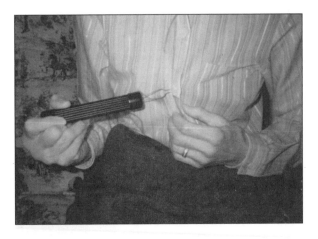

Figure 8.9. Mrs. Doe demonstrates the use of the button hook.

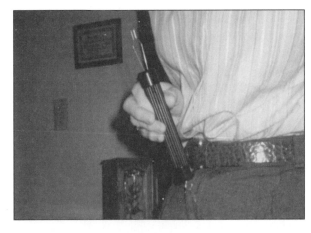

Figure 8.10. Mrs. Doe demonstrates the use of the zipper pull.

Intervention: The therapist recommended exchanging the chair for a stationary one or adapting the existing chair so it does not move. However, Mrs. Doe and her husband did not want to do this, feeling it was easier for her to sit down in a chair that swiveled. No change was made. The therapist will continue to monitor their safe use of the swivel chair.

14. *Problem:* Mr. Doe, as caregiver, appeared to be feeling as though this was a heavy burden, and showed some indications of "burnout."

Intervention: Mr. Doe was given a list of local agencies that provide volunteer companions and respite care. He was also trained in energy conservation techniques and stress management.

Follow-Up

Mrs. Doe had one fall during the time period that the therapist was providing the initial intervention. She had been making the bed, and lost her balance after throwing the bedspread across it. She was not using the walker during this activity. She was instructed to place the bedspread on the bed, then pull the corners of the bedspread to each corner of the mattress. This would eliminate the possibility of rapid body movements, weight shifting, and falls. She was encouraged to use the walker for balance during the activity. The bed is positioned in the room with easy access to all sides.

Mrs. Doe was given the "Nanny Walker" by Walker Works to use for a 5-day trial. This walker has hand grips designed for arthritic hand protection, an excellent braking system activated by applying downward pressure on the hand grips, a seat for resting, and a tray and basket for carrying articles. Since Mrs. Doe has difficulty applying uniform pressure to bicycle-style hand brakes, the downward pressure activated brakes worked better. She was shown how to use this device in her home. She demonstrated independent performance attaching and removing the tray when she needs to sit on the Walker's seat. She needs assistance to attach and remove the basket.

After the trial, a thorough discussion with Mr. and Mrs. Doe took place regarding the benefits of this device. Mr. Doe has concerns regarding the cost of the device ($359.00) and whether Mrs. Doe will be able to use it effectively for a long period. Due to

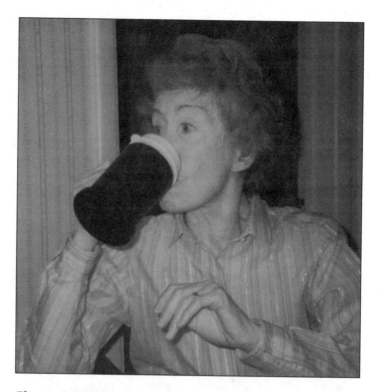

Figure 8.11. Mrs. Doe demonstrates the use of the weighted cup.

the decline in balance and coordination, he expressed concern his spouse may need a wheelchair later on. Then she would own a walker that would go unused. At this time, they are discussing the device with Mrs. Doe's physician to obtain a prescription for Medicare reimbursement.

Mrs. Doe had two more falls in the kitchen following the therapist's initial intervention. The therapist discussed with Mrs. Doe the importance of using her walker in all rooms, including the kitchen. Mrs. Doe had been refusing because, as she stated: "[the walker] makes me look older than I am." Her preferred way of getting about in the house was to hold onto the walls or the furniture.

In summary, Mrs. Doe reflects an elder with multiple challenges, many of which can be addressed with assistive devices and environmental interventions. She also represents a person who had many devices prior to her assessment, and was not using them well, or resisting their use because of the stigma she perceived attached to their use. The assessments and interventions discussed have occurred over an 8-month period. Mrs. Doe will continue to receive follow-up visits at least every 6 months, and phone calls monthly, as part of the comprehensive intervention approach being tested in the research project.

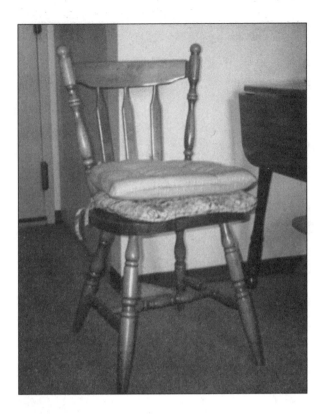

Figure 8.12. Mrs. Blue uses cushions on her dining room chair to make it easier to rise to standing.

Case 2: Mrs. Blue

General

Mrs. Blue is 70 years old and widowed. She was a homemaker and mother for 23 years, raising 5 children. She maintains regular contact with them and other family members. She had worked as a cashier and waitress prior to raising her family. Her education included some college, although she did not attain a degree. Her annual income is well under $10,000, which provides for her needs, but leaves little to spare. Aides provide housecleaning and laundry service 1 hour per day, 4 days per week. Occasionally, the aides accompany Mrs. Blue on shopping trips. Mrs. Blue enjoys working crossword puzzles, listening to music, sewing, and visiting friends in her building.

Assessment: Environment/Housing/Resources

Mrs. Blue lives alone in a subsidized apartment she has been renting for the past 8 years. The apartment is located in an urban area, and Mrs. Blue believes that the neighborhood is safe—she feels comfortable shopping alone in stores nearby. Her apartment building has an elevator, and her apartment is on one

level. She keeps her home neat and orderly, and is conscious of the importance of not having scatter rugs or cords on which she could trip. She uses two floor fans for cooling during the summer, and had a wall lamp installed over her work area. She has two emergency pull cords, one in her bathroom and one in the bedroom, although the one in the bedroom is behind the dresser and inaccessible. The bathroom pull cord is accessible from the toilet, but not from the tub.

Assessment: Medical Status

Mrs. Blue is 5' 3" tall and weighs 82 pounds. She had 8 physician visits in the 6 months prior to the assessment, and had been quite ill—she was unable to carry out daily tasks for about 10 weeks of that 6 month period. She takes 15 medications, and is diagnosed with 8 chronic illnesses. She has had arthritis for more than 30 years. She had scarlet fever as a child and has had heart problems, including pleurisy and arrhythmia, for more than 60 years. She has had digestive problems for 40 years; part of her stomach was removed due to peptic ulcers. She has emphysema, and has smoked for more than 30 years. She has back problems, with a possible lumbar fracture. She drinks little or no alcohol.

Mrs. Blue's medical conditions have had a major impact on her functional status and quality of life. She has little appetite, and has difficulty keeping food down as a result of her digestive and gallbladder problems. She recently lost 20 pounds. Her hyperactive thyroid often causes breathlessness and a choking sensation. Her broken back has affected her mobility and use of upper extremities. She experiences much pain, with a score of 34 (out of 40) on the Jette Pain Index.

Assessment: Physical/Sensory Status

Mrs. Blue describes her hearing and vision as good.

Mrs. Blue scored 42.6% physically disabled on the Sickness Impact Profile. Due to back problems, ROM/strength were not tested thoroughly. Due to back and heart problems, she's not allowed to push, pull, or lift beyond 5 pounds. Due to her broken back, arthritis, and a mastectomy, she does not bend to the floor or twist her trunk.

Assessment: Cognitive/Mental Status

Mrs. Blue demonstrates no cognitive impairment, scoring 30 (out of 30) on the MMSE. She is alert and oriented, and demonstrates appropriate problem-solving and memory skills. She scored 9 on the CESD, indicating no significant depression. She scored 33 (out of 40) on the Rosenberg Self-Esteem Scale, suggesting that self-esteem is moderately high. Mrs. Blue is quite social, and enjoys visiting and assisting other residents in her apartment building. She gets out of her building an average of five times per week, both on her own and with others.

Assessment: Functional Status

As a result of her broken back, Mrs. Blue cannot turn to get out of bed, and getting up and down from chairs and the toilet has become more difficult. It is impossible for her to reach and lift over 5 pounds. Ambulation and transfers are also becoming more difficult for her. She is able to use her toilet independently, but has difficulty sitting down and getting up. She purchased an over-the-toilet commode when she first started having back pain, but her bathroom is small, and the commode legs extend into the doorway, which could cause her to trip.

Mrs. Blue recently bought a new easy chair which is high and firm enough for her to more easily go from sitting to standing. She has placed several cushions on the dining room chair she sits in to raise the seat height (see Figure 8.12). She also finds these cushions more comfortable than sitting without them.

Because Mrs. Blue finds it very difficult to transfer out of bed, she sleeps on the sofa (see Figures 8.13 and 8.14). The bed did not provide something to grasp to help with her turning. On the sofa she positions pillows to keep herself on her side, and then holds onto the coffee table to get up.

On IADL, Mrs. Blue scored 11 (out of 14) on the OARS. She can independently use the telephone, shop within walking distance, prepare her meals, take her medications, and handle her money. However, walking any distance is difficult on some days for Mrs. Blue. She lives in a business area, and enjoys going out to walk and shop. It is difficult for her to carry her purchases home, so she only buys limited amounts on each trip. She is not able to use a cane or walker because of the position they require, and the limitations on lifting due to her back condition. She uses a grocery cart to carry items, but it is heavy and bulky to store and maneuver.

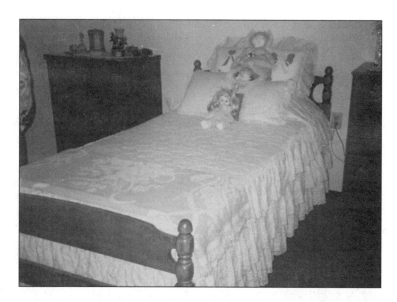

Figure 8.13. Mrs. Blue is unable to turn and transfer in her bed.

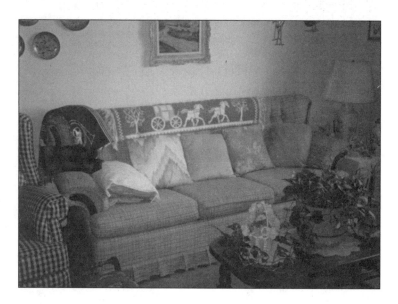

Figure 8.14. Mrs. Blue sleeps on this couch, and holds onto the coffee table to get up.

For meal preparation, Mrs. Blue often uses a microwave oven and a toaster oven. She is unable to reach into her higher cupboards, or lift items out of her lower cupboards. She often asks her aides to get things from these cabinets, but with the limited aide time, this is often not a practical solution.

Mrs. Blue does her own ironing but it is difficult for her to set up and take down the ironing board. She relies on neighbors to help her with this. Mrs. Blue has a phone on her bedroom dresser. On some days she moves very slowly and misses phone calls while trying to get to the bedroom. Other devices she uses include a remote control for her TV, a magnifying glass, and 3 large numbered clocks. She was using 14 assistive devices at the time of this assessment.

On the FIM, Mrs. Blue received a total score of 115 (out of 123). She is able to independently perform grooming, bathing, and dressing, although she fatigues easily and often stops to rest. For bathing, she uses a hand-held shower, long-handled brush, bath mat, shower chair, and grab bar for access into and out of the tub. Her tub area has two grab bars: One is on the end wall and out of her reach, and the other, on the side wall, is mounted at an inverted angle. This second grab bar is unsafe, as it is mounted backwards, and could cause her hand to slide downward when she is getting out of the tub; instead of being able to pull up to a standing position, she must push up to standing (see Figure 8.15). Use of this incorrectly mounted grab bar requires more strength in weaker muscle groups than those required for pulling. This grab bar also protrudes out 3.75 inches from the wall (1.5 inches is the standard), and Mrs. Blue frequently bumps her elbow on it when bathing. If her hand were to slip while pushing up, it could easily get caught between the wall and the bar. Mrs. Blue tends to use her sink for stability when stepping into or out of the tub. As a result the sink has loosened from the wall.

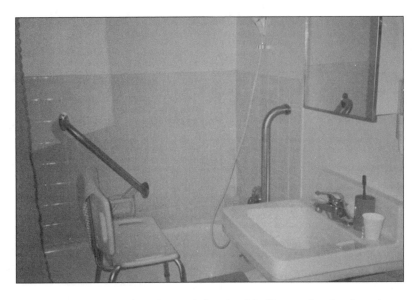

Figure 8.15. Note that the grab bar in this illustration is placed at the wrong angle.

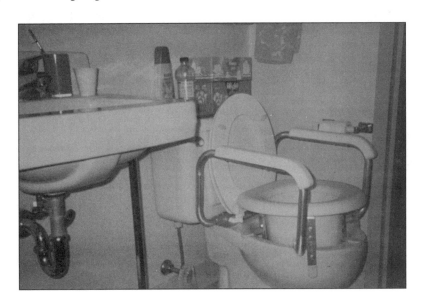

Figure 8.16. Mrs. Blue now has an adjustable raised toilet seat and a safety frame without legs, and legs were added to the sink.

Interventions

The following interventions were recommended:

1. *Problem:* There are a number of safety concerns with the way Mrs. Blue transfers into and out of the tub.
   Intervention: (1) The existing grab bar was replaced with one that extends 1.5 inches from the wall, and installed correctly. (2) A retractable wall-mounted grab bar was installed alongside the sink. This replaced the out-of-reach grab bar, and extends out far enough for appropriate use. With this grab bar, Mrs. Blue no longer needs to grab onto the sink.

2. *Problem:* Sink is coming loose from the wall.
   Intervention: Legs were added to the sink to provide stability, and it was refastened to the wall (see Figure 8.16).

3. *Problem:* Toilet transfers are difficult and unsafe, and the present commode is too large for Mrs. Blue's bathroom.
   Intervention: An adjustable raised toilet seat was provided, and a safety frame without legs was added to the toilet for getting on and off.

4. *Problem:* The pull cords in the tub and bedroom are inaccessible.

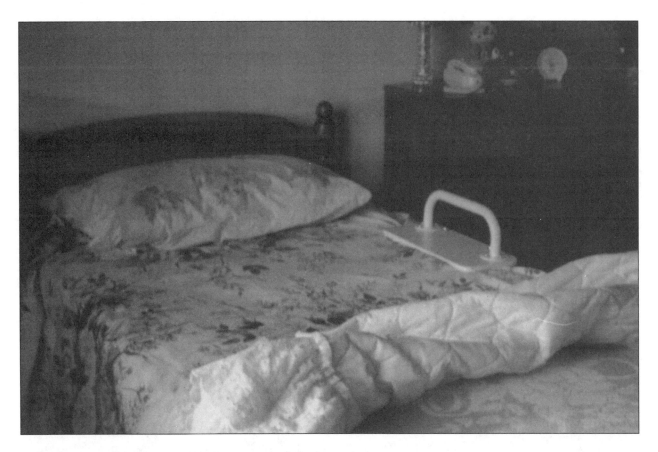

Figure 8.17. A handle was added to Mrs. Blue's bed.

Intervention: The pull cord in the tub was extended with a small pulley and lengthened. An accessible phone was added to the bedroom for emergency use.

5. *Problem:* Mrs. Blue is unable to turn and transfer in bed.

Intervention: A "handle" that fits on the mattress was added to the bed. This provides a place for Mrs. Blue to grasp for rolling over and sitting up (see Figure 8.17).

6. *Problem:* Mrs. Blue has difficulty transferring out of dining room chairs. These chairs are also uncomfortable on the bony prominences, and the two 1 inch cushions she was using tended to slide around.

Intervention: A 2-inch cushion which provides needed comfort without bottoming out, was custom made. This cushion has a "soft spot" in the coccyx area where pain occurred from pressure; softer foam was used in that area. The cushion was upholstered, with ties and Velcro straps sewn into the seams for fastening the cushions to the chair (see Figure 8.18).

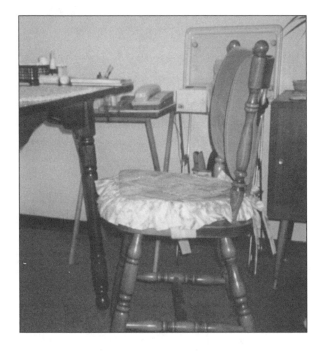

Figure 8.18. A 2-inch custom cushion with soft insert in the coccyx area was provided for Mrs. Blue's dining room chair.

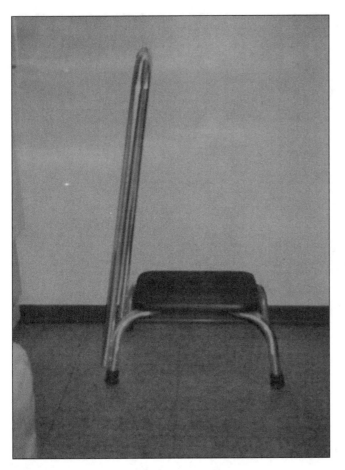

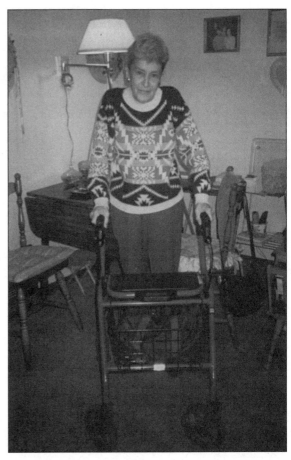

Figure 8.19. This footstool has helped Mrs. Blue reach items in the upper cabinets in her kitchen.

Figure 8.20. Mrs. Blue enjoys using her wheeled walker, with seat and basket.

7. *Problem:* Mrs. Blue has difficulty reaching into upper kitchen cupboards and bedroom closet shelves.

   Intervention: Mrs. Blue was given a footstool with a rail (see Figure 8.19).

8. *Problem:* Mrs. Blue can only reach partway into the lower kitchen cabinets. She cannot pull out and lift anything heavy up to the kitchen counter.

   Intervention: The lower stationary cupboard shelves were replaced with pullout shelves. This eliminated reaching into the cupboard. A height-manageable storage shelf was added in the closet (right off the kitchen) for heavier items such as the crock pot and certain bowls and pans. This solution eliminated the need to bend.

9. *Problem:* Mrs. Blue has difficulty walking distances due to fatigue and leg cramps. She also has difficulty carrying items back home. She has a doctor's order not to use a cane or

walker which would position her forward and require lifting.

Intervention: Mrs. Blue, with physician prescription, was given a wheeled walker with a seat and basket. This walker fosters appropriate posture, does not require lifting, and provides a basket for carrying items and a seat for resting (see Figure 8.20).

10. *Problem:* Placement of Mrs. Blue's one phone resulted in missing many calls.

    Intervention: Her existing phone was placed at her bedside within reach from the bed. She was given a cordless phone which can be kept within reach throughout the day. This has eliminated her problem with missing calls.

11. *Problem:* Mrs. Blue has difficulty reaching to the floor to pick up dropped objects.

    Intervention: Mrs. Blue was given a reacher to grasp dropped objects.

12. *Problem:* Mrs. Blue has difficulty setting up and taking down the ironing board.

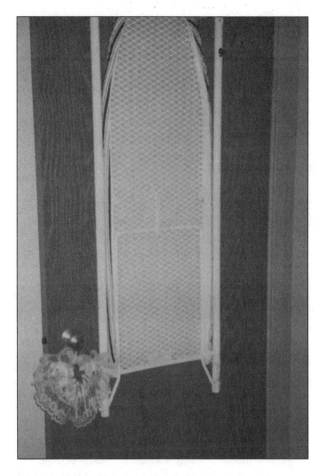

Figure 8.21. Mrs. Blue finds the door hanging fold-out ironing board easy to use.

Intervention: Mrs. Blue was given a door hanging fold-out ironing board, which she is able to manage.

13. *Problem:* Mrs. Blue needs more back support while working at her desk.
Intervention: Mrs. Blue was give a lumbar support for posture and comfort.

Follow-Up

On follow-up visits, additional interventions were provided:

1. The retractable grab bar in bathroom was changed to a floor to ceiling vertical grab bar because Mrs. Blue did not have strength to maneuver the retractable one.

2. A different bed rail was provided, because with the first one the mounting straps around the mattress rubbed on Mrs. Blue's skin. It was also difficult to make the bed with the first bed rail.

3. A body roll pillow was provided so that Mrs. Blue would sleep more comfortably in bed without rolling onto her back (which is a painful position). The body pillow keeps her positioned on her side, and keeps her legs abducted, thus reducing back and sciatic pain after a night's rest.

In summary, Mrs. Blue represents an elder who is remaining active in the face of multiple health problems, and using assistive technology to assist with her functional independence. She also reflects the importance of continued follow-up and an "experimental" approach—trying more than one device for a period of time, then another, until a satisfactory device is identified. Service providers must check back on the success of interventions, and be ready to make changes as needed.

Chapter 8 References

Abyad, A., & Boyer, J.T. (1992). Arthritis and aging. *Current Opinion in Rheumatology, 4*(2), 153–159.

Blasch, B.B., Saltzman, D.M., & Coombs, F. (1989). Evaluation of wandering behavior in elderly persons and interventions: A pilot study. *Rehab Research Progress Reports 25,* 296–297.

Bourgeoris, M.S. (1990). Enhancing conversation skills in patients with Alzheimer's disease using a prosthetic memory aid. *Journal of Applied Behavior Analysis, 23*(1), 29–42.

Broadhurst, M., & Stammers, C.W. (1988). A feeding mechanism for Parkinson's disease patients. *Journal of Medical Engineering & Technology 12*(1), 16.

Farris, D.S. (1988). Dynamic postural sway measurement in elderly fallers. *Rehab R&D Reports, 25,* p. 300.

Fillenbaum, G.G. (1988). *Multidimensional functional assessment of older adults: The duke older americans resources and services procedures.* Hillsdale NJ: Lawrence Erlbaum.

Folstein, M. (1975). Mini mental state: A practical method for grading the cognitive state of patients for the clinician. *Journal of Psychiatric Research, 12,* 189–198.

Fowles D.G. (1988). *A profile of older Americans 1988.* Washington, DC: American Association of Retired Persons.

Glass, L.E. (1986). Rehabilitation for deaf and hearing-impaired. In J. Brody & G.E. Ruff (Eds.), *Aging and Rehabilitation* (pp. 218–236). New York: Springer.

Haworth, E., Powell, R.H. & Mullex, G.P. (1983). Wheelchairs used by old people. *British Medical Journal, 28*(7), 260.

Hotchkiss, D. (1989). *The hearing impaired elderly population: Estimation, projection, and assessment.*

(Monograph Series A, #1). Washington, DC: Gallaudet Research Institute.

Jette, A.M. (1980). Functional status index: Reliability of a chronic disease evaluation instrument. *Archives of Physical Medicine and Rehabilitation, 71,* 108–113.

Labell, T.L., & Glassman, A.H. (1988). An aid for swing-lock partial denture removal. *Prosthetic Dentistry, 59,* 394.

LaPlante, M.P., Hendershot, G.E., & Moss, A.J. (1992). Assistive devices and home accessibility features: Prevalence, payment, need, and trends. *Advance data from vital and health statistics (No. 217).* Hyatts-ville, MD: National Center for Health Statistics.

Long, R.G. (1989). Effects of age and visual loss on independent outdoor mobility. *Rehabilitation R&D Progress Reports, 26,* pp. 364–265.

Mann, W.C. (1992a). Older workers with disabilities: Trends and legislation. *Technology and Disability, 1*(4), 37–46.

Mann, W.C. (1992b). Use of environmental control devices by elderly nursing home patients. *Assistive Technology, 4*(2), 60–65.

Mann, W.C, Granger, C., Hurren, D., Tomita, M., & Charvat, B. (in press). An analysis of problems with canes encountered by elderly persons. *Physical and Occupational Therapy in Geriatrics.*

Mann, W.C., Hurren, D., & Tomita, M. (1993a). Needs of home based older persons for assistive devices. *Technology and Disability, 2*(1), 1–11.

Mann, W.C., Hurren, D., & Tomita, M. (1993b). Comparison of assistive device use and needs of home-based older persons with different impairments. *American Journal of Occupational Therapy, 47,* 980–987.

Mann, W.C., Hurren, D., & Tomita, M. (in press). Assistive devices used by home-based elderly with arthritis. *American Journal of Occupational Therapy.*

Mann, W.C., Hurren, D., Tomita, M., Bengali, M., & Steinfeld, E. (1994). Environmental problems in homes of elders with disabilities. *The Occupational Therapy Journal of Research, 14,* 191–211.

Mann, W.C., Hurren, D.M., & Tomita, M.R. (1994). Assistive device needs of home-based elderly persons with hearing impairments. *Technology and Disability 3,* 47–61.

Mann, W.C., Hurren, D., Tomita, M., & Charvat, B. (1995). An analysis of problems with walkers encountered by elderly persons. *Physical and Occupational Therapy in Geriatrics, 13,* 1–2.

Mann, W.C., Karuza, J., Hurren, D., & Tomita, M. (1993a). Assistive devices for home-based elderly persons with cognitive impairments. *Topics in Geriatric Rehabilitation 8*(2), 35–52.

Mann, W.C., Karuza, J.K., Hurren, D., & Tomita, M. (1993b). Needs of home-based older persons for assistive devices. *Technology and Disability, 2*(1), 1-11.

Mann, W.C., Ottenbacher, K.J., Tomita, M.R., & Packard, S. (1994). Design of hand-held remotes for older persons with impairments. *Assistive Technology 6*(2), 140–146.

Mann, W.C., Tomita, M., Packard, S., Hurren, D., & Creswell, C. (1994). The need for information on assistive devices by older persons. *Assistive Technology 6*(2), 134–139.

Mayo, N.E. (1993). Epidemiology and recovery. In R.W. Teasell (Ed.), *Long term consequences of stroke: Physical medicine and rehabilitation: State of the art reviews* (p. 125). Philadelphia: Hanley and Belfus.

Mortimer, J.A. (1983). Alzheimer's disease and senile dementia: Prevalence and incidence. In B. Reisberg (Ed.), *Alzheimer's disease: The standard reference* (pp. 141–148). New York: The Free Press.

Norrgard, L.E. (1992). *Product report: Canes.* Washington, DC: American Association of Retired Persons.

O'Donnel, P.D. (1989). Electroymyographic incontinence alert device. *Rehabilitation R&D Progress Reports, 25,* 293.

Ottenbacher, K.J., Mann, W.C., Granger, C.V., Tomita, M., Hurren, D., & Charvat, B. (1994). Inter-rater agreement and stability of functional assessment in the community-based elderly. *Archives of Physical Medicine and Rehabilitation, 75,* 1297–1301.

Pawlson, L.G, Goodwin, M., & Keith, K. (1986). Wheelchair use by ambulatory nursing home residents. *Journal of the American Geriatrics Society, 34,* 12.

Prohaska, T., Mermelstein, R., Miller, B., & Jack, B. (1993). Functional status and living arrangements. In *Vital and health statistics: Health data on older Americans: United States, 1992, Series 3: Analytic and epidemiological studies no. 27* (DHHS Publication No. (PHS) 93–1411). Hyattsville, MD: U.S. Department of Health and Human Services.

Radloff, L.S., & Locke, B.Z. (1986). The community mental health assessment survey and the CES-D scale. In M.M. Weissman, J.K. Myers, & C.E. Ross (Eds.), *Community surveys of psychiatric disorders* (pp. 177–189). New Brunswick, NJ: Rutgers University.

Schwartz, R.G. (1989). Investment for an aging population. *Statistical Bulletin, 70,* 3.

Steinfeld, E., & Shea, S. (1993). *HyperHome resource: A technical information manager for home modification services to older people.* Proceedings of the RESNA Conference, Las Vegas, Nevada.

Symington, D.C., Lywood, D.W., Lawson, J.S., & McLean, J. (1986). Environmental control systems in chronic care hospitals and nursing homes. *Archives of Physical Medicine and Rehabilitation, 67,* 36.

U.S. Bureau of the Census. (1986). Disability, functional limitation, and health insurance coverage: 1984/85. *Current Population Reports*, Series p-70, No. 8. Washington DC: U.S. Government Printing Office.

U.S. Senate Special Commission on Aging. (1991). *Aging America trends and projections.* (DHHS Publication No. (FCoA) 91-28001). Washington, DC: U.S. Department of Health and Human Services.

Yelin, E., & Katz, P.P. (1990). Transitions in health status among community dwelling elderly people with arthritis: A national, longitudinal study. *Arthritis and Rheumatism, 33,* 1205–1215.

Yelin, E. (1992). Arthritis: The cumulative impact of a common chronic condition. *Arthritis and Rheumatism 35,* 489–497.

Chapter 8 Study Questions

1. Discuss the consumer perspective in the selection of assistive technology for older persons.

2. Discuss each of the following considerations in assistive technology interventions for older persons:
   a. age
   b. diagnosis
   c. presence or absence of caregiver(s)
   d. setting
   e. roles of elder
   f. environmental factors
   g. disability

3. Describe and provide examples of the use of assistive technology for safety and prevention with elders.

4. Describe how assistive technology can be used to promote independence in the following areas:
   a. mobility
   b. activities of daily living
   c. instrumental activities of daily living
   d. work
   e. leisure

5. Describe the use of assistive devices by elders for the following impairments:
   a. hearing impairment
   b. vision impairment
   c. cognitive impairment
   d. impairment in communication

6. Describe each of the following assessment instruments and their possible use in considering assistive technology for older persons:
   a. FIM
   b. OARS-IADL section
   c. OTFACT

7. Interview an elder you know, perhaps a grandparent. Determine impairments and discuss possible use of assistive technology. For example, if this elder has some hearing impairment, is he or she aware of assistive listening devices available at local electronic stores? Is he or she familiar with the closed captioning feature available on all new televisions? If this elder has moderate to severe impairments, be prepared to make a referral to an appropriate agency for assessment.

Unit IV:
Assistive
Technology
Services

Introduction to Unit IV

A model for assistive technology service provision is presented in Figure IV.1. The five major steps in assistive technology service delivery are:

1. referral
2. screening
3. assessment
4. intervention
5. support

Service delivery programs vary in their procedures and in the personnel involved. Some steps might be combined in certain programs while others follow the sequence of steps. An overview of these five steps is presented in this introduction to Unit IV. More detail on assessment, intervention, and support is provided in Chapters 5, 6, and 7, respectively.

Referrals can come from a number of different sources. Often a person with a disability will learn that assistive technology services are available and will directly contact the provider. In other cases, a family member or friend may contact the assistive technology service provider and schedule an appointment for a screening. Most referrals come from other service providers, such as rehabilitation professionals, special education teachers, physicians, and rehabilitation counselors—especially counselors working in state vocational rehabilitation agencies.

The flow of referrals varies with the type of assistive technology services available. Some providers are very specialized. For example, in New York State, the Commission for the Blind and Visually Handicapped has established technology centers that offer computer assessment and training services exclusively for persons who are blind or have low vision. Some hospital-based rehabilitation programs offer basic services for assistive devices targeted at activities of daily living but are not prepared to offer high-technology services.

To achieve a flow of referrals, publicity about available services is necessary. When promoting your services it is important to be clear about both the breadth and depth of your program. The types of equipment and professionals available, the disability populations served, the types of services offered (assessment, intervention, support)—all must be carefully delineated.

Figure IV.2, entitled "What is the Center for Assistive Technology?" contains the text from a professional services brochure of the Center for Assistive Technology (CAT), an assistive technology service provider connected with the State University of New York at Buffalo. Note that the types of services provided are clearly listed, such as "computer access" and "augmentative communication." The brochure does not list "orthotics and prosthetics," and no one reading the brochure is likely to make the mistake of believing that CAT provides these services.

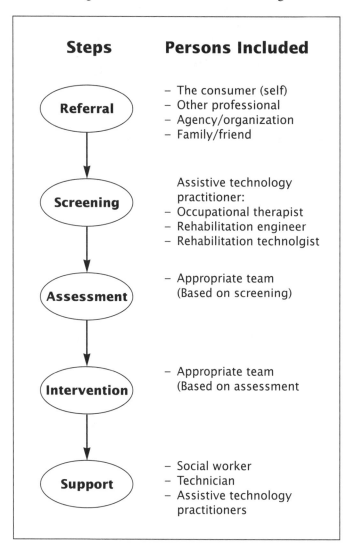

Figure IV.1. Steps in assistive technology service delivery.

What Is CAT?

The Center for Assistive Technology (CAT) conducts service, education and research programs at the University at Buffalo, on assistive technology for persons with disabilities.

CAT has a team of professionals representing multiple disciplines, including the fields of architecture, gerontology, law, medicine, occupational therapy, physical therapy, rehabilitation counseling, rehabilitation engineering, social work, special education, speech pathology, and augmentative communication.

CAT offers personal assessment, and assistive technology evaluation and training services in the areas of seating, positioning and mobility, computer access, augmentative communication, early intervention for infants (birth to 3 years), assistive technology needs for school age children (3 to 21 years), and environment access modifications to home, school, public facilities, and the workplace.

CAT professionals help persons with physical, sensory, developmental or cognitive disabilities, apply technology to achieve their desired outcomes in education, vocation and personal independence.

How Does CAT Provide Services?

CAT is an authorized fee-for-service provider for clients covered by VESID, CBVH, Medicare, Medicaid, Worker's Compensation, and some private insurance.

What Services Does CAT Provide?

CAT professionals provide personal assessments, equipment recommendations, service referrals, device training, and follow-up services for a range of technology-related services such as the following.

• Seating, Positioning and Mobility

CAT's team of rehabilitation engineers, physicians and therapists provides wheelchair seating, positioning and mobility services. It evaluates, prescribes and fabricates systems for pressure relief, postural support, and wheeled mobility.

• Computer Access

Persons with physical disabilities are assessed on appropriate controls, switches, and keyboards for access to computers or environmental control systems. Persons with visual impairments are assessed on devices featuring enlarged print, refreshable Braille, voice ouput and/or voice recognition systems.

• Augmentative Communication

Speech therapists, augmentative communication specialists, and occupational therapists assess client needs, evaluate and recommend appropriate devices, and provide training in their use.

• Office and Home Modifications

Professionals from the disciplines of architecture, design, engineering, occupational therapy, and rehabilitation counseling consult with consumers, counselors, and employers to make the home environment, the workplace, and public facilities more accessible to persons with disabilities.

• Early Intervention for Infants

Parents, caregivers, and service providers of infants (birth to 3 years) participate in team assessments to determine the infant's needs and capabilities related to the applications of assistive technology for infants with special needs. Where appropriate, assistive technology applications are recommended and training in their use is provided.

• Education

Students with disabilities, their parents, caregivers, and education personnel in primary, secondary, and higher education programs participate in team assessments of their educational goals, capabilities, and needs related to seating/positioning, assistive technology devices, and training in the use of assistive technology in their educational programs.

• Vocational Training

Persons with cognitive disabilities receive skills assessments, computer-based vocational training, work internships, job counseling, and referrals for competitive work placement opportunities.

• Information and Referral

CAT is a WNY regional Center in the New York State, Technology Related Assistance for Individuals with Disabilities (TRAID) Program, charged with providing information and referral services on assistive technology devices, services, and resources to consumers, caregivers, and service providers.

The TRAID Program is described in a separate brochure available from CAT.

Figure IV.2. What is the Center for Assistive Technology/University at Buffalo? Figure provided by author.

Screening

Once the referral is received, an appointment is made for an initial screening. Depending on the referral and the service provider, the screening may take place at the service provider's facility, or it may take place at the home, work site, or school of the consumer. Initial screenings are usually conducted by a professional trained in assistive technology, such as occupational therapists, physical therapists, speech pathologists, and rehabilitation engineers.

The purpose of the initial screening is to get an overall sense of the strengths and limitations of the person with a disability, and to determine the tasks with which he or she is having difficulty, the environments within which those tasks occur, and some initial possibilities for assistive devices. Although not always carried out in practice, the person with the disability should play a key role in the screening process—indicating which tasks are difficult, why they are difficult, and discussing areas of interest. With this information, the person conducting the screening will determine three facts:

1. Whether the referral is appropriate or the person should be referred elsewhere.
2. Assuming the referral is appropriate, whether there is a "quick" and obvious solution so that a full assessment is not necessary.
3. Which of the assistive technology team members should be assembled for a full assessment if one is necessary.

Figure IV.3 provides an example of a screening form, showing the kind of information typically collected in an inital screening.

Assessment

Just a decade ago, a therapist was considered the rehabilitation professional responsible for assessing and "prescribing" assistive devices. Times have changed in two major ways. First, today's assistive technology is much too complex for one team member to handle alone. Second, attitudes toward disability have changed considerably, and the person who will use the device—the consumer—is much more at the center of the process of assistive technology selection. New assistive technology professionals, together with the consumer and significant others, form the assessment team. It is very common for the occupational therapist to head the assistive technology team, selecting and organizing the other professionals and technicians who will participate in the assessment process.

The major outcome of the assessment process is a recommendation. The recommendation may take several forms:

1. remediative therapy with no device,
2. therapy with a device,
3. no therapy but a device, or
4. no intervention, but perhaps a referral for some alternate treatment.

If a device or devices are recommended, they are listed in the assessment report. Chapter 5 describes the assessment process in detail.

ASSISTIVE DEVICE SCREENING FORM

NAME _____

ADDRESS _____

CITY _____ STATE _____ ZIP _____

PHONE HOME _____ WORK _____

REFERRED BY _____

REFERRING AGENCY _____

DIFFICULT TASKS _____

POTENTIAL DEVICES/SOLUTIONS _____

SCREENING OUTCOME
_____ Provide Solution Without Further Assesment

_____ Full Assessment - List Team Members Needed:

_____

_____

_____ Refer to _____

FUNDING OPTIONS

_____

_____

Figure IV.3. Assistive device screening form.

Intervention

Once a device is recommended, it has to be either purchased or fabricated. Simple low-cost assistive devices can be bought in quantity and stored on-site in the facility. Unfortunately, this is not true for most assistive technology, which is too expensive and changes too rapidly to permit keeping a supply on hand. Intervention begins with the delivery of the device and setting it up for the person with a disability. Training in the use of the device is a key component of the intervention process, and training may take as much as 6 or more weeks.

Support

Support actually begins after the initial screening. The successful end of training in the use of an assistive devices marks the beginning of a long period of support. Every device must have a maintenance schedule; the consumer must have options for repair of the device if it breaks down or becomes damaged. In addition, the device may need to be modified or replaced with an alternate device as the technology changes and as the consumer changes, grows, gains function, or loses function. Chapter 7 describes support services in more detail.

Chapter 9:
Assessment Services:
Person, Device, Family, and Environment

I. Assessing the Person With Disabilities
  A. Motor Performance
  B. Cognitive Performance
      1. Motivation
      2. Intelligence
      3. Judgment
      4. Attention Span
      5. Problem Solving
      6. Memory
  C. Communication
  D. Sensory
  E. Changes Over Time

II. Assessing the Environment
  A. Home
  B. Work and School
  C. Community

III. Assessing Tasks
  A. Steps in Task Completion
  B. Strengths Needed
  C. Potential for Changing the Task

IV. Assessing Devices
  A. Capability to Assist in Task Completion
  B. Appearance
  C. Cost–Benefit
  D. Off-the-Shelf Versus Custom-Made

V. Person–Environment–Task–Device Interactions
  A. Person–Environment
  B. Person–Tasks
  C. Tasks–Device
  D. Environment–Tasks–Device
  E. Person–Device
  F. Interaction of All Factors

VI. Example of Assessment

9.

Assessment Services: Person, Device, Family, and Environment

William C. Mann, PhD, OTR/L, and Kathleen A. Beaver, BS

Like screening, the assessment process considers the person, the environment, tasks, and devices. Figure 9.1 illustrates these assessment components, the interactions among the components, and the major subcomponents.

Occupational therapists working in acute rehabilitation typically consider assistive devices as part of their overall occupational therapy evaluation, and usually the devices are more traditional activities of daily living (ADL) aids. For assessments that may result in recommendations for more complex and expensive devices, information from a number of sources may be called upon, including the comprehensive occupational therapy evaluation, if available.

Occupational therapists often serve as team leader in an assistive technology assessment. This is due in part to the history of occupational therapy involvement with assistive devices, and in part to the breadth of knowledge that occupational therapists hold in the critical assessment components—knowledge of persons, including psychological, physiological, and sociological factors; knowledge of environments, especially home and work-site evaluations for accommodating persons with disabilities; knowledge of tasks—the skill in conducting activity analyses; and knowledge of assistive devices. This knowledge of assistive devices may be more general than specific. Occupational therapy entry-level curricula are now addressing this training, as are continuing education programs for occupational therapists. This chapter will follow the components and subcomponents as listed in Figure 9.1.

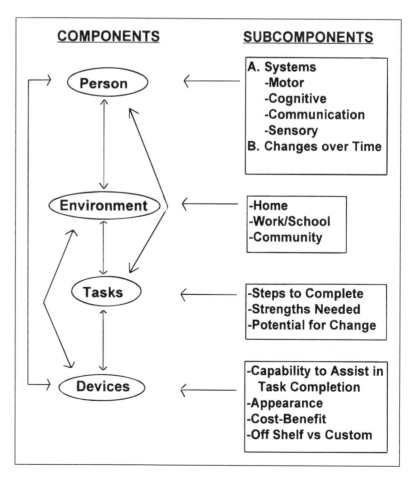

Figure 9.1. Focus of assistive technology assessment.

Assessing the Person With Disabilities

Motor Performance

Occupational therapists are skilled in assessing motor performance and motor performance deficits. Strength, endurance, and range of motion are basic occupational therapy concerns during the evaluation of persons with physical disabilities. In considering assistive devices, occupational therapists are concerned with three major issues related to motor performance: (a) helping the person to achieve the optimal position for using a device; (b) determining the type of controls needed to operate the device; and (c) determining if a device is needed specifically for achieving a motor function (e.g., mobility through a powered wheelchair). A seating and mobility evaluation form is presented in Figure 9.2. A thorough evaluation includes assessing both the person and the environments in which he or she will use the wheelchair.

Cognitive Performance

The assistive technology assessment must consider cognitive function. We include motivation, intelligence, judgment, attention span, problem solving, and memory as components of cognitive functioning. Each of these is considered below.

Motivation

We all have varying amounts of motivation for different activities, and motivation for these specific activities varies over time. It is essential to ascertain the potential consumer's motivation to participate in the tasks that might be assisted by a device. Unless the consumer is motivated, the device will not be used—and in the past, the usage rate of devices has been much too low.

It is difficult to measure motivation—measurement is more of an art than a science. In the course of an assessment, the therapist must ask a number of questions that seek to determine just how motivated the person is. For example, asking people how they enjoy spending their time can be an indirect way of seeking information on interest in employment. In the case of disability sustained through injury, premorbid history can also provide an indication of motivation. It is important not to underestimate a person's potential motivation. An individual with a disability may not realize the potential he or she has to complete tasks, given appropriate assistive technology.

Keep in mind that many people are "shy" about using tools—especially electronic tools such as computers. We may say that they are not motivated to use computers, but this might be giving up too easily. For a person with a disability, who is also shy about using computers, a rigorous training program may make him or her feel more comfortable about using them. The obvious benefits gained, once realized by the person, may serve to eliminate all future shyness.

Intelligence

Standardized tests of intelligence may serve as a measure to judge intelligence. The assistive technology assessment team would review the results of these tests, typically administered by a psychologist outside the team's assessment. The assessment team must recognize strengths and limitations in intelligence, in order to judge just how complex a device can be and still be used successfully. If the device is too simple, the person's full potential may not be realized; conversely, if the device is too complex, it will not be used to its fullest capability.

Judgment

The ability of the consumer to assess correctly his or her own strengths and limitations is itself a strength. If the consumer is overly optimistic about a device, and his or her ability to use it, disillusionment and abandonment of the device may occur. Safety is another important consideration in assessing judgment. Some devices may be dangerous if used incorrectly.

Attention Span

For a person with traumatic brain injury, a learning disability, or mental retardation, the ability to attend to a task for an extended period of time may be limited, and this could have an effect on device use. One of the best ways to assess attention span is to ask the person to complete some tasks; observe how long the person can stay with the task and whether he or she is able to complete it.

Problem Solving

Problem solving is closely related to intelligence and judgment. Many devices, especially those associated with computers, require good problem-solving skills in order to gain the maximum benefit. When a device stops working, problem-solving skills are needed to determine why it is not working and to plan a course of action to correct the problem. The plan should also consider how to substitute for the device, if it should have to go out for repairs.

Wheelchair Seating, Positioning, and Mobility Evaluation

Identification Information
Client _____

Evaluation Date _____

Contact _____

Assessment Team

_____

_____

_____

_____

Background

Referral Service _____

Disability _____

Age _____

Sensory Deficits (Circle):

    Vision   Hearing   Speech

Family/Therapist/Aids Present _____

Seating Mobility Goals

_____

_____

_____

_____

Transportation

Primary (Circle):   Self   Family   Public   Van Service

Secondary (Circle): Self   Family   Public   Van Service

	Vehicle Type	Accessibility	Tie Downs
Primary	_____	_____	_____
Secondary	_____	_____	_____

Home Accessibility

Entrance_____

Width of smallest doorway_____

Bathroom_____

Other issues _____

Work or School Accessibility

(Circle): School Work

Where _____

Distance From Home _____

Accessibility Issues? _____

Restroom Accessibility _____

Width of smallest doorway_____

Leisure Activities/Hobbies _____

Current Equipment

Manual (Circle):   Self-propulsion   Dependent propulsion

Power (Circle):   Joystick   Sip-puff   Switch

Manufacturer (Circle): E&J   Invacare   Quickie   Fortress   Other

Model_____   Age of Equipment_____   Condition _____

Seat (Type)   Sling   Solid

    Width 12" 14" 16" 18" 20"   Depth 14" 16" 18" 20" 22" 24"

Cushion Type _____

Back (Circle):   Sling   Solid   Commercial _____

    Laterals (Circle):   Right   Left   Height _____

    Recline (Circle):   Yes   No   Tilt-In-Space (Circle):   Yes No

Headrest (Circle): Fixed Adjustable   Manufacturer _____

Armrest (Circle):   Std....Desk   Adj. Height   Footrest (Circle) Swingaway Elevating

Hrs/day in chair_____   Transfers (Circle): Independent   Assist   Dependent

Features of current system that are disliked_____

Features needed or desired that aren't present on this chair/seating system _____

(continued)

Figure 9.2. Seating/positioning assessment (developed at the Center for Therapeutic Applications of Technology, University at Buffalo).

Assessment

Medical
    Recent surgeries _____
    Significant medical problems _____
Neuromotor
    Reflexes (Circle)   ATNR   STR   TLRS   EXT THRUST
    Tonal Patterns
                left   right
        UEs   ____   ____
        LEs   ____   ____
        Trunk   ____   ____
Functional (Circle):
        Head control   Poor   Fair   Good
        Trunk control   Poor   Fair   Good
        Mobility   Walk/Stand/Scoot/Crawl
        Hand dominance   Right   Left   Ambidextrous
        Fine motor   Absent   Normal   Poor   Fair   Good
        Gross motor   Absent   Poor   Fair   Good
Orthopedic
    Spine (Circle)   Scoliosis   Kysosis   Lordosis   Fixed   Flexible
    Pelvis
        Tilt   Anterior   Posterior
            Fixed   Flexible
        Rotation   Right   Left
            Fixed   Flexible
        Obliquity   Right   Left
            Fixed   Flexible
    LE ROM _____
    UE ROM _____

Speech (Circle):   Verbal   Nonverbal   Aug.Comm.Device
Sensation (Circle):   Intact   Impaired   Absent
Independent ADL (Circle):   Dressing   Feeding   Bathing   Toiletting
        Transfers
Pressure
    Skin Breakdown History (Circle):   Yes   No
    Location: _____
Positioning Simulation (attach simulator form for each system tried)
Recommendations
    1._____
    2._____
    3._____
    4._____
    5._____
    6.

Figure 9.2. Seating/positioning assessment (continued).

Memory

The ability to remember instructions will determine how complex a device can be and still be used successfully.

Communication

For a person with a communication impairment, the assessment process considers the current and future needs of the person in relation to available augmentative communication devices. Major needs that are considered in the selection process are outlined by Yorkston and Karlan (1986) and presented in Table 9.1.

Sensory

Three very important senses are vision, hearing, and tactile. Most persons referred for assistive technology services who have vision or hearing impairments have already had comprehensive vision and/or hearing examinations, and alternative interventions, such as surgery, have been deemed not appropriate. Given that a person has a hearing or visual impairment, assessment of the other areas (such as motor and cognitive) will determine the type of assistive technology recommended. Tactile sensation may be tested, in consideration of using the sense of touch for receiving information (such as Braille for a person who is blind, or vibration for a person with a severe hearing impairment).

Changes Over Time

The assistive technology assessment team must consider change as part of the assessment process. Many persons with disabilities will show either gains or losses in function. A person who has a progressive degenerative neurological disease will gradually lose function, while a person with a recent traumatic brain injury may show marked improvement in cognitive function. In assessing a person, these potential changes must be noted and considered in recommendations for assistive devices, as well as for the type of follow-up support recommended.

Assessing the Environment

Environments can be modified to accommodate persons with disabilities. Environments are also a factor in the decision to recommend certain types of devices. Three major environments are discussed below.

Home

Occupational therapists have traditionally provided home assessments for persons with disabilities. New standards for housing consider the needs of persons with disabilities, and architects now follow these standards in new construction. Often, therapists find themselves in an older home that requires some structural modification, and an architect may participate in planning these modifications.

The therapist considers entrances to the home, floor coverings, thresholds, access to electrical controls, lighting, furniture, kitchen layout (counters, work area, table, appliances), bed location (type and height), organization of closets and other cabinets, security (locks), door and cabinet handles, stairs, toilets, sinks, bathtub/shower, mirrors, telephones, and the yard or porch. For each of these areas, the therapist is concerned with the question: "Is the environment supportive (or inhibitive) of tasks that occur in this area?"

Work and School

Getting into and out of the facility, as well as access to bathrooms, dining rooms, and break rooms are basic for schools and work sites. The most personal part of the environment is the work area or workstation. For a student, this is the desk, the table in the library, the counter in the lab. For an employee, this may be the station on the assembly line, or the office workstation. The therapist assesses basic facility accessibility issues, as well as the workstation, to determine whether modifications are needed.

Community

Access to parks, theaters, shopping centers, and other community facilities is essential to quality of life for persons who are disabled. The occupational therapist works with the person in determining which community facilities will be used and assesses them for accessibility. If there are problems with accessibility, the therapist will either recommend working with persons in the community facilities for modifications, or recommend devices that can overcome the obstacles to accessibility.

Assessing Tasks

Steps in Task Completion

The occupational therapist works closely with the consumer as well as teachers, employers, and parents in determining the tasks that (a) the person cannot perform or has difficulty performing, and (b) are important in fulfilling a particular role. Once a list of tasks is drafted, prioritizing them will point to the tasks that should receive immediate attention. The occupational therapist breaks down each task into its components. Figure 9.3 is an activity analysis form.

Table 9.1. Examples of Communication Needs Statements.

Positioning

In bed:
- while supine
- while sitting
- in a variety of positions

In adaptive therapeutic positioning:
- side-lying
- in a prone stander
- prone over a bolster

Related to mobility
- carrying the system while walking
- in a manually controlled wheelchair
- with a lapboard

Other equipment:
- eating devices (cups, spoons, feeding devices)
- orally intubated
- with electric wheelchair controls
- with environmental control units
- with adaptive toys or microcomputer work/learning stations

Communication Partners
- someone who cannot read or who has cognitive delays or deficits
- someone who is unfamiliar with the system
- someone who is across the room or in another room
- someone who is an augmentative system user

Locations
- single rooms with multiple activity locations
- noisy rooms
- multiple rooms/settings
- car or van
- workstation

Message Needs
- call attention to/initiate an interaction
- carry on a conversation or take turns in play or social interaction
- take class notes
- respond to teacher's questions
- participate in academic or vocational activities
- construct messages and prepare written text

Modality of Communication
- communicate across a distance
- prepare printed message
- talk on the telephone
- access other equipment (e.g., environmental control units)

Yorkston & Karlan, 1986.

Strengths Needed

Part II of the Activity Analysis form (Figure 9.3) lists potential task requirements.

Potential for Changing the Task

As part of the task analysis, the therapist will determine if there is potential for (a) changing the task so that the person can do it; (b) providing an assistive device to assist in task completion; or (c) determining that it is not possible for the person to complete the task and possibly suggesting alternative tasks. If the task is critical to role performance, it may be possible to have someone else complete it; on the other hand, it may force a reexamination of goals, and possible selection of an alternative that does not include this or similar tasks.

Assessing Devices

Capability to Assist in Task Completion

Members of the assistive technology team must be very familiar with available devices and their features and limitations. This does not mean that every team member must know about every device. It does mean that every team should have at least one expert intimately familiar with the type of device(s) that might be recommended. For example, if the person has a communication problem, a speech pathologist familiar with augmentative communication systems should be a member of the assistive technology assessment team.

Occupational therapists must become familiar with the range of available devices. Depending on the population you work with, your "intimate familiarity" should match the kinds of devices used by persons who are members of that population. Understanding what a specific device can and cannot do is essential information needed in preparing a recommendation to purchase a device. Awareness of similar product offerings, and the different features each offers, will ensure that the best possible device is recommended.

Appearance

Many devices go unused because of their appearance. Persons with disabilities no more want to be seen with a clunky unattractive device than you would with a rusty old car. In considering various features of similar products, appearance must be considered.

ACTIVITY (TASK) ANALYSIS: PART I: ACTIVITY SUMMARY

Name _____ Date _____

A. Name of activity _____

B. Brief description of activity _____

_____

_____

_____

C. Tools/equipment associated with activity

_____

_____

D. Materials/supplies associated with activity

_____

_____

E. Space/Environmental requirements

_____

_____

F. Sequence of major steps, time required for each step

_____

_____

G. Precautions

_____

_____

H. Contraindications _____

I. Special considerations (age appropriateness, educational requirements, cultural relevance, sexual identification, other)

_____

_____

J. Acceptable criteria for completed project

_____

_____

(continued)

Figure 9.3. Activity analysis forms. From *Activity Analysis Handbook* (pp. 2-16–2-24) by N.K. Lamport, M.S. Coffey, & G.I. Hersch, 1989, Thorofare, NJ: Slack, Inc. Copyright© 1989 by Slack. Reprinted by permission.

PART II-OCCUPATIONAL PERFORMANCE COMPONENTS

Indicate the skill components necessary to complete the task.

SENSORIMOTOR COMPONENTS
1. Neurological

____Reflex integration

____Range of motion
>   ___active
>   ___passive
>   ___active assistive

____Gross and fine coordination
>   ___muscle control
>   ___coordination
>   ___dexterity

____Strength and endurance
>   ___building strength, cardio/pulmonary reserve
>   ___increasing length of work period
>   ___decreasing fatigue/strain

2. Sensory integration

____Sensory awareness
>   ___tactile awareness
>   ___stereognosis
>   ___kinesthesia
>   ___proprioceptive awareness
>   ___ocular control
>   ___vestibular awareness
>   ___auditory awareness
>   ___gustatory awareness
>   ___olfactory awareness

____Visual-spatial awareness
>   ___figure ground
>   ___form constancy
>   ___position in space

____Body integration
>   ___body schema
>   ___postural balance
>   ___bilateral motor coordination
>   ___right-left discrimination
>   ___visual-motor integration
>   ___crossing the midline
>   ___praxis

Figure 9.3. Activity analysis forms (continued).

COGNITIVE

____Orientation

____Conceptualization/comprehension

___Concentration
___Attention span
___Memory

____Cognitive Integration

___Generalization
___Problem Solving
___defining or evaluating the problem
___organizing a plan
___making decisions/judgement
___implementing plan
___evaluating decision/judgement

PSYCHOSOCIAL COMPONENTS

____Self-Management

___Self-expression
___experiencing/recognizing a range of emotions
___having an adequate vocabulary
___writing and speaking skills
___use of nonverbal signs and symbols

___Self-Control
___observing own and others' behavior
___recognizing need for behavior/action change
___imitating new behaviors
___directing energies into stress-reducing behaviors

___Dyadic interaction
___Understanding norms of communication and interaction
___Setting limits on self and others
___Compromising and negotiating
___Handling stress
___Cooperating and competing with others
___Responsible relying on self and others

___Group interaction
___Performing social/emotional roles and tasks
___Understanding simple group process
___Participating in a mutually beneficial group

Figure 9.3. Activity analysis forms (continued).

TASK REQUIREMENTS

____Work patterns
   ___Light
   ___Moderator
   ___Heavy

____Method
   ___Structured
   ___Methodical
   ___Repetitive
   ___Expressive
   ___Creative
   ___Neatness
   ___Physical Contact
   ___Protective

PART III OCCUPATIONAL PERFORMANCE MODIFICATION
Indicate ways this activity might be modified to increase independent function

THERAPEUTIC ADAPTATIONS

____Orthotics
   ___Static or dynamic positioning
   ___Relieve pain
   ___Maintain joint alignment
   ___Protect joint integrity
   ___Improve function
   ___Decrease deformity

____Prosthetics

____Assistive/Adaptive Equipment
   ___Architectural modification
   ___Environmental modification
   ___Assistive equipment
   ___Wheelchair modification

PREVENTION

____Energy conservation
   ___Energy-saving procedures
   ___Activity restriction
   ___Work simplification
   ___Time management
   ___Environmental organization

____Joint protection/Body mechanics
   ___Proper body mechanics
   ___Avoiding static/deforming postures
   ___Avoiding excessive weight bearing
   ___Positioning
   ___Coordinating daily living activities

Figure 9.3. Activity analysis forms (continued).

Cost–Benefit

Many assistive devices are expensive. "Expensive," of course, is simply a concept that varies with the amount of money available to a person. For our purposes, when devices start costing over a few hundred dollars, they can be considered expensive. For persons purchasing devices with their own funds, it is important that they understand just what a device can and cannot do in assisting them in completing tasks. For third-party payers, it is essential that the assistive technology assessment team carefully document the expected benefits along with the cost of the device. Public policy on what is "fundable" through public sources of funds is in a relatively early stage for most assistive technology, and thorough documentation may make the difference between funding and not funding a particular recommendation.

Off-the-Shelf Versus Custom-Made

Whenever possible, commercially available devices are preferable. They are almost always less expensive; they usually come with a warranty and some system for maintenance and repairs; and they often offer consultation support in the operation of the device. However, there are many excellent devices that have never made it to market because of low demand, or have not yet been invented. It may be necessary to design a very individualized solution to a person's task needs, and part of this solution may be modifying of an existing device, or designing and building an entirely new device.

Person–Environment–Task–Device Interactions

Assessment of the person, environment, tasks, and devices cannot be done in isolation from each other. Therapists cannot simply assess the person, then the environment, then the tasks, and then the devices. Ultimately, assessment must consider the person–environment–task–device interaction simultaneously. Experienced therapists grasp this interaction with little effort. A useful exercise—very helpful while gaining experience—is to consider the interactions of each possible combination of two components and then put them together.

Person–Environment

In considering the person, one must consider the environment in which he or she lives. What supportive resources are available in the environment? These resources include facilities, such as grab bars in the bathroom, and people, such as a spouse or parent who can provide certain kinds of assistance.

In considering the environment, the therapist considers the person in that environment. What does the person need from the environment that may be missing? If the person has difficulty coming to a standing position, then grab bars may need to be added. If the person is also weak, then a modified chair may be needed to help the person come to a standing position.

In summary, the therapist considers the strengths and limitations of the person and the environment and looks for an optimal fit between the two. This may require modification of the environment, or—in extreme cases—a change in environment.

Person–Tasks

At first glance, this interaction seems simplistic: What tasks does the person do? But assistive technology practitioners take a much closer look at the person and the tasks. Which tasks does the person *need* to do (such as activities of daily living and school- or work-related tasks) and which does the person *want* to do (such as skiing or going to concerts)? Which aspects of these tasks are difficult or impossible for the person to do? Why are they difficult or impossible?

An essential skill of the assistive technology practitioner is this understanding of person and task. The practitioner does not simply conclude, "This person has low vision." Instead, the analysis is, "This person has been working as a copy editor, a job that has required reading fine print for most of each 8-hour day. At this point, the person's vision is significantly impaired, making it impossible to read print."

Tasks–Device

Continuing with the example above, the task is to read fine print for most of each 8-hour work day. A second task is to mark up the copy with editorial corrections. Is there a device that can change fine print to large print—print large enough for someone with low vision to be able to read it? There are such devices.

Are the tasks associated with copy editing done in one place (at one desk), or does the copy editor move from place to place in carrying out the job? This latter question raises the issue of portability of equipment. A copy editor will most likely be able to use heavy "desktop" devices. This is not so for a college student with low vision who must move from class to class, taking notes. In this case, a portable device is needed. Portability is closely associated with durability. Will the equipment hold up if it is jarred when being moved from place to place?

How much does the device cost? For the copy editor, the employer may be able to cover the cost of the device. For the college student, the state vocational rehabilitation agency may cover the cost of the device. What about an elderly person with low vision, for whom there is no employer, no vocational goal or state agency, and no savings or income to draw upon?

Environment–Tasks–Device

It is difficult to consider the environment and tasks without also considering the devices that might be used. This section considers the environment–task–device interaction.

Where will the tasks be performed? Is the environment supportive of performing the tasks? For the person with low vision who may need to use an enlarged print system, lighting will be an important consideration. If external light is too bright, it will be more difficult to see the screen. The therapist might recommend moving the copy editor's desk away from the direct sunlight at a window.

The environment must support successful task completion. In considering the task, consider the effect of distractions such as noise; consider "clutter" that may get in the way of task completion; consider lighting that could enhance or detract from task completion; consider comfort.

Person–Device

The device must be able to help the person to do the task. But that is just the basic level. The device must be right for the person. The person must want the device. Therefore, it is essential to include the person with a disability in the assessment process. The most basic question is whether the idea of using a device is acceptable to the potential user. Is the appearance of the device acceptable to the person? If the device resembles devices used by nondisabled persons—such as a computer—it may be accepted more easily. Motivation is a complex concept, but the therapist must feel certain that the person is motivated to use the device to complete the tasks for which it was designed.

Interaction of All Factors

After each of the components—person, environment, tasks, and device—has been assessed and the interactions considered, the therapist is likely to still have several possible choices. One may be to recommend no device. A device may not be appropriate for the person, at least at present. Many individuals who are receiving therapy realize gains in performance that eliminate the need for a assistive device.

If a device is considered necessary and appropriate, there may be several choices. Wheelchairs are a good example; there are many manufacturers with similar products. It is often useful to provide the consumer and/or third-party payer with several possible vendors if the products are essentially identical. However, if there are differences, including differences in warranties, repair, and maintenance policies, then these should be considered in the recommendation.

Example of Assessment

The following 6 pages provide an actual example of a person who was assessed for a mobility and seating system. The assessment is divided into three sections. Section 1 of the assessment was done by a physician; section 2 was done by rehabilitation engineer; and section 3 was done by an occupational therapist.

Chapter 9 Reference

Yorkston, K., & Karlan, G. (1986). Assessment procedures. In S.W. Blackston & D.M. Bruskin (Eds.), *Augmentative communication: An introduction.* Rockville, MD: American Speech-Language-Hearing Association, pp. 163–196.

Assessment Example

Section 1: Physician Assessment

Center for Assistive Technology
J.L.
Wheelchair Medical Component Assessment Summary
3/11/91

Mr. J.L. is a 64-year-old black male with a history of C4-C5 subluxation secondary to a fall on June 3, 1986. He was reportedly neurologically intact after the injury, and underwent spinal fusion with bone grafting on June 9, 1986. Postoperatively he was noted to be quadriplegic.

Mr. J.L. has had a long history of multiple complications, including an aseptic necrosis and dislocation of the left hip, heterotopic ossification in the hips on both sides and in the left shoulder, thoracic scoliosis and recurrent pressure sores in the sacral and ischial areas.

Despite his disability, Mr. J.L. lives an active life. He propels his own power wheelchair which he uses for the greater part of the day. More recently however, he has been unable to tolerate sitting in his wheelchair for more than 2 hours at a time.

Previous Medical History:
1. As above.
2. Neurogenic bowel and bladder secondary to quadriplegia.
3. Severe spasticity.
4. Pulmonary insufficiency (restrictive and obstructive).

Social History: Mr. JL lives with his wife in a wheelchair-accessible dwelling. He has 24-hour aide service. He is dependent in all his activities and requires a Hoyer lift for transfer.

Examination: Mr. JL is an elderly, slightly obese black male in no distress. Musculoskeletal examination was remarkable for moderate to severe contractures of the neck, shoulders, wrists, digits, and hips bilaterally. He had a marked pelvic obliquity with his left hip obviously dislocated and internally rotated. He had a moderate mid-thoracic scoliosis with convexity to the right. His neck was deviated to the right and he had minimal active, voluntary neck movement.

Assessment Example (continued).

His neurologic examination was remarkable for severe tone in all his extremities. On sensory examination he had intact pinprick on the right (sacral area not tested) and intact to T-10 dermatome on the left. On motor examination he had limited range of motion in the left deltoids (up to approximately 95°), 5-/5 biceps, 4/5 triceps, approximately 3/5 wrist extensors, and no intrinsic finger motion. In the right upper extremity, his deltoids were 3-/5, biceps 4-/5, wrist extensors approximately 3/5 (severe contractures limiting exam), triceps 0/5. He had some thumb oppostion on the left.

Impression:

1. C6 incomplete quadriplegia.
2. Moderate thoracic scoliosis and pelvic obliquity.
3. History of recurrent pressure ulcerations.
4. Severe contractures.

Recommendation:
1. Wheelchair replacement as per attached specifications.

L.R., MD

Section 2: Rehabilitation Engineer Assessment

Center for Assistive Technology
Seating and Positioning Assessment
Rehabilitation Engineer Assessment Summary

1.0   Referral Information

J.L. was seen on March 11, 1991, for a seating and position evaluation. He was referred to this clinic by S.M., OTR.

Those participating in the assessment were
        J.L. Client
        J.L.'s Attendant
        L.R., MD
        O.T., ECMC
        S.M., OTR
        N.S., Rehabilitation Engineer, RTS
        R.D., Adaptive Equipment Specialist, RTS

J.L. uses an E&J Premier 18" powered chair, however he is experiencing difficulties with this chair including positioning, pressure, and repair problems.

Powered Chair:
E&J Premier 18", undetermined age (probably 4-5 years old)
Left mounted joystick
PinDot products, Contour-U Seating system with gel pad and sheepskin.
Powered recline, driver-operated, switch mounted on joystick box.

2.0   Posture

    2.1   J.L. leans heavily to his left and was not adequately supported by the lateral supports of the back component. He has put on approximately 25 lbs. since the system was fitted, several years ago, and this may be the main factor that has rendered the current system inappropriate. Sitting tolerance has decreased from all day to 3 hours. He has one incident of tissue breakdown related to this system- (RIT).
    2.2   Head control. He is unable to hold his head upright and will need additional support to rest his head.
    2.3   Recline. The powered recline mechanism fitted to J.L.'s chair is operated by a switch or his attendant operates to enable access to his van, transferring, resting etc.
    2.4   Leg positioning. J.L. has a problem with fatigue and discomfort of his lower legs. This is not relieved by the recline mechanism.
    2.5   Foot positioning. J.L. uses adjustable angle, foot platforms for correct foot positioning.
    2.6   Arm positioning. J.L. uses an Otto Bock arm trough for his right arm.

3.0   Mobility

    3.1   J.L. was able to drive the wheelchair using joystick control.

Assessment Example (continued).

4.0   Evaluation

During the evaluation of J.L.'s positioning requirements, a seating simulator, pressure evaluation pad, bead system, Memphis and Otto Bock, and Jay cushions were used.

4.1   Contouring and Pressure
      4.1.1   A significant contribution of J.L.'s spinal curvature is his pelvic positioning; correct pelvic positioning appeared to reduce leg length discrepancy and enabled increased upright positioning. It was found that a standard Otto Bock Slim Line Pommel cushion provided good pelvic and thigh positioning. However, pressure readings obtained contraindicated this cushion. Use of standard Jay cushion relieved pressure but did not allow controlled pelvic and thigh positioning. See attached information.

      4.1.2   Using a Bead Back (Vacuum Consolidation) insufficient support was available to hold J.L. against the curve to the left. However, the use of Memphis Back (mechanical lateral supports combined with vacuum consolidation for accommodation of spinal deformities) provided good support characteristics, with the support provided in areas of normal sensation.

4.2   Gross Positioning
      4.2.1   See attached information on Seating Simulation and pressure distribution.
      4.2.2   Once established on a contoured surface providing good support, it was found that changing the tilt of the seat between 15 and 25 degrees provided:
      -a good working position
      -a good resting position for pressure relief

5.0   Recommendations

5.1   Support surfaces
      5.1.1   Pelvis. Large Bead Seat 20" molded to allow a 2" Roho Insert to be used for pressure relief of IT's
      5.1.2   Back. Adult Memphis Back with 3 large thoracic brackets, combined with a large Bead Cushion
      5.1.3   Head. Otto Bock
      5.1.4   Feet. Miller Special Products adjustable angle foot platforms

5.2   Gross Positioning.
      5.2.1   Powered tilt in space is necessary to relieve gravitational forces exacerbating curvature of spine while remaining a close fit in seating system, during reclining for pressure relief. Tilt interface for Fortress 760 FS.
      5.2.2   Powered Back Recline for accessing van. Power recline for Fortress 760 FS.

5.3   Mobility
      5.3.1   Fortress 760 FS left hand control mounting.
      5.3.2   Frame requirements, S500, no cushion:
                  Back Frame Welded Mount Assembly; Seat Frame; Seat Mount
      Adaptor

Section 3: Occupational Therapist Assessment

Occupational Therapy
J.L.
Center for Assistive Technology
Wheelchair/Seating Assessment Summary
3/11/91

Recommended the following:

1. **Powered wheelchair** is needed as patient has nonfunctional wheelchair propulsion capabilities. It is required to provide functional mobility for access to essential medical, rehabilitation, and community services. Independent mobility provides the ability to exit from home quickly in emergency situations.

2. **Tilt in space** feature is required in this wheelchair as patient has no ability to provide independent pressure relief and a Hoyer lift cannot be accomplished on a frequent enough schedule to make the procedure practical. Patient is overweight, and motor is dominated by extensor tone that is exacerbated by recline mechanism alone. Tilt feature allows for maintenance of proper body alignment while position is being adjusted. Patient has history of decreased skin integrity (now healed) which this feature will help to maintain.

3. **Power recline** feature to allow patient to lie supine when necessary without being transferred back to bed and to allow for pressure relief through the recline mechanism.

4. **Memphis bead back** as custom molded system provides necessary support and stabilization of the trunk needed for upper-extremity control, prevents progression of scoliosis with resultant pulmonary compromise.

5. **Otto Bock firm support base with ROHO insert as needed** to provide necessary base of support to allow for pelvic obliquity and provides pressure relief through ROHO insert-solid base provides anterior/posterior wedge to assist with hip flexion and in decreasing spastic extensor tone. Solid base of support provides even weight distribution and prevents further pelvic obliquity. Allows for addition of pommel effect and necessary addition of pelvic laterals to normalize seating position.

6. **3 Memphis laterals (large)** provides lateral support to the spine for midline positioning, and decreasing tendency for further scoliosis and compromised respiration and functional ability.

Assessment Example (continued).

Occupational Therapy   Page 2
J.L.
Center for Therapeutic Applications of Technology
Wheelchair/Seating Assessment Summary
3/11/91

7. **Otto Bock arm rests** from current wheelchair to assist with upper-extremity upright
    posture and weight bearing and allow for fixed position caused by contractures and
    tonal changes.

8. **Miller (90°) footplates** to provide stable base of support for full weightbearing on the
    feet to decrease pressure areas-will also accommodate patient's inability to fully
    plantar flex at the ankles (already in place on current wheelchair).

9. **Toe straps** to secure feet to the foot pedals as safety feature and provide
    weight-bearing in seated position.

10. **Otto Bock head rest** from current wheelchair if possible to maintain head upright and
    provide stabilization for the head/neck, assisting in respiration and swallowing.

S.M., OTR

Chapter 9 Study Questions

1. List the five steps in assistive technology service delivery.

2. List four sources of referrals for assistive technology services.

3. Describe two major changes in assistive devices that have occurred over the past 2 decades.

4. List the four major components of an assistive technology assessment.

5. Do a task (activity) analysis for preparing a term paper on assistive technology.

6. List and describe the factors associated with device selection that a therapist must consider.

Chapter 10:
Intervention Services: Implementation and Training

I. Overview
- A. Device Delivery
    1. Macro Level
    2. Micro Level
    3. Case Studies
- B. Device Fitting
    1. Case Studies
- C. Training/Adaptation
    1. Training
    2. Adaptation
    3. Case Studies
- D. Documentation
    1. Case Studies

II. Assistive Technology Intervention Providers

III. Treatment Versus Training
- A. Nature of the Technology
- B. Marketing System
- C. Assistive Technology Team

10.

Intervention Services:
Implementation and Training

William C. Mann, PhD, OTR, and Kathleen A. Beaver, BS

Once the assessment process is completed and the equipment with the proper specifications is ordered, the assistive technology service process moves into the next phase—assistive technology intervention.

Overview

The intervention phase includes the period beginning with the initial contact between the consumer and the assistive device. It starts with the *delivery* of the assistive technology and continues through the consumer's *training* process for device use, initial *adaptations* to the device and environment, and maintaining proper *documentation* of the entire process for future reference. Figure 10.1 illustrates the steps in the intervention process.

In considering assistive technology intervention, we will follow three case studies through each phase. Each of these case studies represents a different area of assistive technology.

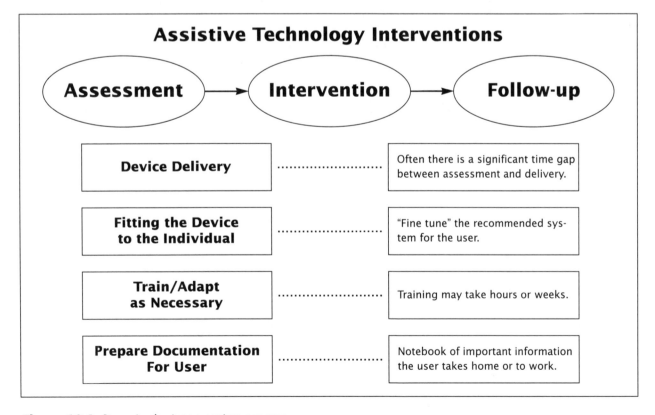

Figure 10.1. Steps in the intervention process.

- *Case Study #1. John: Requires Computer Access Technology.* John is a 30-year-old man who worked in a chemical company as an inspector until 1 year ago. His employment as an inspector with this company ended after he suffered total loss of vision in a chemical spill accident. Both he and his employer want him to return to work, but he will need to consider a different position within the company.
- *Case Study #2. Mary: Requires Environmental Control Technology.* Mary is an 80-year-old widow, living alone in a three-bedroom apartment. Her daughter, who lives in the same town, visits daily and assists with shopping, meal preparation, and personal hygiene. Mary has arthritis, with contractures in both hands, and limited fine motor movement. She walks using a cane and has difficulty coming to a standing position. Mary is alert, enjoys reading, and wants to remain in her apartment.
- *Case Study #3. Susan: Requires Seating and Positioning System.* Susan is a 12-year-old student with developmental disabilities. She also has a severe scoliosis. Susan uses a manual wheelchair for mobility and uses pillows as positioning supports. She attends school and travels from home to school on a bus, with the family car used for all other travel.

Device Delivery

Assistive technology service delivery has a macro and a micro level. The macro level is the organizational structure in which the professional functions—the business of service delivery. The micro level is the actual delivery of services to a consumer.

Macro Level

At the business level, service delivery professionals are concerned with the environment in which they work and the resources this environment provides to them. Some professionals work within larger organizations such as rehabilitation centers in medical facilities, university research centers, state-funded service agencies, or companies that supply durable medical equipment. Others work as members of private practices, community agencies, or not-for-profit groups. To a greater or lesser extent, depending on the size and health of the organization, all professionals must be concerned with the business aspects of service delivery, such as developing and implementing service programs, administration and resource management, marketing services, and funding issues.

A discussion of the service delivery business falls outside this book's mission. Fortunately, several excellent publications have compiled instructive information on relevant aspects of establishing and maintaining a service delivery business. A RESNA publication, *Rehabilitation Technology Service Delivery: A Practical Guide* (1987), is indeed a practical guide to understanding the business of service delivery. Professionals can use the publication to better understand their own work environments and to improve their business practices.

Another publication, *Provision of Assistive Technology: Planning and Implementation* (Electronic Industries Foundation, 1989), describes methods and experiences in planning and implementing assistive technology service programs. The report explains that the availability of assistive devices preceded the development of an adequate service network, impeding widespread dissemination of products and information. In response, the report compiles workshop presentations by experts on various service delivery topics and presents the output of workshop focus groups addressing specific issues of planning new technology services for a community, a regional area, and at a statewide level.

Micro Level

The micro level of service delivery—service to consumers—starts with the arrival of assistive technology devices or materials. The members of the service team and the consumer decide upon the point of delivery for the devices or materials ordered. Possible destinations are the place where equipment assembly and training occurs, the location selected for training, the consumer's home, or even the work site. Equipment ordered through third-party payment systems may be shipped to a central receiving point at the agency making payment, then reshipped to the service team and consumer.

The point of delivery is an important consideration because it determines who has access to the device or materials, whether it must be transported to other locations, and who holds ownership for purposes of insurance claims and equipment warranties. Any equipment or materials received must be carefully inspected for damage and to ensure that all components are correct and complete.

Several factors enter into the decision on where to have the device delivered. For therapists in private practice, or practicing home- and work-based services, the device will likely be delivered to the place where the consumer will use it. For many high-tech devices, especially computer-based systems, a period of training will be essential. It is often much more effective and efficient to deliver the equipment to the center where the person will receive the training. Center-based training provides the opportunity for several team members to participate in the set-up, fitting, training, and adaptations that may be needed. Following training, with all adaptations in place, all "bugs" worked out, and the consumer no longer needing a high level of equipment support, the device can be delivered to the site where it will be used (see Figure 10.2).

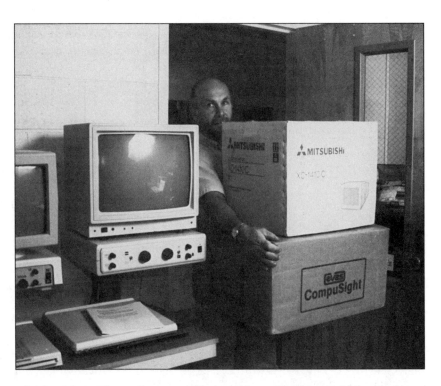

Figure 10.2. The equipment may be delivered either to the work site or to an assistive technology center.

Assembling and testing devices immediately upon receipt protects the recipient. Damage suffered during shipment—if it is not detected until after modifications are made—may reasonably be blamed on the modification process. Assembling and testing all components also verifies that components from different sources that are combined to perform a specific function are fully compatible. For example, an enlarged keyboard may not be compatible with a specific computer make or model; or an alternate switch may require adaptation to fit the electrical connection to a powered wheelchair base.

Once the professional team determines that all components function properly, the consumer should examine and test the basic device. If the consumer finds the basic device inappropriate, then it is pointless to spend time and resources on modifications. The professional team should explain how the device will be modified to accommodate the consumer's needs, but the consumer should retain the right of first refusal. Accepting the basic device reduces the likelihood of future abandonment by the consumer.

The service professionals review the modification process, if any, and the timetable in which they are operating. Consumers have a right to know how long the service delivery process will last and when they can expect to be using the device independently. The professional should provide a realistic time frame for assembly, modification, training, and adjustment.

Case Studies

John: The assistive technology (AT) assessment determined that John's new job title was "technical writer" and that he would be using a computer on his new job assignment primarily for word processing. He would also need to tie in with the company's mainframe computer for database management work, and occasionally he would be using spreadsheets. The AT practitioner recommended an IBM-compatible PC with a terminal emulation package (to tie in with the mainframe), a large hard drive (to store the many technical manuals John would be writing and calling up for his writing), a monitor, and a voice output package. The system also included a laser printer, as John had to prepare high-quality print documents for the company. A braille printer was not recommended. John—as with many persons who have recently become blind—had not learned how to read Braille, and felt it was not necessary with the voice output feature.

The voice output package was the major "assistive" component to this computer system. Voice output packages often suffer compatibility problems with terminal emulation (i.e., tie-in to the mainframe). The AT practitioner tested the recommended voice output package with the company's terminal emulation system, using an assessment computer

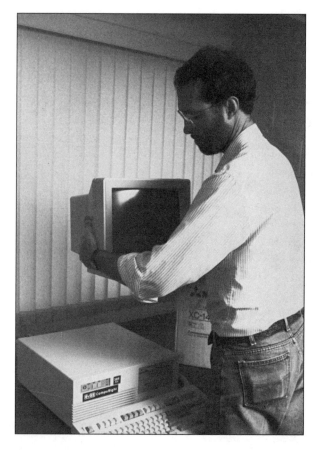

Figure 10.3. Unpacking and assembling the components of John's computer access system.

from her center. In addition to the terminal emulation compatibility, the voice output system also required compatibility with the word processing program used, the database program, and the spreadsheet program. The voice output package included a computer board and software. It provided the user with the capability to define areas of the screen that could be read.

The system was delivered to the assistive technology center where the practitioner was employed. Technicians unpacked and assembled the computer, monitor, keyboard, printer, and cables (see Figure 10.3). After all cables were connected, the computer was turned on, and left on for several hours, to make sure all components were working. The computer was delivered to the center with the operating system already installed. The technician tested all components of the system, including the printer.

After being certain that the basic computer system was fully operational, the voice synthesizer board was installed. This required opening the computer and plugging in the card as a first step.

Software also had to be installed for the voice output program. All other software was installed. In the installation process, the technician was prompted for information such as type of printer and type of monitor that would be used with the system.

After installing the business software, the voice program was configured to work with each of the programs.

If any of the hardware had not been in working order when it arrived, it might have been necessary to return it to the company from which it was purchased. Usually the technical support personnel at a center will contact the company to determine if there is something that can be tried to fix the problem before returning the equipment. With good technical support at an assistive technology center, and a close working relationship with a company's product support department, many problems can be handled over the phone within a couple of hours, or the problem component can be isolated and replaced with an overnight shipment of a new part. Technical support, both at the assistive technology center and at the companies from which equipment is purchased, is essential to any successful assistive technology program.

Mary: Mary was assessed by an occupational therapist working for a home health care agency. The therapist recommended an X-10 type remote control device for Mary to operate her radio and her lights, and a phone that stores up to 16 phone numbers that can be dialed by pushing one button. The therapist indicated in her assessment report that modification of the device buttons might be necessary; she further recommended that the remote control device be attached to the cane with Velcro so that it would always be with Mary as she moved within her apartment, but could be removed when she went out or if she chose to remove it while sitting. The memory-phone and the X-10 remote control device system could each be purchased for less than $100, and Mary's daughter agreed to buy them at the local electronics store (Radio Shack carries several models of each type of device, and most other electronics stores offer comparable models and value). Mary's system is pictured in Figure 10.4.

After Mary's daughter delivered the equipment to her mother's apartment, the occupational therapist installed the phone and remote control system. The phone installation required a simple plug-in connection, followed by "keying in" telephone numbers that would later be retrieved by Mary with the push of one button. The X-10 system required plugging in lamp and appliance modules to wall outlets and then plugging in lamps and the radio to the modules. The whole process took less than 1 hour to complete.

Susan: Susan received a seating, positioning, and mobility assessment which revealed that Susan has sufficient intelligence to use a powered mobility platform and that she has the fine motor skills for operating a joystick control. Physically, Susan has a pelvic obliquity (tilted pelvis) and a difference in the length of her legs. Based on Susan's scoliosis and age, the assessment team determined that she required a custom support system for her seat and back and a head support for transporting in her wheelchair. The seating/mobility components are shown in Figure 10.5.

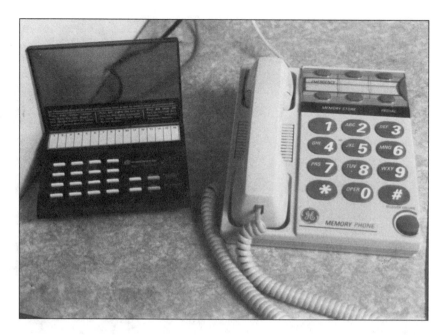

Figure 10.4. Mary's environmental control device system (left) and telephone (right).

The powered platform would be used at home and at school so the selection criteria for the platform required that it be lightweight, foldable, able to accommodate a tray, and accept the custom support system for Susan and the tie down straps for transportation on a school bus. The assessment team determined that Susan's support system should be designed to alleviate the long-term effects of her scoliosis and stop it from worsening. The team selected a custom-contoured bead seat and a Memphis Back bead back with padded metal lateral supports. The support system also includes a seat belt, a butterfly harness for Susan's chest, and a removable head support. The custom-contoured components will provide the required positioning and support, and they form the type of system that lends itself to inexpensive modifications as Susan grows. The lateral restraints will constrain Susan's trunk movement, adding further justification for the powered mobility platform. The assessment team decided that Susan's youth and energy level precluded the need for a base that tilted in space like a recliner. The joystick control will be placed to help Susan maintain the appropriate position in the seating system while operating the joystick.

The assessment team members wrote a detailed prescription for Susan's system to justify acquiring Susan's seating/mobility system to a third-party source of payment.

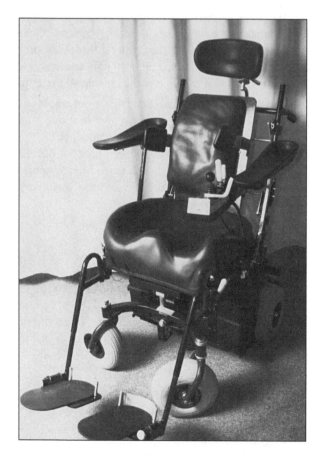

Figure 10.5. Susan's powered mobility base, joystick controller, and seating support materials.

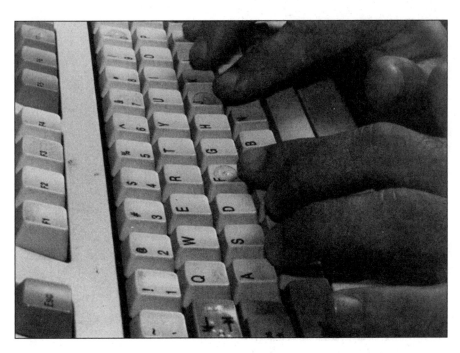

Figure 10.6. Raised symbols placed on the keyboard helped John orient his fingers.

definable," and the AT practitioner taught John how to set these features as part of his training. Because John could not see the keyboard, the practitioner placed raised dots on the "F" and "J" keys so John could orient his hands to the keyboard. Figure 10.6 shows John's keyboard.

Mary: As the therapist determined during the assessment, Mary had difficulty with the buttons on the phone and remote control. The therapist adapted the device by gluing large washers (using Super Glue) on each of the buttons that Mary would use. This worked well for Mary. The therapist also added Velcro to the remote controller and the cane to make transport of the controller easier and ensure that it would always be close by. The radio was tuned to Mary's favorite station, and the volume was set, as the X-10 device simply turned the radio on and off but did not control station or volume. (Radios with remote control devices are available that offer on-off, station selection, and volume control. They are somewhat more expensive—typically well over $200, and the buttons are usually even smaller than those on an X-10. Since Mary listens almost exclusively to one radio station, she was quite satisfied with the simple on-off feature afforded by the X-10.)

The report established that the system was medically appropriate for Susan, described Susan's functional needs and the outcomes expected from the prescribed system, and detailed the materials and supplies needed to assemble and deliver the prescribed system.

Once the service team received prior approval from the third-party payer, the clinic sent out purchase orders to vendors for all components on the list. All components arrived at the clinic within 90 days. The mobility platform was assembled to specifications and tested. Then the service team was ready to custom-fit the system to Susan.

Device Fitting

Case Studies

Service delivery next moves to fitting the device to the person. This will vary with both the type of device and the person. Many devices require little or no initial fitting. Others require minor, or in some cases major, adaptations. The three case studies illustrate well the fitting process.

John: The main assistive technology component of John's system was the voice output feature. This required a certain amount of "fitting." The voice could be adjusted for John in the following ways: the speed at which words are read, the tone and pitch of the voice, and the volume. These features are "user

Susan: Susan and two family members attended the fitting session. In the last step, the service team showed them all the parts of the system, demonstrated the mobility platform's operation and special features, and described characteristics of this bead system process for creating a custom seating system.

Once the service team created the final forms for the bead seat and bead back supports, both were temporarily fastened to the mobility platform. With the seating supports in place, the service team determined the positioning of the joystick controller, set the proper height for the tray, and checked the points of contact between Susan and the seat and harness straps. The service team then made the necessary adjustments to the original specifications and completed the fitting process.

Training/Adaptation

Training

Ideally, the delivery and training steps will occur in the same location, which may or may not be the actual site where the equipment will be used. If assembly and training at the final destination are not feasible, then the training program should take account of differences between the training site and the final use site. These differences should either be recreated in the training site or worked through with the consumer. A training program that neglects the constraints of the actual use site fails to prepare the consumer with options that can mitigate those constraints.

The training program includes familiarization and practice with basic functions, an introduction to any advanced functions that may be available, and instruction on performing the specific functions for which the device was obtained. The length of training will vary according to the consumer's ability, the device's complexity, and the level of mastery required to perform the intended tasks.

Adaptation

Even with great care and attention during the initial assessment process, many devices require some adaptation during the intervention phase. The many variables in the person's abilities, the device's capabilities, and the context in which the two come together, often require an individualized approach.

The delivery phase will expose any obvious problems requiring major adaptations, such as recommending a different device, although a careful assessment should preclude such drastic changes. However, the training phase will reveal less serious problems that are amenable to minor adaptations.

Minor adaptations include adjustments in the position of the person, the assistive device, or other equipment in the environment; altering the operational characteristics of switches and controls; and modifying the procedures involved in using the device. If the new device does not fit within the existing space, rearranging furnishing or adding adjustable bases may suffice. Workstations at the office or at home are particularly suited for multiple minor adjustments.

A very useful publication on modifying the workplace is entitled *The Workplace Workbook: An*

Illustrated Guide to Job Accommodation and Assistive Technology (Mueller, 1990). It shows more than 30 sets of modifications to a standard workstation. This publication is especially useful because it shows both major and minor modifications. The specific modifications depend on the person's impairment and the particular equipment that must be accommodated within a workspace.

The book has three sections:

1. The Universal Workspace;
2. Seating, Storage, and Work Stations; and
3. Computers, Information Displays, Communication Devices, and Controls.

Each section of the book includes a full-page picture of a standard office space with the example's specific devices and adaptations highlighted. The devices and adaptations have a number that corresponds to descriptive narrative on the adjoining page. The book is a useful guidebook for consumers, employers, and professional service providers.

Thoroughly accommodating the assistive device is a critical step of "debugging" in the delivery of effective services. Adjustments considered minor by the professional may create major problems in device use for the consumer. A faulty contact point in a switch is quickly corrected by the professional, but to the consumer it would represent a broken device rendered unusable.

Training and adaptations go hand in hand. During training on the use of the device, the practitioner or trainer is spending considerable time with the user. The trainer will determine if any additional modifications are needed beyond those made during the initial fitting. The training/adaptation phase of interventions is illustrated in our three case studies.

Case Studies

John: John first practiced using the keyboard with a word processor. After several hours of practice, he felt comfortable using the keyboard. The practitioner fastened some additional raised symbols to certain keys on the keyboard to further assist with finger orientation.

The practitioner next worked with John on the basic operating system of the computer (MS-DOS), the menu system for choosing the software packages used on the PC, use of the modem, and connecting to the company's mainframe computer. This was followed by more intensive work with the word processor and its special features, the database program,

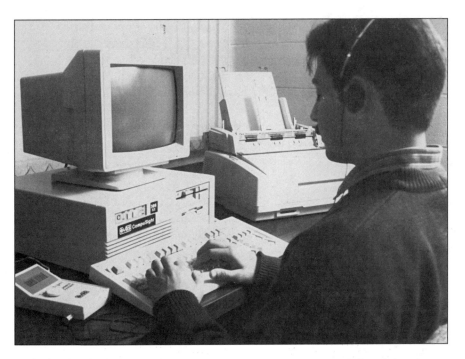

Figure 10.7. John in training receiving instructions through headphones.

Susan: Susan and her family members learned how to operate the mobility platform, how to maintain the platform and the seating components, and how to disassemble the system for transportation in the family vehicle. Susan operated the mobility platform under close supervision, then independently. She practiced moving forward and in reverse, accelerating and slowing down, turning and maneuvering in tight spaces. She also practiced passing through doorways and moving around objects in her path. The training session lasted 2 hours.

The family members were also trained to help Susan through the initial period of learning and adjustment. Susan's schedule for using the system started with brief uses. The family members were to look for signs of discomfort or irritation during use. Sore spots or skin redness indicated a problem in fit or positioning. Each successive use lasted a bit longer until Susan reached full-time use.

and the spreadsheet program. As shown in Figure 10.7, John practiced using both a headphone and a speaker system (the headphone provides privacy and limits distractions to others).

Much of what John was learning is taught in business schools, high schools, and some college courses. The difference was that John used a computer with a special feature (voice output) to access a machine that was otherwise not accessible. The practitioner was acting as a teacher, but a teacher of assistive technology that could be used in the workplace.

Other than some fine tuning of the speed and volume of the voice output, some adjustments in the desk and chair to increase comfort, and the added key markings, John's system did not require any additional adaptations. After 6 weeks of training, John's computer was packed up, delivered to the company, and set up by the assistive technology center's technician. It was given a final on-the-worksite test to be sure everything was still working.

Mary: Mary required little training in the use of her new devices. She practiced using the different buttons of the X-10 for the various lamps and the radio she wished to operate. She also practiced using the automatic dialing phone. No further modifications were needed to these devices. Training took about 1 hour.

Documentation

The professional service team must take a long-term perspective on the assistive device. An appropriate device may be in use for years, long after the team members have lost contact with the consumer. The device will require maintenance and repair—as described in the next chapter—without the benefit of the team's presence. Documentation provides an information map that other people can follow.

Proper documentation explains what equipment or materials were acquired; it details how and why they were modified; and it records the history of maintenance and repair. Documentation includes original order forms, purchase receipts, manufacturer's warranties, and standard instructions. The professional and consumer work together to determine if the commercial documentation is sufficient to operate the equipment, answer questions, and provide information on access to additional materials (Cohen & Frumkin, 1987). Follow-up calls to the manufac-

Table 10.1. Table of Contents for John's "Documentation Manual."

Important telephone numbers	This includes the Assistive Technology Center, and the technical support numbers for each of the equipment components and each of the software companies.
Description of hardware	A one-page summary describing all of the equipment. (When a problem arises with one component, a technical support person may need to know about all components of the system—not simply the one that appears to be not working.)
Description of software	List of software and the key features.
Rationale	The practitioner should document why each component of the system was purchased.
Order forms, receipts, warranties	Originals or copies of all purchases and warranties that came with the equipment and software.
Standard instructions	For a computer system with so many parts, this became too large for one notebook, so a list of each manual that came with the system was put in the notebook. The place where John kept the standard instructional manuals was listed.

turer or vendor for clarification should be documented in an annotated telephone log for future reference.

Beyond the commercial documentation, detailed information on all modifications is essential. Devices that are custom-designed and developed require extensive documentation from the people originally making modifications. Anyone involved in future maintenance or repair will need access to blueprints, wiring diagrams, and schematics on the device. Even if a device does not require repairs, it may need additional modifications as the consumer, task, or environment change over time. The three case studies illustrate the documentation phase.

Case Studies

John: The practitioner set up a table of contents for John's "Documentation Manual," which is shown in Table 10.1. The information in the Documentation Manual is also available to John on audiotape

Mary: The documentation for Mary's system included the phone number for the therapist's agency, the rationale for the choice of system, the purchase receipts and warranty information, and the instructions that came with the devices. Compared with John, Mary's system required much less documentation.

Susan: Documentation for the seating/mobility system contained vendor instructions and warranties, the device prescription reports, and instruction sheets from the clinic. The instruction sheets included a list of names, addresses, and telephone numbers for vendors and Service providers involved in Susan's seating/mobility system. A description of the seating orientation parameters established for Susan and achieved through the seat and back supports were provided for reference. Two checklists were furnished. One covered the care and maintenance of the seating/mobility system; the second explained the process for monitoring Susan's progress during the breaking period. The service team kept a copy of this documentation and the service schedule record in a secure, confidential location in the clinic.

Assistive Technology Intervention Providers

Assistive technology interventions are provided by skilled persons who gain their skill through either professional training or work experience. Professional service providers are trained in traditional disciplines and hold licensure or certification in a recognized field. As described in Chapter 1, therapists, educators, and architects fit this definition.

Many skilled persons who provide assistive technology services have not pursued academic training to obtain professional certification in a recognized discipline. Their roles vary depending on their backgrounds; some are called "trainers," others "technicians," and others simply "consultants." Some of these providers have undergraduate degrees in applied sciences like engineering, computer science, or allied health. Others lack a degree but have extensive experience working with particular technologies such as electronics, computer systems, or mechanics.

Certified professionals, technicians, trainers, and consultants from multiple disciplines and backgrounds provide technology-related services to consumers. There have been recent efforts to establish mechanisms to ensure that each assistive technology service provider is indeed qualified to provide the service. These recent efforts address several issues of concern. How do consumers, professionals, and reimbursement agencies know when someone is qualified to provide technology-related services? What controls are needed to ensure that consumers receive services of good quality? What standards currently exist?

These issues are beyond the scope of this text. RESNA, the leading interdisciplinary organization for technology-related services, is deeply involved in developing formal positions on these issues. The third issue of the journal *Technology and Disability* focuses on the topic of credentialing and quality assurance for assistive technology services. For the reader's purpose it is important to note that there are very few standards and methods of quality assurance at present. Persons who are certified professionals and those with less traditional backgrounds may all make valuable contributions to the service delivery team. The occupational therapist must evaluate the expertise and capabilities of each member of the service team. The therapist should not discount the potential contribution of any person simply because the person lacks formal professional certification, nor embrace someone as an assistive technology expert simply because he or she has traditional certification.

Treatment Versus Training

Assistive technology services often fall outside the medical and rehabilitation systems. While occupational therapists have been "prescribers" of assistive technology for decades, typically in medical settings, there have been many changes in the past 10 years. These changes include the nature of assistive technology, the marketing system for assistive technology, the practitioners of assistive technology services, and the attitudes and perspectives of consumers and caregivers.

Consider first consumer attitudes and perspectives. In many cases consumers do not want to have assistive devices "prescribed"; they consider the process one of "selection," with strong consumer involvement. They do not consider themselves "sick"

and do not feel they need a doctor or a therapist to "treat" them. On the other hand, they recognize the complexity of the emerging applications of technology and know they have much to learn, both about what is available and about the use of specific devices and systems. Given this perspective, the practitioner often participates in an *assessment* (not diagnosis) with the consumer, helps in the *selection* (not prescription) of a device or system, and provides *training* (not treatment) with the consumer.

The authors of this book share this consumer perspective, with one caution. Medical oversight is essential for certain areas of assistive technology. This includes the area of seating and positioning. For other areas, such as computer access and environmental control, having a physician as part of the assistive technology team is rarely necessary or cost-effective. Keep in mind that not all therapists, physicians, and other assistive technology team members share this view. We indicated in this chapter and other chapters that for many aspects of assistive technology intervention, an occupational therapist is not the appropriate service provider, either because different expertise is needed, or because a technician is the more appropriate level for the type of service. In addition to sharing the consumer perspective on this issue, there are other reasons for taking this view.

Nature of the Technology

Is a computer with a voice output system a medical device? Is an X-10 type environmental control device a medical device? Complex and simple technology both need to be selected carefully. Viewed as tools, therapists can assist individuals in selecting the best tools for the jobs they need to do. Therapists, assisted by trainers, can help individuals learn to use those tools, adapt them for the "perfect" fit, and select new or different tools as the individual and/or the technology change.

Marketing System

Most assistive devices can be purchased through mail order without a medical prescription or any other formal assessment. This approach is not recommended. A single consumer or caregiver lacks the experience or training to know which device will be the right tool or if a tool is the best path to take in providing services. A team of service providers, on the other hand, does have the training and experience in selecting devices that have a high likelihood of being used. Its members also know whether to recommend therapy to improve function or suggest a device to assist function.

Assistive Technology Team

Is an occupational therapist the only professional team member who should assess persons with visual impairments for a computer system? This question reflects a change in service provision. New professions have emerged with the new technology, (e.g., rehabilitation engineering). The need for adaptation of devices and individualized solutions required the materials and design expertise of an existing field (engineering) applied in a new specialty area (rehabilitation technology).

In conclusion, we recommend that you consider the setting in which you work, the licensure requirements in your state, and the nature of the intervention when deciding whether or not a particular intervention is "selection" or "prescription"; "treatment" or "training."

Chapter 10 References

Cohen, C.G., & Frumkin, J.R. (1987, May). Service delivery systems: Administrative and clinical issues in augmentative communication. *Seminars in Speech and Language.*

Electronic Industries Foundation. (1989). *Provision of assistive technology: Planning and implementation.* Washington, DC: Electronic Industries Foundation Rehabilitation Engineering Center.

Mueller, J. (1990). The workplace workbook. *An illustrated guide to job accommodation and assistive technology.* Washington, DC: The Dole Foundation.

RESNA. (1987). *Rehabilitation technology service delivery: A practical guide.* Washington, DC: RESNA Publishers.

Chapter 10 Study Questions

1. What are the four steps in the intervention process? Explain the importance of each.

2. Why are there macro and micro levels to service delivery?

3. How are training and adaptation related to documentation?

4. Discuss the issues of credentialing and quality assurance in the delivery of assistive technology services.

5. Describe the issues in "treatment versus training."

Chapter 11:
Support Services: Device Funding, Maintenance, Repair, and Modification

I. Funding Options
    A. Recent Federal Legislation
    B. Medicare Reimbursement Regulations
    C. Medicaid Reimbursement Regulations
    D. State Vocational Rehabilitation Services
    E. Nongovernment Funding Options
    F. Role of Technologists in Obtaining Funding

II. Professional Follow-Through Services
    A. Preventive Maintenance, Repair, and Replacement
    B. Device Modifications or Improvements
    C. Supplemental Training Programs
    D. Providing Follow-Through Services
    E. Implications for Occupational Therapists

11.

Support Services: Device Funding, Maintenance, Repair, and Modification

Joseph P. Lane, MBPA, and Kathleen A. Beaver, BS

As described in the introduction to Unit III, support services actually begin immediately after the consumer's initial contact with assistive technology practitioners. Following the first screening interview to determine the consumer's likely needs, a professional begins to explore the consumer's options for financing the necessary assistive technology and technology-related services.

Identifying funding to obtain devices and to pay for the assessments and training is the first type of support service involving members of the service provision team. After successfully completing training in the device's use, the consumer enters a period when protracted support services are essential to the long-term value of assistive devices. These support services include a schedule of regular maintenance for the device, a procedure for obtaining repair services, and a method of periodic follow-through by professionals to evaluate the device's utility on a continuing basis. The follow-through assessments may result in device modifications or replacement as the consumer's needs change. Changes occur as the consumer ages, grows, gains or loses function, or alters skill level in device use. Failing to provide support services results in inappropriate device use, device abandonment, or a waste of support funding. Inappropriate devices are also a threat to the consumer's health, safety, or functions.

The long-term consequences of device use are critical. The assistive technology practitioner must assist in setting up a preventive maintenance schedule and in identifying a permanent source of repair support for the user. Moreover, the practitioner must plan for increased user proficiency or decreased user capabilities, depending on conditions and expectations. The assistive device is viewed as a new dynamic component of the person's everyday life.

Funding Options

If a consumer is unable to pay for a device, then the device is essentially not available to that person. Therapists must understand the potential for device purchase through existing systems and how to ensure payment for devices. On the other hand, practitioners must understand the limitations to funding and consider this in the assessment and prescription process.

If an assistive device or technology-related services must be obtained, the individual has numerous options for acquiring the funding (see Table 11.1).

Recent Federal Legislation

Recent actions at the federal government level are developing new avenues for funding assistive devices. For example, the General Services Administration has implemented portions of Public Law 99-506. The GSA adopted a policy covering all federal agencies that makes federal employees with disabilities eligible to receive adaptive devices (hardware and software) that make electronic office equipment accessible. The policy also includes training in the use of these adaptive devices (Mallik, 1990).

The Technology-Related Assistance for Individuals With Disabilities Act of 1988 & 1992 (P.L. 100-407) provides funding on a competitive basis to establish statewide, consumer-responsive networks of technological assistance. A basic element of "Tech Act" funding involves efforts to identify sources of funding for assistive

Table 11.1. Assistive Technology Financing Options.

PUBLIC PROGRAMS **Medicare** • Part A • Part B **Medicaid** • Required and Optional Services • Intermediate Care Facilities for Persons Who Are Mentally Retarded (ICFs/MR) • Early and Periodic Screening, Diagnosis and Treatment (EPSDT) • Section 2176 Home and Community Based (HCB) Waivers • Community-Supported Living Arrangements **Maternal and Child Health** • Maternal and Child Health Block Grant • Children with Special Health Care Needs • Special Projects of Regional and National Significance (SPRANS) **Education** • Individuals With Disabilities Education Act (IDEA) State Grants (Part B) • IDEA: Programs for Infants and Toddlers With Disabilities and Their Families (Part H) • State-Operated Programs (89-313) • Vocational Education • Head Start **ALTERNATIVE FINANCING** • Revolving Loan Fund • Lending Library • Discount Program • Low-Interest Loans • Private Foundations • Service Clubs • Special State Appropriations • State Bond Issues • Employee Accommodations Program • Equipment Loan Program • Corporate-Sponsored Loans • Charitable Organizations	**U.S. TAX CODE** • Medical Care Expense Deduction • Business Deductions • Employee Business Deductions • ADA Credit for Small Business • Credit for Architectural and Transportation Barrier Removal • Targeted Jobs Tax Credit • Charitable Contributions Deduction **PRIVATE HEALTH INSURANCE** • Health Insurance • Worker's Compensation • Casualty Insurance • Disability Insurance **Vocational Rehabilitation** • State Grants • Supported Employment • Independent Living Parts A, B, and C **Social Security Benefits** • Title II: Social Security Income (SSI) • Work Incentive Programs **Developmental Disability Programs** **Department of Veterans Affairs Programs** **Older Americans Act Programs** **CIVIL RIGHTS** The Americans With Disabilities Act Rehabilitation Act • Section 504 **UNIVERSAL ACCESS** Rehabilitation Act, Section 508 Decoder Circuitry Act **TELECOMMUNICATIONS** Telecommunications for the Disabled Act of 1982 Telecommunications Accessibility Enhancement Act of 1988

devices and disseminating that information to consumers. Several of the state programs are also developing some form of consumer loan program under which persons with disabilities can borrow money from a revolving loan fund.

In addition to funding individual states, the Technology-Related Assistance for Individuals With Disabilities Act of 1988 funded RESNA, an interdisciplinary association for the advancement of rehabilitation and assistive technology, to provide technical assistance to the collective group of funded state-

level projects. One product is the publication *Assistive Technology: A Funding Workbook* (Morris & Golinker, 1991).

RESNA's workbook has two parts. The first part, "A Road Map to Funding Sources," describes existing federal streams of funding for assistive devices and it offers a structure by which the funded states can chart the various funding sources in existence and under development there. The second part, "Outline of Federal Laws and Rules," presents the content and scope of regulations governing the three principal sources of federal money for assistive technology: Medicaid, Special Education (including early intervention), and Vocational Rehabilitation. States are encouraged to use the federal regulations as a standard by which to compare their own approaches to funding assistive technology.

The RESNA workbook is written primarily for state-level agencies, but the content is useful for anyone involved in securing funding for persons with disabilities. The workbook is designed to help participating agencies better understand, and therefore explain to consumers, what funding options exist and how to obtain them. The very presence of this book suggests that each state represents a different process, and that identifying sources of funding and securing payment for devices or services is a challenging task for consumers and professionals alike.

Medicare Reimbursement Regulations

The Medicare system was established in 1965 through Title XVII of the Social Security Act. Medicare has two programs: the Hospital Insurance Program (Part A) and the Supplementary Medical Insurance Program (Part B). Medicare pays for physician's services in nonacute treatment settings, including home health, rehabilitation, ambulatory surgical, and outpatient centers.

In 1992, the Health Care Financing administration (HCFA) issued rules to improve Medicare administration and service delivery. The rules set minimum standards for suppliers and changed the jurisdictions for payment of claims. In 1993, Medicare phased in contracts with four major insurance companies as regional carriers to process claims for durable medical equipment (DME). These four Durable Medical Equipment Regional Carriers (DMERCs) process all claims for durable medical equipment, prosthetics, orthotics, and supplies eligible under Medicare Part B.

Rehabilitation technologists may submit claims to these DMERCs as a qualified supplier. A supplier is defined as an entity or individual that provides, sells, or rents durable medical equipment to Medicare beneficiaries and meets Medicare's standards.

Medicaid Reimbursement Regulations

Another study illustrated the complexity of funding reimbursement for assistive technology and the wide variation in reimbursement regulations among states. The Electronic Industries Foundation's Rehabilita-

tion Engineering Center examined a single funding mechanism—Medicaid reimbursement—in detail across the entire nation (Markowicz & Reeb, 1988).

The Medicaid system was established in 1965 through Title XIX of the Social Security Act to meet the basic health care needs of persons who are "categorically needy." Eligible people include those who qualify for the Aid to Families with Dependent Children (AFDC) program, or the Supplemental Social Security Income (SSI) and Social Security Disability Income (SSDI) programs for persons who are older or have disabilities. Medicaid is a joint federal and state program. Each state is responsible for developing and administering its own program, with the federal government sharing part of the cost with the Health Care Financing Administration (HCFA). While all states must provide a common, core set of benefits, each state has the option of providing additional benefits and covering a broader range of services. State services vary because of these optional services. The Electronic Industries Foundation's study revealed that Medicaid reimbursement coverage for 40 different types of equipment varied widely among the 50 states and the District of Columbia.

The authors of the Medicaid reimbursement study concluded that professionals and consumers must develop good lines of communication with Medicaid personnel in order to understand their own state's rules and exceptions. Medicaid personnel involved with prior authorization of services and with policy decisions were viewed as particularly important because the agency guidelines typically contain some room for discretionary decisions on a case-by-case basis. Good communication with these personnel, who may not have a thorough background in the service provider's area of expertise, helps them understand the clinical basis for an intervention that in turn helps justify payment for the intervention.

State Vocational Rehabilitation Services

The need to understand the specific requirements of each funding source cannot be overemphasized. The Stout Vocational Rehabilitation Institute conducted a similar survey of state regulations in which it examined the methods used by state vocational rehabilitation agencies to purchase facility-based rehabilitation services for clients (Thomas, 1986). As the study's report explains, state vocational rehabilitation agencies grew from federal government initiatives to offer vocational rehabilitation services first to disabled veterans, then to persons disabled in industry and other circumstances. Due to limited funding allocations, state agencies were encouraged to develop cooperative relationships with private and public not-for-profit agencies in order to deliver the authorized services. The state vocational rehabilitation agencies developed close ties with private rehabilitation facilities.

The Vocational Rehabilitation Act Amendments of 1965 provided federal funds to build facilities and conduct state-wide development of sheltered workshop programs and other rehabilitation facilities. The Council of State Administrators of Vocational Rehabilitation summarized the six basic functions of state vocational rehabilitation agencies (Baxter, 1972):

1. Evaluate the needs of disabled and other disadvantaged individuals and provide comprehensive vocational rehabilitation to those eligible for services.
2. Conduct statewide planning to continuously assess the needs of persons with disabilities and to determine how best to meet their needs.
3. Provide leadership in developing rehabilitation facilities and programs.
4. Develop and maintain cooperative relationships with public and private agencies within the state's communities.
5. Perform functions related to other federal assistance acts, such as providing minor medical services under the Manpower Development and Training Act; make disability determinations for the Social Security Administration; and develop certifications to the Department of Labor under the Fair Labor Standards Act.
6. Exercise leadership in research and in the training of vocational rehabilitation personnel.

The presence of new programs and services resulted in new referrals by schools, private corporations, and local and county agencies. These referrals expanded the number and type of collaborative agreements between vocational rehabilitation agencies and other entities within each state. Each state developed its own particular approach to service provision. The Stout Vocational Rehabilitation Institute's survey of 41 state vocational rehabilitation agencies and 11 agencies serving persons who are blind and visually impaired revealed that the practices of state agencies varied within each of eight areas related to service provision.

These eight areas of variability are:

1. methods for establishing working relationships with facilities
2. determining cost reimbursement rates
3. methods of purchasing service elements
4. monitoring facility costs
5. renegotiation of costs
6. other purchasers of services
7. the extent of facility services purchased by state agencies
8. the diagnostic and therapeutic services purchased

The implication for therapists and consumers is to clearly communicate expectations and understand the particular practices of the funding source within that particular state.

Nongovernment Funding Options

A report from the Electrical Industries Foundation entitled *Subsidy Programs for Assistive Devices* is another source of information. It lists organizations and programs that subsidize the purchase of assistive devices (Ward, 1989). Subsidy programs either lower the purchase cost of a device or provide the device free of charge. The subsidy may be a cash grant or a discount or rebate on the purchase price. Each subsidy program has its own eligibility criteria. The report lists 21 subsidy programs, organized under the following headings. More programs probably exist today:

- competitive subsidies to individuals offered by private, nonprofit organizations
- competitive subsidies to institutions offered by assistive device manufacturers
- subsidies offered through collaboration between business and voluntary organizations including formal partnerships, volunteer organization initiatives, membership discounts, and nonprofit entities created to market discounted assistive devices
- rebates on equipment purchases
- discounts on telecommunications devices and services
- manufacturer discounts offered for special events

The report's classification scheme is useful for understanding the types of subsidy programs that exist. Therapists can use the list as a starting point to inquire about the subsidy programs for which their clients might be eligible.

Two additional reports from the Electronic Industries Foundation address two other potential sources of funding: revolving loan funds and private insurance reimbursement. The report on revolving loan funds describes the concept and explains how to establish such a program (Reeb, 1987b). According to this report, there are two basic types of revolving loan funds: (1) self-perpetuating funds, and (2) loan guarantees.

1. Self-perpetuating revolving loan funds involve a direct loan to a borrower from a fixed amount of resources. The loan payments replenish the principal fixed cash reserve. They may also pay some portion of the associated lending costs. The self-perpetuating loan fund is limited by the amount of cash available to lend and must cover the administrative costs of the loan program.

2. Loan-guarantee loan funds do not use the cash available in the loan fund for direct loans to consumers. Instead the funds are used to leverage or underwrite loans acquired from other sources such as commercial banks. In this system, the administration of loans is conducted by a third party. Further, the loan program can underwrite loans in excess of the actual cash amount available in the loan fund. The loan fund is replenished by payments to the third-party lender, which allows the loan fund to underwrite new loans.

The second Electronic Industries Foundation report—on private insurance reimbursement—describes the insurance industry, the method of determining reimbursement, and the types of insurance involved (Reeb, 1987a). Insurance is described as an economic, legal, and sociopolitical method for sharing the risk of potential harm or loss. The insurance payment process has two steps:

1. Establish the presence of an obligation and the extent of that obligation.
   a. Verify that a loss or harm has occurred.
   b. Determine the cost of the loss or harm.
   c. Identify the parties involved in sharing the cost of the loss or harm.
2. Fulfill the obligation.
   a. Pay a monetary settlement.
   b. Provide or purchase a reasonable amount of equipment or services. The insurance payment process for rehabilitation equipment or services may result from any one of the following four categories of insurance policies:
      i. *Health insurance* guards against the loss of health through injury or illness and pays to restore health. Health maintenance costs are sometimes included.
      ii. *Disability insurance* agrees to pay a portion of income lost over time when a person suffers a loss of income due to a disability.
      iii. *Workers' compensation* insurance is a special type of disability insurance that covers employees for medical and disability costs resulting from injury or illness incurred on the job.
      iv. *Liability insurance* pays for harm or loss caused by the policyholder acting in a negligent manner.

All types of policies involve key decisions made by insurance company employees, health care professionals, and others. It is important to provide the decision-makers with the data needed to make an informed decision regarding payment and to expedite the payment process.

Many other payment or reimbursement options do not necessarily represent whole industries but may be the best source of funding for a particular need. A recent book, *Financial Aid for the Disabled and Their Families,* provides detailed information on sources and requirements for scholarships, fellowships, loans, grants, awards, and internships designed primarily for persons with disabilities and their families (Schlacter & Weber, 1990). The book defines the following sources of funding:

- *Scholarships* support undergraduate education with no obligation for service or repayment.
- *Fellowships* support graduate or postgraduate education or research.
- *Loans* provide money that must eventually be repaid, with or without interest.
- *Grants and Grants-in-Aid* support research, innovative work, travel expenses, or emergency needs.
- *Awards* recognize innovative work or exemplary public service.
- *Internships* are work experience programs involving paid positions.

The same book lists about 950 funding sources categorized by general, orthopedic and developmental, hearing, visual, and communication/other disabilities. It also lists state sources of information on financial aid, guaranteed student loan programs, vocational rehabilitation services, services for the developmentally disabled, and social services.

Role of Technologists in Obtaining Funding

While a range of options for funding assistive devices exist, not all options are appropriate for every individual. Every funding source has a particular mission and specific qualifications for individuals who apply for funding. Therapists cannot be thoroughly versed in every funding option, but they should be aware of resource materials that can help individuals identify appropriate sources of funding support.

A good reference for information on sources of funding—as well as all other issues pertaining to assistive technology—is the *Assistive Technology Sourcebook* (Enders & Hall, 1990). The Sourcebook compiled and updated much of the existing literature on assistive technology resources. The section entitled "Funding for Assistive Technology and Related Services" reviews the payment systems for assistive devices, discusses methods of finding and justifying funding for devices, and describes options for acquiring needed technology. The section also includes an annotated bibliography on more than 150 publications addressing the issue of funding assistive devices and services.

The Sourcebook highly recommends one particular publication to anyone in the field of assistive technology, *Financing Adaptive Technology: A Guide to Sources and Strategies for Blind and Visually Impaired Users* (Mendelsohn, 1987). Although the book focuses on one disability group, the author relates the information to the needs of other consumers. The author describes the various systems involved in funding and reimbursement. These systems include the Vocational Rehabilitation System, the Social Security Administration's payment systems, the monetary credit system through which money is loaned and purchases are financed, the tax code system of expenses and deductions, and the education system. The book also contains a section on miscellaneous sources of funding.

To summarize the support issue of funding, the technologist is one member of the team delivering assistive technology devices and services to the consumer. All members of the service delivery team have some knowledge of funding sources and reimbursement methods. The technologist should understand the role of government agencies, be aware of funding options, and know where to obtain further information.

Once the issue of funding devices or services is resolved and the devices or services are delivered, the support system shifts its focus from the professional providing competent services to the consumer's long-term use of the assistive technology.

Professional Follow-Through Services

Funding is the first support service invoked in the delivery of assistive technology. Once funding is received or a mechanism for reimbursement identified, the professional team involves the consumer in the assessment, delivery, and training components of assistive technology. What happens then? Most professionals use the term "follow-up" when describing the period after direct service delivery is completed. This section of the book will instead use the term "follow-through" as used by Enders and Hall (1990). They make a very important point about support services:

> For most individuals, the use of assistive technology is an ongoing process, and continuing services such as system integration, basic and ongoing training, repair and maintenance will, in many instances, be as important as the devices themselves. These services might not be provided in the same place, but they must be available. If follow-through services are not available, provision of the equipment may need to be reconsidered. (Enders & Hall, 1990, p. 122)

Thinking about the support services process as follow-through rather than as follow-up places the support services component as equal in importance to the components of assessment and device delivery. As the final sentence of the preceding quote concludes, a lack of support services may require rethinking the technology solution.

Consequently, the service providers should think of the assessment and delivery of assistive technology as only portions of the service delivery continuum. A major portion—and probably the most prolonged portion—consists of the follow-through services. Follow-through services can be summarized in three components, each described separately in the following pages:

1. preventive maintenance, repair, and replacement programs
2. device modifications or improvements
3. supplemental training for changes in device, person, or context of use

Follow-through services do not necessarily require the time and expense of professional service teams. One study reports that videotapes of training programs are useful to consumers, because the consumer can replay and review the training program as needed (Mortola, Kohn, & LeBlanc, 1990). Videotapes for maintenance and repair might also be useful yet inexpensive methods for providing follow-through support services.

Preventive Maintenance, Repair, and Replacement

The maintenance, repair, and replacement of assistive devices does not fit any typical pattern. Some vendors of large-market assistive devices such as wheelchairs have literature available for establishing regular maintenance programs. These programs are typically geared to high-volume operations, such as long-term-care facilities and institutions, so the information is less relevant to individual consumers. *The Assistive Technology Sourcebook* (Enders & Hall, 1990) lists five publications about maintaining and repairing wheelchairs, but it lists no publications about maintaining assistive devices that use integrated circuits or computer-based technology.

A preventive maintenance program is appropriate for a mechanical or simple electrical device but is of little use to a computer-based device that has complex components that either work or must be replaced. However, even complex mechanisms can benefit from basic rules of keeping the device clean and dry, avoiding temperature extremes and bumps, and turning off when not in use. In the case of high technology, preventing damage is more in the user's control than is maintaining the device's operation.

Many devices have warranties that cover the cost of repairs for 30 days to 1 year. While traditional warranty programs are useful for standard goods, they are less appropriate for assistive technologies. Warranties are typically valid only for the original owner, although many assistive devices go through several lifespans of ownership. Further, suppose a device is purchased by a third party (e.g., vocational rehabilitation agency), through a value-added retailer (e.g., durable medical equipment supplier), delivered to a service provider for setup and training (e.g., an occupational therapist in a clinical site), then moved to the consumer's home or workplace. Who is the warranty made out to and who has the paperwork? When does the warranty begin and end? Such questions should be answered for the consumer during the follow-through process.

Some manufacturers and suppliers offer service contracts on their devices. Service contracts extend the lifespan of warranties or provide a warranty where none existed. If the consumer purchases the service contract, the device will be repaired by the contracted party during a specified future length of time. Of course, such contracts start when the device is new and least likely to experience problems. The consumer must weigh the cost of the service contract against the likelihood of having no problems with the device during the contract's lifespan. When receiving repairs through warranties or service contracts, the consumer will probably forego use of the device for the time period of shipment, repair, and return. As the number of devices in use increases, the number of people in the business of equipment repair will also increase. In the interim, the consumer is left with few options when the device requires repair or replacement.

There are not enough repair facilities to accommodate all the assistive devices in operation, nor do all devices have extended warranties or service contract options. Many consumers must pursue alternative sources of maintenance and repair. Skilled tradespeople such as mechanics and electricians probably provide the majority of informal repair services. One consumer became so dissatisfied with the wait for reimbursement and services through formal channels that he opened his own mobile repair service for wheelchairs. That consumer transferred his expertise at car restoration to the area of assistive devices. The professional service provider may also be making repairs or modifications to an assistive device.

The biggest issue concerning warranties that professionals must face is whether or not to repair or modify an assistive device. A small repair to a circuit board, such as resoldering a connection, may save the money and time of returning the device to the vendor. But opening the device and making the repair will probably void the warranty and eliminate the consumer's only free option for receiving major repair work at a future date. Making major modifications to any device automatically voids the manufacturer's warranty. After all, the modification may make the device perform in a manner not intended, or it may cause the device not to function at all. The professional may not wish to modify the internal workings of a device such as a control device for operating an alternate computer keyboard but may want to adapt the switch to fit the consumer's needs. Will the alteration void the warranty? The professional should be familiar with the explicit and implied aspects of warranties and service contracts before attempting to make any repairs, and before modifying a device in any way.

Device Modifications or Improvements

Service providers report in the literature that devices must be evaluated and modified during the period of consumer use. In 1987 the Trace Research and Development Center described its service delivery program in terms of four major activities; one was the reevaluation, monitoring, and revision activity (Smith, 1987). An interdisciplinary program that develops assistive devices for people with disabilities reported on the significance of monitoring the use of devices and making adjustments to meet the consumer's needs (Reavis, Hensley, Dudek, Jones, & Sparling, 1989).

Why is it important to monitor and revise devices? Numerous variables are involved in evaluating, selecting, and delivering an assistive device. The consumer has opinions as well as abilities. Those opinions and abilities change over time. The technology itself also changes rapidly over time. Computer-based devices produced less than 10 years ago bear only the slightest resemblance to those in the marketplace today. Someone has to keep track of the emerging technologies and compare them to the device the consumer is using. Last year's optimal solution may be hopelessly antiquated compared to current capabilities. A third reason for professionals to monitor the use of a device over time is that the consumer's abilities change. They may become more proficient in device use, or they may lose some function important to device use. For all of these reasons, the professional may consider the device in use a temporary solution in the consumer's long-term quest to maintain function.

Consumer feedback on the device's value is the single most important source of information available to the service providers. Regardless of the technical capabilities or the fit between ability and function, if the consumer does not like the device, it will not be used. A relatively new area of study in assistive technology is "technology abandonment." Technology abandonment explores the question: Why does a perfectly useful device end up in the closet?

Publications and conference proceedings address the issue of technology use and abandonment. They explore the process by which a consumer selects or receives a device, finds the device inappropriate, and either stops using the device or seeks improvement through modifications or different devices (Batavia, Dillard, & Phillips, 1990; Batavia & Hammer, 1989;

Mallik & Elder, 1993; Mortola, Kohn, & LeBlanc, 1989; Tewey, Barnicle, & Perr, 1994). According to these publications, the value of an assistive device is not intrinsic in the device but in the consumer's level of satisfaction with its performance. These studies of technology use and abandonment identified five common reasons why consumers stop using an assistive device:

1. The device compromises the consumer's performance in other areas.
2. The consumer is no longer interested in performing the function.
3. The device does not perform in a reliable manner.
4. The device is too difficult to operate.
5. Maintenance and repair is unavailable or too expensive.

Technology abandonment is a costly outcome for all parties. The consumer loses the opportunity to gain functional abilities. The consumer or some other funding source expends resources that could have been applied more constructively. The professionals involved lose the opportunity to deliver other forms of assistive technology. The professional's follow-through process should identify instances of abandonment and perhaps intervene before the opportunity is lost.

Since the decision to accept or reject an assistive device rests with the consumer, some studies are exploring the variables that will influence the consumer's decision. By understanding the consumer's perspective, the professionals may avoid making an inappropriate recommendation, or at least understand what modifications are needed to make the device acceptable.

According to one study, the variables relevant to device acceptance or rejection fall into four categories (Scherer, 1989):

1. Disability: type, age at onset, degree or severity.
2. Person: cognitive abilities and aptitude, personality traits, judgments and preferences, outlook.
3. Psychosocial set: exposure and opportunity, expectations, social support.
4. Assistive device: design factors, service delivery.

Another study identified 17 different criteria used by consumers to evaluate their assistive devices (Batavia & Hammer, 1989). These criteria are: affordability, compatibility, consumer repairability, dependability, durability, ease of assembly, effectiveness, flexibility, learnability, maintenance, operability, personal acceptability, physical comfort, physical security, portability, securability, and supplier repairability. The relative ranking of these criteria depended on the consumer's disability and the type of technology under evaluation. Overall, the four most important criteria across all disability and technology classifications were effectiveness, affordability, operability, and dependability.

Regardless of the number or type of criteria involved, the professional should understand that the consumer will react to the assistive device once it is in use. By understanding the consumer, anticipating likely reactions and performance outcomes, and selecting the most appropriate device for that consumer and for those outcomes, the professional can minimize the likelihood of abandonment. The follow-through process should provide ample warning about problem areas for professionals to make modifications or substitutions before the consumer loses faith in the technology's value.

Beyond the consumer's own experience with an assistive device, technical advances in commercial products may require upgrading a device or obtaining an improved model. You may be reading this book 6 months to 1 year after these words are written. In that time span, some of the devices described may become obsolete and some of the companies may go out of business. New advances in materials, components, and devices will drive the marketplace and improve the options available. The service provider should consider the likely lifespan of the equipment not only in terms of physical performance but also in terms of advances in the marketplace. How long has the device been in the marketplace? How often is the product line upgraded or replaced? What are the vendors working on? Exploring these questions before making a final purchase will minimize the upgrading required and perhaps avoid purchasing a nearly obsolete item. However, the pace of technological change will still require upgrades and replacements. The first choice made will ease or complicate future options during the follow-through period.

Not all modifications result from a poor match between the user and the device. A consumer with a very useful device will gain greater proficiency with the device. A device with a keyboard becomes more useful as the person becomes a better typist. The same is true for headpointers, scanning systems, and other devices. As consumers' abilities improve, they may outgrow the capabilities of the device. The professional should take this learning curve into consideration during the initial evaluations. The person may need a planned migration to increasingly sophisticated devices. The professional can consider the potential of available systems to accommodate increased proficiency and perhaps choose the system that allows the greatest improvement over time.

Supplemental Training Programs

Information about the initial training process for consumers new to an assistive device also holds true after a device is altered. The device may be modified, upgraded, or replaced. The consumer may have gained great proficiency in device use or may have lost some of the function previously used to operate the device. The consumer may also be preparing to use the device in a new context such as school, work, or an institution. Different environments place new conditions on optimal device use.

In all of these circumstances, the consumer must be trained in the new or different aspects of the device. In addition, the consumer must unlearn the old or familiar aspects of operating the previous device. Unlearning old behaviors and learning new ones is a more complicated process than simply learning with no prior knowledge. The professional should ensure that the training process recognizes both aspects of learning, and should budget enough time and resources to achieve effective results.

Providing Follow-Through Services

Although all three components of follow-through services seem rational and important, the question remains: How many of these follow-through services can the professional afford to provide? In general, it is easier to obtain funding or reimbursement for devices than for services. Further, it is probably most difficult to obtain funding or reimbursement for services provided after the assistive device is delivered and in use—especially services extended over a prolonged time period.

Enders and Hall (1990) commented on the dearth of resources and written documentation concerning follow-through. They believe there is little incentive to prepare written documentation on the follow-through process because there are few mechanisms for receiving payment for support services. However, they do point out some novel approaches that may signify greater interest in long-term support. For example, some device manufacturers and suppliers are offering service contracts on their products. Also, funding agencies are accepting bills for original service costs that include an additional amount for follow-through services.

Either professionals must include the cost of some "average" expected amount of follow-through work into the initial billing for services, or the funding and reimbursement systems must be educated about the importance of follow-through services to the overall success of assistive technology applications. Perhaps a combination of both approaches will have the best results. The occupational therapist's knowledge of funding policies and practices is as useful in the follow-through phase as in the initial acquisition of the assistive device.

Implications for Occupational Therapists

The technologist's role in follow-through services for assistive technology was the topic of a recent paper by Mortola, Kohn, & LeBlanc (1991). The authors reason that an occupational therapist has basic assessment and evaluation skills that are applied in the decision to provide assistive technology. The therapist's objective is to provide functional gains to the consumer through the application of assistive devices. Once the technology is delivered, the occupational therapist can again apply those assessment skills by assessing the consumer's new level of functioning while using the assistive device.

Thus, the therapist is now concerned with the functional gains achieved by the combined efforts of the consumer, the device, and the environmental context in which the device is being applied. The results of follow-up assessments will provide the assistive technology service team with important feedback on the service outcome. This information may lead to minor or major modifications to the technology provided. It should also reduce the likelihood of technology abandonment by the consumer.

Preliminary findings from this reported follow-up study show that the group of consumers with seating systems who received the highest level of follow-up services were seated more comfortably, were comfortable for longer periods of time, and were more pleased with their device's appearance than the group of consumers receiving less follow-up service. These findings can be generalized to all types of assistive devices. The therapist has a critical role in the delivery of follow-through services that is not yet widely recognized.

Chapter 11 References

Batavia, A., Dillard, D., & Phillips, B. (1990). How to avoid technology abandonment. *Proceedings of the 5th Annual Conference on Technology and Persons with Disabilities*. Los Angeles, CA, 55–64.

Batavia, A., & Hammer, G. (1989). Consumer criteria for evaluating assistive devices: Implications for technology transfer. *Proceedings of the 12th Annual RESNA Conference*. New Orleans, LA, 194–195

Baxter, R. (1972). *Guidelines for working relationships between VR agencies and rehabilitation facilities* (pp.1–2). Washington, DC: Council of State Administrators of Vocational Rehabilitation.

Enders, A., & Hall, M. (Eds.). (1990). *Assistive technology sourcebook*. Washington. DC: RESNA Press.

Mallik, K. (1990). Rehabilitation engineering: Who pays for it? *Proceedings of the 13th Annual RESNA Conference*. Washington, DC, 317-318.

Mallik, K., & Elder, G. (1993). Consumers who choose use... *Proceedings of the 16th Annual RESNA Conference*. Las Vegas, NV, 39–40.

Markowicz, A., & Reeb, K.G. (1988). *An overview of Medicaid reimbursement for rehabilitation equipment in the United States*. Washington, DC: Electronic Industries Foundation.

Mendelsohn, S. (1987). *Financing adaptive technology: A guide to sources and strategies for blind and visually-impaired users*. New York, NY: Smiling Interfaces.

Morris, M.W., & Golinker, L.A. (1991). *Assistive technology: A funding workbook, 1991 edition*. Washington, DC: RESNA Press.

Mortola, P., Kohn, J., & LeBlanc, M. (1989). Implementation and follow-up of rehabilitation technology. *Proceedings of the 12th Annual RESNA Conference*. New Orleans, LA, 202–203.

Mortola, P., Kohn, J., & LeBlanc, M. (1990). Follow-up and videotape in rehabilitation technology. *Proceedings of the 13th Annual RESNA Conference*. Washington, DC, 29–30.

Mortola, P., Kohn, J., & LeBlanc, M. (1991). A follow-up plan for rehabilitation technology: An occupational therapist's role. *Proceedings of the 14th Annual RESNA Conference*. Kansas City, MO, 24–26.

National Council on Disability. (1993). *Study on the financing of assistive technology devices and services for individuals with disabilities*. Washington DC: Author.

Reavis, D., Hensley, O., Dudek, R., Jones, J., & Sparling, C. (1989). Individualized technology. *Proceedings of the 12th Annual RESNA Conference*. New Orleans, LA, 356–357.

Reeb, K.G. (1987a). *Private insurance reimbursement for rehabilitation equipment*. Washington, DC:

Rehabilitation Engineering Center, Electronics Industries Foundation.

Reeb, K.G. (1987b). *Revolving loan funds: Expanding equipment credit financing opportunities for persons with disabilities.* Washington, DC: Rehabilitation Engineering Center, Electronics Industries Foundation.

Scherer, M.J. (1989). But will the assistive technology device be used? *Proceedings of the 12th Annual RESNA Conference.* New Orleans, LA, 356–357.

Schlacter, G.A., & Weber, R.D. (1990). *Financial aid for the disabled and their families 1990–1991.* San Carlos, CA: Reference Service Press.

Smith, R.O. (1987). *Service delivery and related issues at the Trace Research and Development Center.* Madison, WI: Trace Research and Development Center.

Tewey, B.P., Barnicle, K., & Perr, A. (1994, October). The wrong stuff. *MAINSTREAM,* 19–23.

Thomas, D.F. (1986). *Fees for services: Principles and practices among state vocational rehabilitation agencies and facilities.* Menominie, WI: Stout Vocational Rehabilitation Institute, University of Wisconsin-Stout.

Ward, C.A. (1989). *Subsidy programs for assistive devices.* Washington, DC: Rehabilitation Engineering Center, Electronic Industries Foundation.

Chapter 11 Study Questions

1   What are five options for funding assistive devices?

2. Describe the funding implications of two federal programs.

3. Identify and describe the three components of follow-through services.

4   What are the roles of equipment vendors and consumers in the follow-through process?

5. How do occupational therapists support the follow-through process?

Unit V: Assistive Technology Information

Introduction to Unit V

This unit provides information on methods and resources to remain current in the field of assistive technology. If one thing is certain, it is that the devices we select today will be replaced by improved devices tomorrow. Practitioners must keep up-to-date on what is available.

In addition to keeping current, practitioners need a place to go with questions. If you experience some difficulty in installing software or a computer board, there may be others who have experienced the same problem and who can share the solution.

This unit provides information on organizations that relate to disability and technology, publications on disability and technology, and electronic resources—information that is available via computer.

Chapter 12:
Organizations, Publications, and Electronic Resources

I. Organizations

    A. Professional Organizations/Conferences

    B. Interdisciplinary Professional Organizations

    C. Interdisciplinary Professional Conferences

    D. Consumer-Oriented Organizations

        1. Organizations for Persons With Vision Impairments

        2. Organizations for Persons With Hearing Impairments

        3. Organizations for Persons With Physical Disabilities

        4. Organizations With a Focus on Developmental Disabilities

        5. Organizations With a Focus on Older Persons

        6. Organizations With a Cross-Disability Focus

II. Publications

    A. Resource Guides

    B. Books

    C. Journals/Magazines

    D. Newsletters

III. Electronic Resources

    A. Networks

    B. Online Databases

    C. Bulletin Boards

IV. Helpful Reference Works

12.

Organizations, Publications, and Electronic Resources

Joseph P. Lane, MBPA

Organizations

Professional Organizations/Conferences

American Occupational Therapy Association (AOTA)

4720 Montgomery Lane
P.O. Box 31220
Bethesda, MD 20824-1220
(301) 652-2682; (800) 843-2682 (toll-free number for members only)

Each year at the AOTA national conference, three major components on assistive technology are offered: (1) Technology Forum, where papers are presented; (2) Technology Lab, where products and new devices are displayed and personnel are available to discuss the latest developments; and (3) the Exhibitors Hall, which is not limited to assistive devices but does include many vendor displays with the very latest assistive technology. In addition, AOTA members have the opportunity to join a Technology Special Interest Section (SIS) that publishes a quarterly newsletter and a new book (in press), *The Pictorial Dictionary of Low-Tech Assistive Devices*.

American Physical Therapy Association (APTA)

1111 N. Fairfax Street
Alexandria, VA 22314-1488
(703) 706-3395

APTA has special interest groups, workshops, and publications addressing assistive technology. The annual conference includes sessions and exhibits on technology and disability.

American Speech-Language-Hearing Association (ASHA)

10801 Rockville Pike
Rockville, MD 20852
(301) 897-5700 or (800) 638-8255 or (800) 638-6868

ASHA publishes a booklet targeted primarily at consumers, entitled *Augmentative Communication*, which provides an overview of the topic and includes brief case studies. ASHA also has a packet of information on assistive listening devices.

IEEE Engineering in Medicine and Biology Society

The Institute of Electrical and Electronics Engineers
345 East 47th Street
New York, NY 10017-2394
(212) 705-7900

IEEE members with principal professions in biomedical engineering are increasing their focus on assistive technology and rehabilitation. They now publish the journal *IEEE Transactions on Rehabilitation Engineering* (see Figure 12.1).

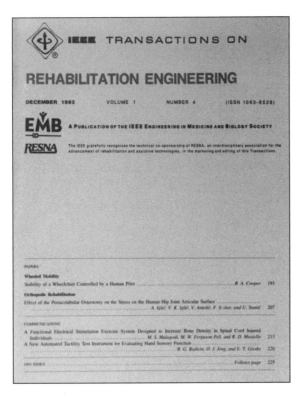

Figure 12.1. IEEE *Transactions on Rehabilitation Engineering.*

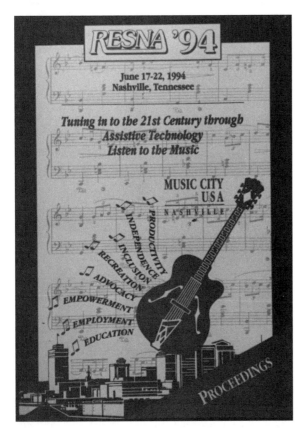

Figure 12.2. *RESNA '94.*

Interdisciplinary Professional Organizations

Interdisciplinary Society for the Advancement of Rehabilitative and Assistive Technology (RESNA)

1700 N. Moore Street
Suite 1540
Arlington, VA 22209
(703) 524-6686

Originally named the Rehabilitation Engineering Society of North America, RESNA changed its name to reflect the diversity of professional groups among its members, but it maintained the same acronym—RESNA. This is the premier organization focused on assistive technology. RESNA holds an annual conference devoted entirely to assistive technology (see Figure 12.2). Conference proceedings are available for purchase. It publishes a journal called *Assistive Technology,* which is described in this chapter. In addition, RESNA offers a number of other publications on assistive technology. For any person whose focus is assistive technology, RESNA membership is a must.

Human Factors and Ergonomics Society

1124 Montana Avenue, Suite B
Santa Monica, CA 90403

The Human Factors and Ergonomics society is an interdisciplinary association for people involved in the characteristics of human beings that are applicable to the design of systems and devices of all kinds. It publishes the quarterly journal Human Factors, and two monthly bulletins.

International Society for Augmentative and Alternative Communication (ISAAC)

428 East Preston Street
Baltimore, MD 21202-3993

ISAAC publishes a journal entitled *Augmentative and Alternative Communication.* It also holds a biennial conference and publishes the proceedings in its journal.

Interdisciplinary Professional Conferences

Technology & Persons With Disabilities

Center on Disabilities
California State University, Northridge
18111 Nordhoff Street
Northridge, CA 91330-8340
(818) 885-2578

The "CSUN" conference is held each spring in Los Angeles. It features strong international representation, multidisciplinary breadth, and substantial consumer orientation. CSUN offers workshops, presentations, demonstrations, and the most comprehensive exhibit on the west coast. CSUN also includes mini-conferences on selected topics such as virtual reality and the information superhighway. Conference proceedings are available for purchase.

Closing the Gap

> P.O. Box 68
> Henderson, MN 56044
> (612) 248-3294

Closing the Gap offers an annual conference that is held in Minneapolis each year. This conference attracts a number of both therapists and educators. Thus, the focus of Closing the Cap is mainly, though not exclusively, on assistive technology for education. Closing the Gap also offers workshops that are held around the country. Contact their office for details. It offers a bimonthly newspaper. One does not become a member of Closing the Gap, but rather subscribes to its newspaper. For school-based occupational therapists, a subscription to *Closing the Gap* is a very helpful information source.

Council for Exceptional Children (CEC)

> 1920 Association Drive
> Reston, VA 22091
> (703) 620-3660

The national association for teachers, special educators, and consulting teachers. CEC supports the Center on Special Education Technology, and the Technology and Media (TAM) Conference. It publishes the journal *Exceptional Children.*

European Conference on the Advancement of Rehabilitation Technology (ECART)

> Conference Secretariat
> The Swedish Handicap Institute
> Box 510
> S-162 15
> Uallingby, Sweden
> +4686201700

The ECART conference is the European equivalent of RESNA. It presents the work of researchers, practitioners, and consumers on all aspects of rehabilitation and assistive technologies. Like RESNA, the conference proceedings are organized into special-interest categories (see Figure 12.3).

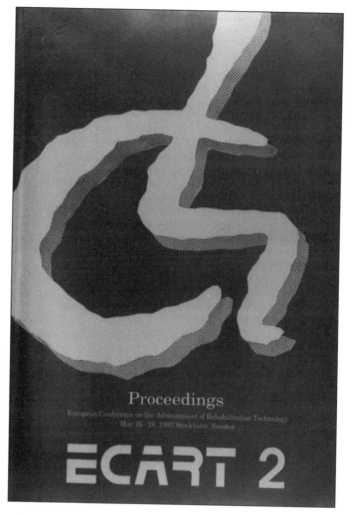

Figure 12.3. *ECART.*

Consumer-Oriented Organizations

The following organizations offer information on assistive devices for specific disability groups. This information may be helpful to you as a therapist, but you can also recommend that the people you serve contact the appropriate organizations below. Typically, the information is written in a style that is understandable and informative for consumers.

Organizations for Persons With Vision Impairments

American Foundation for the Blind

> 15 West 16th Street
> New York, NY 10011
> (212) 620-2000

Offers a free publication entitled *Public Education Materials Catalogue.*

Association for Macular Diseases

210 East 64th Street
New York, NY 10021
(212) 605-3719

Offers a hot line for information on macular degeneration and produce a newsletter.

Blinded Veterans Association

447 H Street, N.W.
Washington, DC 20001
(202) 371-8880

Publishes the *Bulletin,* offering information on a variety of topics including funding issues.

National Library Service for the Blind and Physically Handicapped

1291 Taylor Street, N.W.
Washington, DC 20542
(800) 424-8567 or 424-8572

Provides a number of services, including *Talking Books,* publications on audio cassettes, and computer discs. Each state has at least one regional library.

Resources for Rehabilitation

33 Bedford Street, Suite 19A
Lexington, MA 02173
(617) 862-6455

Provides information and training on resources for people with vision loss.

Organizations for Persons With Hearing Impairments

Alexander Graham Bell Association for the Deaf

3417 Volta Place, N.W.
Washington, DC 20007-2778
(202) 337-5220

This association provides information on hearing aids and lip-reading.

National Technical Institute for the Deaf (NTID)

1 Lamb Memorial Drive
Rochester, NY 14623
(716) 475-6400

A national resource center for technical services, devices, and information for persons who are deaf or hard of hearing.

American Deafness and Rehabilitation Association

Box 55369
Little Rock, AR 72225
(501) 868-8850

Publishes a journal and newsletter on hearing impairment.

American Tinnitus Association

P.O. Box 5
Portland, OR 97207
(503) 248-9985

Provides information on tinnitus and support research and education.

National Association for Hearing and Speech Action

10801 Rockville Pike
Rockville, MD 20852
(800) 638-8255 or 638-6868

This association offers "HELPLINE," which helps consumers locate service providers.

National Captioning Institute

5203 Leesburg Pike
Falls Church, VA 22041
(703) 998-2400; (800) 533-9673

The National Captioning Institute offers help in locating TeleCaption decoder retail outlets.

National Information Center on Deafness

Gallaudet University
800 Florida Avenue, N.E.
Washington, DC 20002
(202) 651-5051 (voice); (202) 651-5052 (TDD)

Provides information on hearing impairments and makes referrals to local community service providers.

Self Help for Hard-of-Hearing People

7800 Wisconsin Avenue
Bethesda, MD 20814
(301) 657-2248 (voice); (301) 657-2249 (TDD)

This organization and its local chapters provide information, referrals, and support.

U.S. Veterans Administration

Prosthetics Division
All Local VA Medical Centers

Provides hearing aids to eligible veterans and TeleCaption decoders free if the hearing loss is service-related.

Organizations for Persons With Physical Disabilities

TASH (The Association for Persons With Severe Handicaps)

7010 Roosevelt Way N.E.
Seattle, WA, 98115

(800) 482-TASH

TASH provides information on severe disabilities and disseminates materials through an active publications department.

National Spinal Cord Injury Association

600 West Cummings Parkway
Woburn, MA 01801
(301) 565-0433

They are involved with the direct care rehabilitation and independence of persons who have paraplegia or quadriplegia. They also publish newsletters and other materials.

National Autism Society of America (ASA)

1234 Massachusetts Ave, N.W., Suite 1017
Washington, DC 20005
(202) 783-0125

ASA is a national parent, professional, and advocacy organization for people with autism. ASA provides services at a local level, information on developments in the field of autism, public policy advocacy, and referral services.

Organizations With a Focus on Developmental Disabilities

United Cerebral Palsy Association (UCPA National Headquarters)

1522 K Street N.W., Suite 1112
Washington, DC 20005
(202) 842-1266; (800) 872-5827

A research, information, and advocacy agency for persons with cerebral palsy and their families. UCPA has 2,215 local affiliated agencies throughout the country.

Association for Retarded Citizens (The ARC)

2501 Avenue J
Arlington, TX 76006
(817) 640-0204

Focuses on assistive technology development, delivery, and use by persons with mental retardation or other developmental disabilities.

American Association on Mental Retardation (AAMR)

1719 Kalorama Road, N.W.
Washington, DC 20005
(202) 387-1968

The AAMR is a major source of information on developmental disabilities. They publish two journals: *Mental Retardation* and *American Journal on Mental Retardation,* as well as several books. They sponsor an annual convention and state and regional meetings. Members of AAMR can also join special interest groups (i.e., aging, Down's syndrome, sexual/social concerns, health promotion) and divisions (i.e., education, psychology, occupational and physical therapy, communication disorders, etc.).

Developmental Disabilities Bureau

Department of Health and Human Services
330 C Street, S.W.
Washington, DC 20201
(202) 245-0870

This organization provides support and advocacy services.

Organizations With a Focus on Older Persons

American Association of Retired Persons (AARP)

1909 K Street, N.W.
Washington, DC 20049
(202) 434-2277

AARP offers a variety of membership programs, publications, and advocacy. AARP is increasingly interested in the role of assistive technology in the lives of older persons.

American Society on Aging (ASA)

833 Market Street, Suite 511
San Francisco, CA 94103-1824
(415) 974-1824

The American Society on Aging is taking an active role in exploring the value of assistive technology. ASA established a special interest group on "Aging, Disability and Rehabilitation," and linked it to a focus on "Technology and Aging."

The Gerontological Society of America (GSA)

1275 K Street, N.W., Suite 350
Washington, DC 20005-4006
(202) 842-1275

The GSA's emphasis on improving functional independence in later life includes an interest in rehabilitation and assistive technology.

Organizations With a Cross-Disability Focus

Technology Related Assistance for Individuals With Disabilities Act

Every state operates an information and referral program on assistive technology devices and services. Unfortunately, the programs have different adminis-

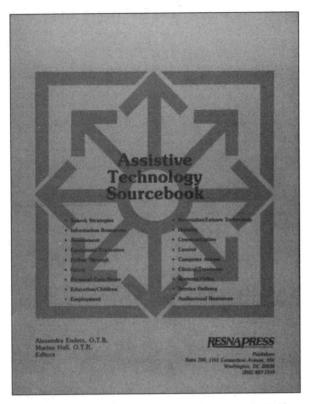

Figure 12.4. *Assistive Technology Sourcebook.*

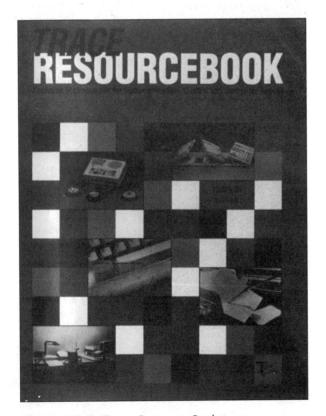

Figure 12.5. *Trace Resource Book.*

trative locations, different names, and different contact numbers. Call the RESNA Technical Assistance Project at (703) 524-6686 for contact information in your state.

National Council on Independent Living (NCIL)

3607 Chapel Road
Newton Square, PA 19073
(215) 353-6066

The national organization for independent living centers, with approximately 400 members. Each state also has an organizing board and a state-level membership.

PUBLICATIONS

Many publications are available to help you identify products and learn more about how to use them. The four types described here are:

A. Resource Guides
B. Books
C. Journals/Magazines
D. Newsletters

Resource Guides

Assistive Technology Sourcebook (1990)

Alexandria Enders & Marian Hall, Editors
RESNA
1700 N. Moore Street
Suite 1540
Arlington, VA 22209
(703) 524-6686

A thorough review of information acquisition, personal assessment, technology evaluation, applications, policy issues, service delivery, and resources (see Figure 12.4). Buy this resource guide first, followed by the *TRACE Resource Book* described below (see Figure 12.5).

Trace Resource Book: Assistive Technology for Communication, Control and Computer Access (1993-94 Edition)

TRACE
S-151 Waisman Center
University of Wisconsin, Madison
1500 Highland Avenue
Madison, WI 53705
(608) 262-6966

This 937-page book is complied and updated to help professionals, consumers, and family members understand and locate useful tools. The book emphasizes functions, not disabilities, so the products are organized under "communication," "control," "computer access," and "special software." It includes 50 pages of small type on information resources much more complete than this chapter. The RESNA and TRACE guides will be your critical resources.

Directory of National Information Sources on Disabilities (1992)

> National Institute on Disability and
> Rehabilitation Research
> U.S. Department of Education
> Washington, DC 20202
> (202) 732-5800

This directory is a reference tool for organizations and people providing information, referrals, and direct services relating to disabilities. It contains 550 pages of national program descriptions in alphabetical order, and a list of databases, directories, and hot lines in the field. It also contains an index organizing agencies by subject. Very useful (see Figure 12.6).

Resources for Elders With Disabilities (1990)

> Resources for Rehabilitation
> 33 Bedford Street, Suite 19A
> Lexington, MA 02173

This 168-page resource guide includes chapters on hearing loss, vision loss, diabetes, arthritis, stroke, and osteoporosis. Each of these chapters includes lists of: (1) publications and tapes on the disability area; (2) assistive devices and other special equipment; and (3) organizations that provide information and/or services. The last chapter is entitled "Aids and Devices That Make Everyday Living Easier."

The Accessible Housing Design File: Barrier Free Environments (1991)

> Ronald L. Mace, FAIA
> Van Nostrand Reinhold
> 115 Fifth Avenue
> New York, NY 10003

This 200-page book is based on the work of Barrier Free Environments, Inc., combined with findings from work funded by the National Institute on Disability and Rehabilitation Research (NIDRR). It contains designs for accessibility that are readily integrated into housing. It includes designs addressing accessibility of vehicles and transportation, entrances, doorways and windows, kitchens, bathrooms, and bedrooms (see Figure 12.7).

Beautiful Barrier-Free: A Visual Guide to Accessibility (1993)

> Cynthia Leibrock and Susan Behar
> Van Nostrand Reinhold
> 115 Fifth Avenue
> New York, NY 10003

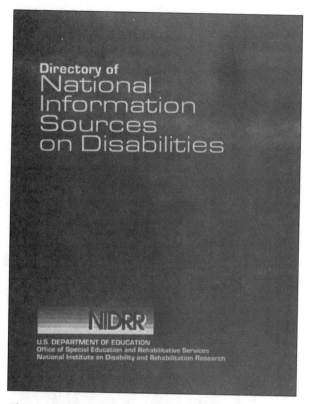

Figure 12.6. *Directory of National Information Sources on Disabilities* (1992).

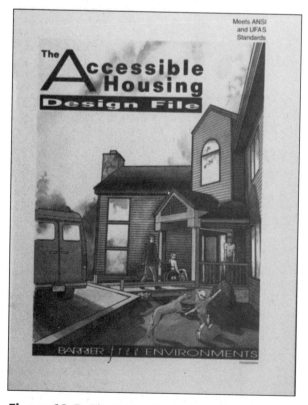

Figure 12.7. *The Accessible Housing Design File: Barrier Free Environments* (1991).

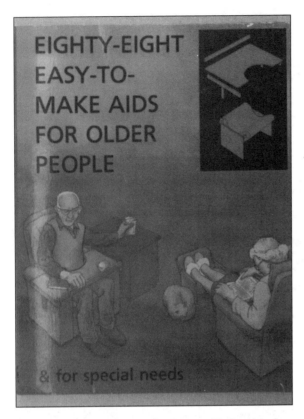

Figure 12.8. *Eighty-Eight Easy to Make Aids for Older People* (1990).

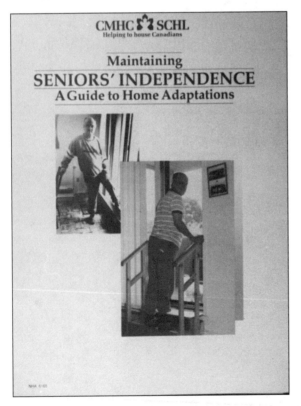

Figure 12.9. *Maintaining Seniors' Independence in the Home: A Guide to Home Adaptations* (1989).

A 200-page book of full-color photographs and detailed text demonstrating that accessibility is both readily achievable and quite attractive. The book shows adaptable products for the exterior and entrances; the mechanical, electric, and acoustic infrastructure; the ceiling and wall finishes; windows and doors; floor covering options; furniture of all types; accessories and equipment; then a final focus on hardware for the kitchen and bathroom. Although many of the products have a high price, the ideas they represent can be adapted. Accessibility concepts have reached product designers and manufacturers.

Eighty-Eight Easy to Make Aids for Older People (1990)

> Don Caston
> Hartley & Marks, Inc.
> P.O. Box 147
> Point Roberts, WA 98281

This 108-page book contains detailed steps and drawings so people can make or participate in making and installing helpful devices and gadgets for the home. The book opens with a chapter on tool use, followed by device plans for the kitchen (e.g., foot stool, cutting aid), dining and living room (e.g., backrest, trolley table), bedroom (tray, step), and bathroom, and yard and garden items. Although many of these devices can be purchased, building them may offer more reward as a consumer or family project (see Figure 12.8).

Maintaining Seniors' Independence in the Home: A Guide to Home Adaptations (1989)

> Danielle Maltais, Program Director
> Public Affairs Centre
> Canada Mortgage and Housing Corporation
> Montreal, Canada

This 100-page workbook presents an assessment tool for identifying needed home improvements or adaptations that are easy or inexpensive to perform. It works through a wide range of activities. If the senior reports difficulty with an activity, the workbook branches off to identify specific functional limitations, present likely problem areas in checklists, then present multiple recommendations for consideration (see Figure 12.9).

Special Education Technology: Classroom Applications (1993)

> Rena B. Lewis
> Wadsworth, Inc.
> Belmont, CA 94002

This 550-page book covers the role of assistive technology within the domain of special education. It has chapters on the technology in the classroom, adapting and using computers, selecting software, technology for the youngster, the severely impaired, and integrating technologies. It also addresses the access technologies, including augmentative communication, physical barriers, and sensory impairments. The book is easy to follow and contains hundreds of device photos and computer screen examples.

The Source Book for the Disabled (1979)

Glorya Hale
Saunders Press
W.B. Saunders Company
Philadelphia, PA

While this book is somewhat dated for a publication on assistive devices, it is included because it goes beyond a listing of available products and provides a very useful resource for consumers. This book begins by listing and describing, with illustrations, product types and product features. Thus, though the book was written in England, an awareness of these product types and features provides the consumer with information upon which a search for specific products could be undertaken. Product descriptions are provided for eating and drinking, bathing, dental care, shaving, hair care, nail care, cosmetics, menstruation, incontinence, clothing, dressing, hosiery and footwear, aids to sexual pleasure, furniture and equipment, lifting and carrying, bathing a baby, dressing a child, leisure, and recreation. Resource lists of organizations and a few product companies are provided in the last section of the book.

Coping With Daily Life: Handbook of Technical Aids (1988)

Les Editions Papyrus
745, Avenue Eymard
Quebec, Canada G1S3Z9

The uniqueness of this handbook is that all of the technical aids included are "buildable," and this publication describes how they can be made (see Figure 12.10). The purpose of the book is described by the authors in their introduction:

> In spite of the numerous devices and technical aids available on the market, it may sometimes become necessary to make an adaptation from scratch. This guide shows how to make widely used adaptations not

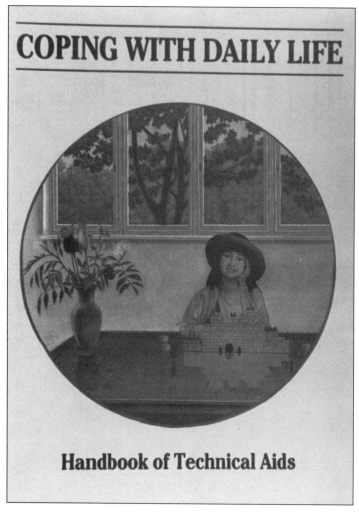

Figure 12.10. *Coping With Daily Life: Handbook of Technical Aids* (1988).

available elsewhere. Major categories covered include personal care, home management, vocational and educational management, mobility, seating, transportation, communication, recreation, and ambulation.

Resource Inventory: Assistive Devices

Center for Special Education Technology
1920 Association Drive
Reston, VA 22091

The Center for Special Education Technology is a project of The Council for Exceptional Children. It publishes a list, updated annually, of organizations that offer services in assistive devices, augmentative communication, and other resources. The listings appear alphabetically by state. The listings are simply organization name, address, phone number, type of services, and contact person. Beyond this basic information, there is no descriptive or evaluative data.

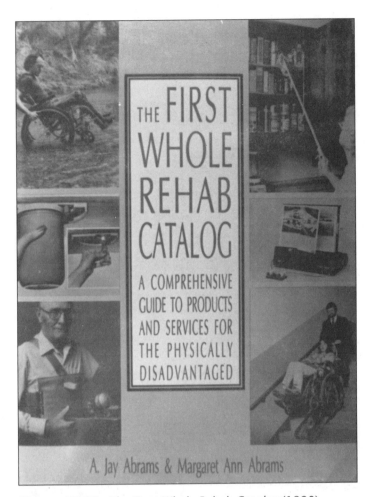

Figure 12.11. *The First Whole Rehab Catalog* (1990).

The First Whole Rehab Catalog (1990)

> Jay Abrams & Margaret Ann Abrams
> Betterway Publications, Inc.
> Box 219
> Crozet, VA 22932

Targeted at consumers, this publication "can help you find out what commercial products are available, where and how to get them and, in many instances, what you can expect to pay for them." It contains many helpful pictures and uses short case studies for examples of who would use certain kinds of equipment. The descriptions of products are much more detailed than you would find in a vendor's product catalog (see Figure 12.11).

Visual Aids and Informational Material (1987–1988)

> National Association for Visually Handicapped
> 22 West 21st Street—6th Floor
> New York, NY 10010

This publication provides pictures and descriptions of a variety of products for people who are blind or have low vision. Some of the products are available from the National Association for Visually Handicapped. Categories of devices include magnifiers, lamps, clocks and watches, writing aids, personal items, and miscellaneous items.

Specialized Audio, Visual, and Tactile Alerting Devices for Deaf and Hard of Hearing People (1989)

> Carl J. Jensema
> Technology Assessment Program
> Gallaudet University
> 800 Florida Avenue, N.E.
> Washington, DC 20002

This 36-page publication lists sound, vibration, and light alerting devices, and provides comparative information on features and prices among different products. Addresses of companies that sell these products are listed on the last page.

Cognitive Rehabilitation Resources for the Apple II Computer

> Jeffrey S. Kreutzer, Mark R. Hill,
> Catherine Morrison
> NeuroScience Publishers
> 6555 Carrollton Avenue
> Indianapolis, IN 46220

This 117-page book provides an overview of cognitive rehabilitation, information on basics of computer operation and selection of a computer system, definitions of cognitive rehabilitation terminology, and reviews of software in these areas: arithmetic, attention and concentration, auditory discrimination, auditory memory, concept formation, funding information, hand–eye coordination, motor coordination/dexterity, nonverbal memory, reaction time, reading comprehension, reasoning, sequencing, spatial orientation, spelling, verbal memory, verbal skills, visual discrimination, visual scanning, and visuospatial abilities.

Resource Guide for Persons With Mobility Impairments (1989)

> IBM National Support Center for
> Persons With Disabilities
> P.O. Box 2150
> Atlanta, GA 30055
> (800) IBM-2133 (Voice/TDD); 404-238-4760

This directory provides product descriptions and

basic ordering information for computer access equipment, including keyboard modification, alternate input devices, switching devices, voice recognition, environmental control devices, alternatives to printed documentation, word processing, and an IBM PC voice-activated keyboard utility. Information is also included on agencies and associations related to assistive technology.

The Lighthouse Low Vision Catalog: Optical Devices, Products, Services (1990)

> 36-02 Northern Boulevard
> Long Island City, NY 11101

This catalog lists products assembled by the Lighthouse for resale, most of which are low-tech. Sections include spectacles, hand magnifiers, stand magnifiers, telescopes and adaptive devices, absorptive lenses/sunwear, electronic magnification, nonoptical devices, lighting, frames and accessories, and test materials.

Technology and Employment of Persons With Disabilities (1989)

> Leonard G. Perlman and Carl E. Hansen, Editors
> National Rehabilitation Association
> 633 South Washington Street
> Alexandria, VA 22314-4193

This 84-page monograph is subtitled "A Report on the 13th Mary E. Switzer Memorial Seminar." It includes papers by eight authors, focusing on issues related to applications of technology for employment of persons with disabilities.

Books

Technology and Aging in America (1985)

> Congress of the United States
> Office of Technology Assessment
> for sale by: U.S. Government Printing Office
> Washington, DC 20402

This 496-page book reports on a national study of older Americans and ways in which technology can help in maintaining independence and quality of life. It discusses aging, chronic conditions, prevention, nutrition, medications, cost of health care, and many other topics that serve as background information for discussing technology applications. This is more of a policy-level analysis than a description of how to use specific devices (see Figure 12.12).

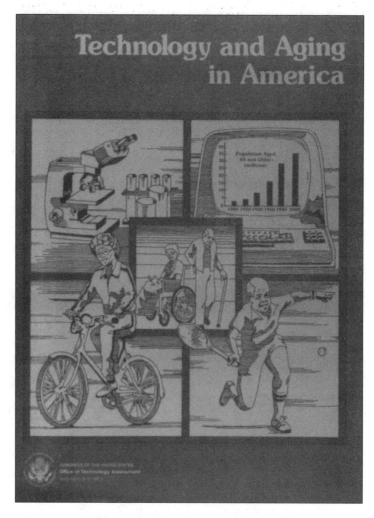

Figure 12.12. *Technology and Aging in America* (1985).

Selected Readings on Powered Mobility for Children and Adults With Severe Physical Disabilities (1986)

> RESNA
> 1101 Connecticut Avenue, N.W.
> Suite 700
> Washington, DC 20036

This book describes the evaluation and prescription process for powered mobility and the application of various options for persons with physical disabilities. It includes articles on issues related to powered mobility, a listing of products available, descriptions of control options, case studies, and listings of other resources.

Colleges That Enable (1989)

> Prudence K. Tweed and Jason C. Tweed
> Park Avenue Press
> Oil City, PA

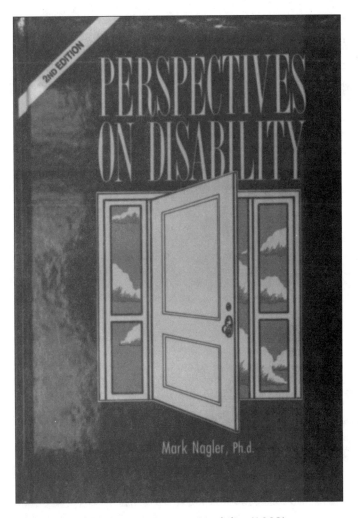

Figure 12.13. *Perspectives on Disability* (1993).

Subtitled "A Guide to Support Services Offered to Physically Disabled Students on 40 U.S. Campuses," this publication evaluates campuses on the types and levels of services for students with disabilities. It is not limited to an evaluation of assistive devices but includes information about books on tape, adapted computer labs, voice-controlled computers, financial counseling, and special equipment for the sensory and hearing impaired. Check to see if your campus (or your alma mater) is listed as an adapted campus. If not, consider becoming an advocate for accessibility!

Rehabilitation Engineering (1990)

Raymond V. Smith and John H. Leslie, Jr.,
Editors
CRC Press
Boca Raton, Ann Arbor, Boston

This is a 533-page book, with 26 contributing authors. While a very expensive publication, the level of detail on many engineering aspects makes this worth considering as a resource. It addresses the topics of assessment, measurement, selection criteria, accessibility, and applications of assistive technology.

Technology and Handicapped People (1982)

Congress of the United States
Office of Technology Assessment
[Out of Print]

This 214-page report examined the specific factors affecting the research and development, evaluation, diffusion and marketing, delivery, use, and financing of assistive devices. The review is in the context of federal public policy. An update report is in development for publication in 1995.

Managing End User Computing for Users With Disabilities (1989)

General Services Administration
Information Resources Management Service
for sale by: U.S. Government Printing
Office
Washington, DC 20402

This book was written to provide personnel managers in federal government jobs with information on the application of computer and related information technology to accommodate users with disabilities. It offers a short overview of available technology, followed by "assessment forms" for determining environmental and equipment availability and limitations, and user needs. All of the above is covered in 16 pages. The remainder of the book contains resource lists and policy and regulatory information.

From Toys to Computers: Access for the Physically Disabled Child (1988)

Christine Wright and Mari Nomura
Box 700242
San Jose, CA 95170

This book, written by two occupational therapists, is based on experience in working with more than 200 children with orthopedic disabilities. The focus is on physical disabilities, particularly motor impairments of the extremities. It does not address the needs of children with auditory, visual, or cognitive disabilities, although some of the adapted toys would be useful for other populations. This book includes directions for adapting toys, complete with illustrations. It also describes how to set up a lending library, switches, positioning, and microcomputers. Resource lists are included as appendixes.

Perspectives on Disability (1993)

> Mark A. Nagler, Editor
> Health Markets Research Publishers
> 851 Moana Court
> Palo Alto, CA 94306

This 550-page book of small type addresses the spectrum of concerns that are considered crucial in understanding the issues related to the study of disability and people with disabilities (see Figure 12.13). It contains 52 different articles, each with references, organized under seven headings: "What it Means to be Disabled," "Society and Disability," "The Family and Disability," "Sexuality and Disability," "Medical and Psychological Issues and Disability," "Education, Employment, Social Planning and Disability," and "Legal and Ethical Issues in Disability."

Living in the State of Stuck:
How Technology Impacts the Lives of
People With Disabilities (1993)

> Marcia J. Scherer
> Brookline Books
> P.O. Box 1046
> Cambridge, MA 02238-1046

The author presents the experiences of being born with a disability or acquiring a disability through the words and daily lives of people with different disabilities. The chapters focus on the role of assistive technology in these peoples' lives. The main message is that assistive devices can be helpful, but the consumers must be prepared to use the technology. Technology users also need continuing consultation as their technology use changes with their life circumstances (see Figure 12.14).

Disabled Village Children (1988)

> David Werner
> The Hesperian Foundation
> P.O. Box 1692
> Palo Alto, CA 94302

The 650-page book introduces the reader to the concept of "appropriate" interventions—including assistive devices. The book addresses those primary and secondary disabilities most common throughout the world, particularly in developing countries. The three sections, "Working With the Child and Family," "Working With the Community," and "Working in the Shop," all demonstrate the remarkable achievements possible by understanding, respecting, and involving the local community's culture. The text, photos, and illustrations are engaging. Every page draws the reader into the message (see Figure 12.15).

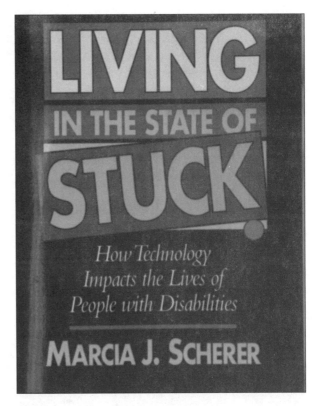

Figure 12.14. *Living in the State of Stuck: How Technology Impacts the Lives of People With Disabilities* (1993).

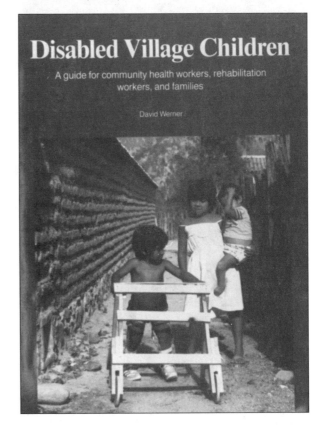

Figure 12.15. *Disabled Village Children.*

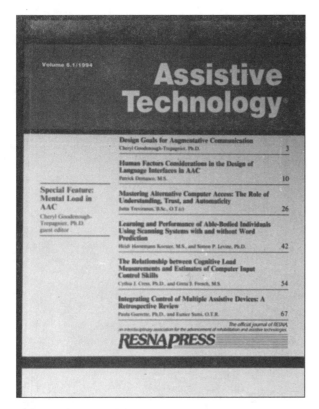

Figure 12.16. *Assistive Technology.*

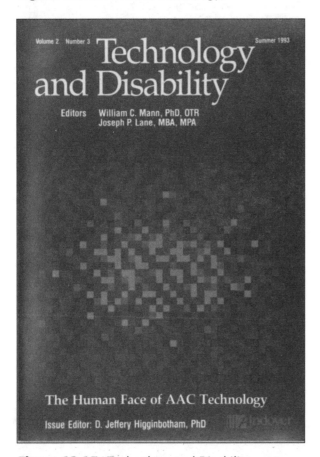

Figure 12.17. *Technology and Disability.*

Journals/Magazines

Assistive Technology

RESNA Press
1700 North Moore Street, Suite 1540
Arlington, VA 22209-1903

This journal is published twice per year and focuses on practitioners in assistive technology service delivery. Articles fall into the following categories: (1) applied research; (2) review papers summarizing the work of several investigators; (3) perspectives on issues in assistive technology by recognized authorities; (4) practical notes or papers that describe new methods; and (5) case studies that present work in progress or studies where there are only a few subjects (see Figure 12.16).

Technology and Disability

Elsevier Science Ireland Ltd.
Bay 15
Shannon Industrial Estate Co.
Clare, Ireland
t35361 471944

This journal covers the application of rehabilitative and assistive technology by persons with disabilities. It considers both low- and high-technology devices designed to improve human function. Each issue focuses on one specific topic. *Technology & Disability* is concerned with the application of technology to the performance of major life roles: education, employment, and recreation (see Figure 12.17).

IEEE Transactions on Rehabilitation Engineering

IEEE Headquarters
345 East 47th Street
New York, NY 10017-2394

This quarterly, peer-reviewed journal publishes basic and applied papers on rehabilitation engineering and assistive technology. It includes clinical applications, and experimental science and technological developments. This publication has a hard science emphasis.

Journal of Rehabilitation Research and Development

Superintendent of Documents
U.S. Government Printing Office
Washington DC 20402

This journal is published quarterly by the Rehabilitation Research and Development Service, Department of Veterans Affairs. It is a "scientific engineering publication in the multidisciplinary field of disability rehabilitation. General priority areas are prosthetics and orthotics, spinal cord injury, sensory aids, and gerontology. Only original scientific/engineering papers are published."

OSERS

> U.S. Department of Education
> Office of Special Education and Rehabilitative Services
> Room 3129
> Switzer Building
> 330 C Street, S.W.
> Washington, DC 20202-2524

This quarterly magazine is published by the U.S. Department of Education. Each issue focuses on a specific topic (e.g., independent living, vocational rehabilitation). The government, service agencies, funded grants, and unaffiliated people contribute articles to address the topic from various perspectives. Available free of charge (see Figure 12.18).

TEAM REHAB REPORT: For Professionals in Assistive Technology

> P.O. 8987
> 23815 Stuart Ranch Road
> Malibu, CA 90265
> (310) 317-4522

This is a monthly business magazine devoted to the assistive technology marketplace. It presents feature topics (e.g. aging and assistive technology), brief case studies of successful programs and technologies, advice columns for practitioners, new product and product line information, and current events. Free to long-term-rehabilitation professionals who purchase, prescribe, or recommend products. $24.00 per year for others (see Figure 12.19).

Independent Living: Connecting Dealers and People With Special Needs

> 150 Motor Parkway
> Suite 420
> Hauppauge, NY 11788-5145

The magazine is published seven times per year, including the *Resource Directory* and *Buyer's Guide.* Like *TEAM REHAB,* the magazine addresses topics, case studies, and new products. *Independent Living* focuses on the interactions between equipment suppliers and the end users. $18.00 per year (see Figure 12.20).

Mainstream: Magazine of the Able-Disabled

> 2973 Beech Street
> P.O. Box 370598
> San Diego, CA 92137-0598

Published 10 times per year, *Mainstream* covers a range of topics of interest to consumers. It provides

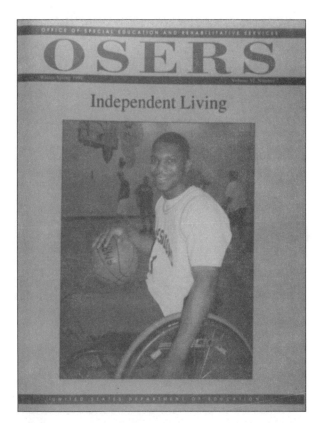

Figure 12.18. *OSERS.*

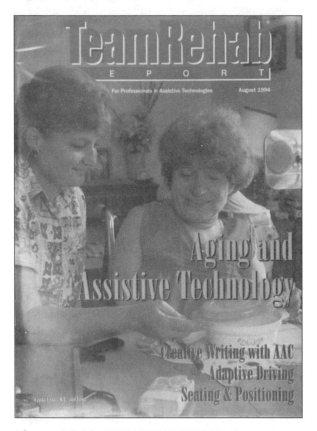

Figure 12.19. *TEAM REHAB REPORT: For Professionals in Assistive Technology.*

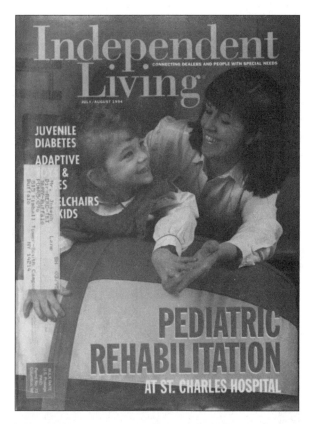

Figure 12.20. *Independent Living: Connecting Dealers and People With Special Needs.*

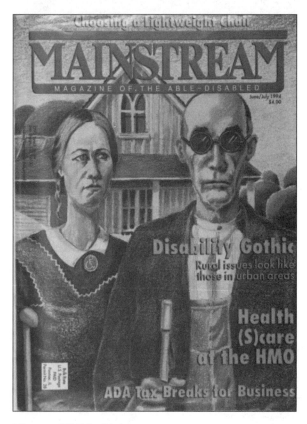

Figure 12.21. *Mainstream.*

updates on legislation, funding and politics, travel and fitness, new products, current vendors and manufacturers, and current events. $24.00 per year (see Figure 12.21).

Exceptional Parent: Parenting Your Child With a Disability

> P.O. Box 3000
> Dept. E.P.
> Denville, NJ 078342

A national, monthly magazine for parents of children and young adults with disabilities or special health care needs. It includes articles by parents and professionals, and information on products and resources. $24.00 per year.

Paraplegia News

> Paralyzed Veterans of America (PVA)
> 5201 North 19th Avenue, Suite 111
> Phoenix, AZ 85015
> (602) 246-9426

Monthly magazine advancing independent living for persons with paraplegia or quadriplegia. It features articles on the PVA organization research, and pertinent legislation.

Sports 'n Spokes

> PVA Publications Dept.
> 5201 North 19th Avenue, Suite 111
> Phoenix, AZ 85015
> (602) 246-9426

A bimonthly publication covering wheelchair competitive sports, recreation, equipment, and people. Includes calendar of sports events and features on recreational opportunities.

Accent on Living

> Cheever Publishing Company
> Box 700
> Bloomington, IL 61702
> (309) 378-2961

A guide to services and information on daily living and assistive technology. Articles focus on personal experiences of persons with disabilities and their ideas for improving daily living.

T.H.E. Journal Source Guide of High-Technology Products for Education

> Information Synergy, Inc.
> 2626 S. Pullman
> Santa Ana, CA 92705

T.H.E. Journal (T.H.E. stands for Technological Horizons in Education) is published monthly and is free for anyone having any connection with education. While not focused on disability or special education, the annual *Source Guide* includes computers and systems, input/output devices and enhancement boards, telecommunications, administrative and general-purpose software, courseware, furniture and accessories, CAD and robotics, and video and interactive video. In addition to individual product descriptions, the *Source Guide* includes comparative products for a given product line.

Newsletters

A.T. Quarterly

RESNA TA PROJECT
1700 N. Moore Street
Suite 1540
Arlington, VA 22209

The Technology Related Assistance for Individuals With Disabilities Act of 1988 provides funding to every state for establishing information networks that respond to consumer requests for information on assistive technology. See Chapter 1 for a description of related legislation. RESNA has a contract to provide technical assistance to states. This newsletter provides excellent summaries of important issues and excerpts of state program initiatives of interest to others.

Rehab Brief: Bringing Research Into Effective Focus

PSI International, Inc.
P.O. Box 5186
Arlington, VA 22205

This newsletter is funded through the U.S. Department of Education. Each issue takes a particular topic (e.g. vocational rehabilitation, assistive technology) and provides four to eight pages of summary information, examples, and references. It is written in a clear, informative style (see Figure 12.22).

Breaking New Ground: Cultivating Independence for Farmers and Ranchers With Disabilities

Breaking New Ground Resources Center
Purdue University
1146 Agricultural Engineering Building
West Lafayette, IN 47907-1146
(317) 494-5088

A quarterly newsletter offering features on helpful techniques and technologies, both low-tech and high-tech. Includes a calendar of events, a list of new resources, and opportunities to network.

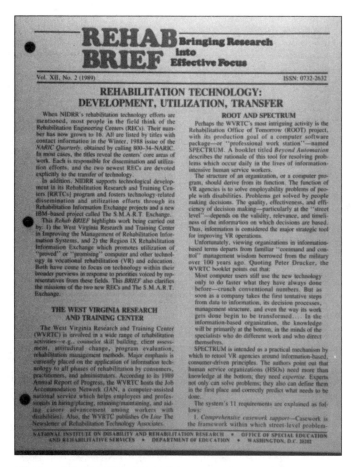

Figure 12.22. *Rehab Brief: Bringing Research into Effective Focus.*

Electronic Resources

The past 100 years have seen tremendous advances in our ability to communicate information. Consider that until the time of the telegraph, you either had to be in the same location as the person or group you were communicating with, or send a letter, smoke signal, or light signal. After the telegraph came the telephone. Then came radio communication to large groups and the television. Only very recently have we had computer technology and the communication capabilities it affords.

The term *telecommunications* is used for electronic information processing. Electronic pathways are used to channel data, voice, or even pictures, graphs, and video information. These electronic pathways consist of wires, which just within the past 100 years have been laid down around the world like a web. More recently we have fiber optic systems that include the use of microwave, and satellites.

We used to think of the telephone as a tool for voice communication—one person talking with another person. Now we use the telephone system to transfer other kinds of information. We can send data from one computer to another or to several others. We can also use the telephone system to "fax" letters and pictures across the country or around the world.

When we use computers to communicate—some people would say when we get computers to talk to each other—we are "networking." Networking requires some special hardware that is added to the computer and software to provide a meaningful interface for the people using the system. Networking can be as simple as linking two computers, or several in close proximity (called a local area network or LAN), or large numbers in a wide area network.

Current network developments are concerned with linking the huge and growing number of computer-based resources that already exist. In a sense, the "information highway" is already built. The Internet is an international network of interconnected computer networks that descend from a defense-related network called ARPAnet. Through the Internet, a computer with a modem can access the World-Wide Web (W3), developed by researchers at CERN in Switzerland.

The World-Wide Web defines itself as a "distributed heterogeneous collaborative multimedia information system" that permits anyone anywhere to disseminate or receive information in text, audio, and full-motion video through the Internet. To learn more about the Internet and the World-Wide Web, go make a friend in the computer sciences. These disciplines are bringing the future to you in ever-easier formats, offering more information access than space allows for discussion here.

The beauty of networking is the ease and speed with which large amounts of information can be transferred, combined with the computer's ability to search through large amounts of information (usually in databases) for precisely what is needed.

Electronic networks may offer three (or more) valuable features: bulletin board services, electronic mail, and access to databases. Bulletin boards are used for "posting" messages. A person looking for information on where to get a certain part for a computer could post this question on an appropriate electronic bulletin board such as SpecialNet. Someone reading the question could then post the answer. With bulletin boards, a person or agency can post messages about training opportunities, meetings, and other items of interest to several people at once and immediately.

Electronic mail is used for private communication, usually between two or a few people. The communication or message can be sent almost instantly, and sits in an "electronic mailbox" until the receiver calls up the message on his or her computer. Consider that two people, one in New York and one in Hong Kong, could send 20 or more electronic letters back and forth in a morning. What could be faster?

A third major use of networks is access to databases. A database is simply a collection of information carefully organized. A person can search through a database usually using one or a few "sort" variables. For example, a database of equipment for persons with disabilities could have the sort variable "type of equipment" and one could select among "mobility," "sensory," "environment control," and so forth. If the person selected "mobility," this category could be further focused into one of the following: "wheelchairs—powered," "wheelchairs—nonpowered," "walkers and canes," or "other." By using databases accessible on networks, a person can quickly receive information.

Networks

There are a number of networks that offer services and information relating to access issues and technology. They are described in the following section. Some of this information was collected and published by the RESNA Technical Assistance Project and is reproduced here with their permission.

World-Wide Web (W3)

To access W3 you need a computer (terminal, PC, MAC, or workstation) with a direct connection to the Internet, and a copy of a suitable client browser program such as Mosaic, Cello, Lynx, or WWW.

The World-Wide Web connection gives you access to hundreds of networks, databases, bulletin boards, and directories, in addition to links to discussion, news, and information groups under development through other networks.

Cooperative Electronic Library on Disability

Trace Center, University of Wisconsin
1500 Highland Avenue, Room 5-151
Madison, WI 53705
(608) 262-6966

This on-line or CD-ROM version library contains extensive compilations of resources on assistive technology, disabilities, and reference materials including:

- HyperAbleData—more than 19,000 products,
- Cooperative Services Directories—Eleven directories of services,
- Publications, Media, and Materials—books, videos, and REHAB DATA, and
- Text-Document Library—full text of 34 key documents.

CompuServe Disability Forum

CompuServe Information Service
5000 Arlington Centre Boulevard
P.O. Box 20212
Columbus, OH 43220
(800) 848-8990; (614) 457-8600

Description: An electronic network with many bulletin boards and databases. Information can be found on a number of subjects, such as the weather, the stock market, sports, child care, health care, and personal airline tickets, as well as educational and recreational computer programs. CompuServe services that provide information on assistive technology and/or disabilities include the Handicapped Users Database, Disabilities Forum, Rehabilitation R&D Database, and the Education Forum.

Target audience: Individuals interested in telecommunication services such as electronic mail, bulletin boards, and on-line conferencing.

Hardware/software needs: Telecommunications software and modem.

How to access: Subscription to CompuServe; 1200 or 2400 baud.

Cost: $39.95 to join, which includes a $25 usage credit, a free subscription to Compu-Serve magazine, and a user's guide. There is also a $1.50 monthly fee plus a connect charge of $12.50 an hour or 12 cents a minute.

Deaftek. USA

International Communications Limited
P.O. Box 81
Fayville, MA 01745
(508) 620-1777

Description: An electronic mail service that offers private communication and a bulletin board service.

Target audience: Designed for, but not limited to, persons who are hearing impaired.

Hardware/software needs: Telecommunications software and modem.

How to access: Via Telemail.

Cost: Standard phone charges.

SCAN (Shared communication and assistance network)

8630 Fenton Street, Suite 410
Silver Spring, MD 20910
(301) 588-8252

Description: A wide-ranging electronic network with local, state, regional, and national levels that offers mail, file transfers, bulletin boards, and databases.

Target audience: Persons interested in the developmental disabilities field.

Hardware/software needs: Telecommunications software and modem.

Cost: A one-time setup fee of $35.00; a monthly service fee of $6.95; an hourly charge of $17.50 for prime time, and $12.50 nonprime time.

How to access: Call SCAN to get set up. Access can be local via a telephone network service.

SpecialNet

GTE Education Services
8505 Freeport Parkway
Irving, TX 75063
(800) 634-5644

Description: An electronic network devoted to the information needs of special education teachers and administrators. The network includes electronic mail, bulletin boards, databases, and conferencing. The use of SpecialNet hookups for professional interchanges within several local agencies is also possible.

Target audience: Special educators and administrators.

Hardware/software needs: Telecommunications software and modem.

How to access: Via local Telenet number.

Cost: Several types of subscription plans are available. The basic plan is $200 a year, with subscribers billed monthly for connect time. Connect rates vary from $4 per hour at night (9:00 p.m.–7:00 a.m. daily) to $13 per hour during business hours (7:00 a.m.–6:00 p.m. Monday through Friday).

Online Databases

A database is a set of documents organized for easy search and retrieval. The purpose of the database is to archive information and provide a comprehensive search of information on a particular topic.

Abledata

National Rehabilitation Information Center
8455 Colesville Road, Suite 935
Silver Spring, MD 20910
(301) 588-9284 or (800) 346-2742

Description: An information source on disability-related products, this database contains more than 19,000 commercially available products from approximately 2,500 manufacturers. Detailed information is provided for products in all aspects of independent living, personal care, transportation, communication, and recreation.

Target audience: Individuals interested in assistive technology devices and equipment.

How to access: The database is accessible online.

Apple Solutions

Apple Computer, Inc.
20525 Mariani Avenue
MS 435
Cupertino, CA 95014
(408) 974-7910; (408) 974-7911 (TDD)

Description: Database of products and resources for Apple computers. The database contains more than 1,000 entries, which are updated on a regular basis.

Target audience: Persons interested in products for the Apple computer that can be used by persons with disabilities.

Hardware/software needs: Telecommunications software and modem.

How to Access: Apple Solutions is accessible via AppleLink or SpecialNet.

Cost: Standard phone charges.

CTG Solutions

Closing the Gap, Inc.
P.O. Box 68
Henderson, MN 56044
(612) 248-3294

Description: A relational database containing information on current products and how to use them. The database can be customized for local use so that information relating to student/client activities, administrative considerations, and so forth, can be linked to existing product information.

Target audience: Special education and rehabilitation professionals.

Hardware/software needs: Macintosh computer.

How to access: The database is Macintosh-based. Searches are conducted by the subscriber with documentation provided on strategies for searching.

Cost: Annual license fee is $975 including updates.

Developmental Disabilities Technology Library

Association for Retarded Citizens of the U.S.
2501 Avenue J
Arlington, TX 76006
(817) 261-6003 (voice); (817) 277-6989 (computer)

Description: A database of information on publications related to rehabilitation technology, resource agencies in the field of disabilities, experts and users of assistive devices, and commercial vendors of assistive technology products.

Target audience: Individuals interested in the applications of technology for children and adults with disabilities.

Hardware/software needs: Telecommunications software and modem.

How to access: Via the DD Connection on the OPUS Network, (817) 649-2857; OPUS Net 130, Node 10.

Cost: Standard telephone charges.

Handicapped Users' Database

CompuServe, Inc.
Rear 4
Furry Court
Lancaster, OH 43130

Description: Database containing information about technology for persons with disabilities.

Target audience: Individuals interested in the use of technology for persons with disabilities.

Hardware/software needs: Telecommunications software and modem.

How to access: Via CompuServe.

Cost: Standard phone charges; subscription to CompuServe.

HyperAbledata

Trace Research and Development Center
Waisman Center
1500 Highland Avenue
Madison, WI 53705-2280
(608) 262-6966

Description: A microcomputer-based version of Abledata listing more than 17,000 assistive technology products.

Target audience: Anyone interested in assistive technology products.

Hardware/software needs: Computer with hard disk of at least 26 megabytes to run tape and disk version; or CD-ROM and Macintosh computer.

How to access: Searches are conducted by the individual via disk tape or CD-ROM.

Cost: $50 for the CD-ROM Macintosh-based database, which includes a 6-month update; $199 for floppy disks (33 total); $122 for tape backup.

Rehabdata

National Rehabilitation Information Center (NARIC)
8455 Colesville Road
Suite 935
Silver Spring, MD 20910
(301) 588-9284 or (800) 346-2742

Description: A database of more than 16,000 disability-related documents that allows for custom searches.

Target audience: Individuals interested in the field of rehabilitation.

Hardware/software needs: Telecommunications software and modem.

How to access: Accessed within BRS Information Technologies.

Cost: Standard phone charges and a subscription to BRS.

Specialware Database

LINC Resources, Inc.
4820 Indianola Avenue
Columbus, OH 43214
(614) 885-5599 or (800) 772-7372

Description: Contains information on descriptions of software programs for special education ranging from early childhood to adult education; mildly disabled to severely disabled persons; and from reading to word processing to administration. Database also available on disk and in print formats.

Target audience: Individuals interested in software programs for persons with disabilities.

Hardware/software needs: Telecommunications software and modem. How to access: Dial (614) 433-0851 and follow directions.

Cost: Check with LINC Resources.

Bulletin Boards

Bulletin boards are public message systems that are used by individuals or agencies to post information. The purpose of a bulletin board is to provide access to current information and the latest developments that may be of interest to multiple users. Information is displayed in a user-friendly "menu" format and grouped by subject matter. Depending on what network you use, there are hundreds of bulletin boards available. SpecialNet lists more than 50 bulletin boards containing information on topics such as special education software, technology, current legislation, and assessment of students with disabilities. Bulletin boards are usually operated on microcomputers, and many are available at no cost to the user when accessed through a local phone call. School systems and public agencies have supported specialized bulletin boards (BBSs), and some of these have become so popular that they receive calls from all over the country. Most boards are dedicated for 24-hour access, and users often call late at night when long-distance charges are lowest. Although membership fees are sometimes required, many BBSs are free and are operated by hobbyists or groups of computer users.

Equal BBS

Michael Bowen
3535 S. Wilmington Street
Office 205
Raleigh, NC 27603
(919) 851-6806 (computer)

Description: A bulletin board on adaptive hardware and software, and resource information.

Target audience: Anyone interested in using technology with disabled persons.

Hardware/software needs: IBM-compatible; FlDO/SEAdog software.

How to access: Dial (919) 851-6806; FIDO Net 151, Node 101.

Cost: Standard phone charges.

4 Sights Network

National Information System for the Visually Impaired
16625 Grand River
Detroit, MI 48227
(313) 272-3900

Description: A bulletin board and database providing information on rehabilitation and educational technology resources including information about hardware and software products.

Target audience: Blind and visually impaired and those who work with this population.

Hardware/software needs: Telecommunications software and modem.

How to access: Dial (313) 272-7111; if you are a new user, log on as "new user" and assign yourself a password. Then you become a registered user.

Cost: Standard telephone charges.

Fidoracer

Murray State University
2004 University Station
Murray, KY 40271
Contact: Bill Allbritten
(502) 762-6861; (502) 762-3140 (Computer)

Description: An electronic mail and bulletin board system on the use of computers by persons with disabilities. There is also some public domain software that users can download.

Target audience: Persons interested in the use of technology by persons with disabilities.

Hardware/software needs: Telecommunications software and modem.

How to access: Dial (502) 762-3140; FIDO Net 11, Node 301.

Cost: Standard phone charges. No subscription fee.

ED Board

400 Maryland Avenue, S.W.
ROB, Room 3616
Washington, DC 20202-4726
(202) 708-6775

Description: ED Board is a bulletin board in the U.S. Department of Education (USDE), broadcasting information about grant and contract opportunities.

Target Audience: Persons interested in new grant and contract opportunities offered by USDE agencies. Information includes *Federal Register* announcements, a guide to doing business with USDE, and Request for Proposals in detail.

Hardware/Software needs: Telecommunications software and modem.

How to Access: Dial (202) 260-9950, log in as new user. Use UT 100 terminal emulation. Do not request no line feeds.

Cost: Standard telephone charge. No subscriber fee.

Project Enable/Rehabilitation Information System

Rehabilitation Technology Associates
West Virginia Research and Training Center
One Dunbar Plaza, Suite E
Dunbar, WV 25064-3098
(304) 759-0716

Description: This bulletin board has information on computer use in administration and management of rehabilitation programs. The system has several hun-dred discussion groups available. Public conferencing is also available. The Rehabilitation Information System component lists information on government grant activities including mission, resources, and activities.

Target audience: Persons interested in vocational rehabilitation, rehabilitation engineering, and government-funded programs

Hardware/software needs: Telecommunications software and modem.

How to access: Dial (304) 759-0727 and follow the instructions.

Cost: Standard phone charges. No subscription fee.

RESNA

RESNA Technical Assistance Project
1700 Moore Street
Suite 1540
Arlington, VA 22209
(703) 524-6686

Description: Bulletin board providing an opportunity for states and organizations to share information of interest as they develop and administer assistive technology services. The RESNA Technical Assistance Project is funded by the National Institute on Disability and Rehabilitation Research under the Technology-Related Assistance for Individuals With Disabilities Act of 1988 (P.L.100-407).

Target audience: States and organizations interested in assistive technology services.

Hardware/software needs: Telecommunications software and modem.

How to access: Access is via SpecialNet.

Cost: Standard phone charges; subscription to SpecialNet

TECH.LINE

Center for Special Education Technology
The Council for Exceptional Children
1920 Association Drive
Reston, VA 22091
(703) 620-3660; (800) 873-8255

Description: Just one of many national boards on SpecialNet that offer news and information about technology in special education. A different technology topic is highlighted each month.

Target audience: Persons interested in special education technology.

Hardware/software needs: Telecommunications software and modem.

How to access: Via SpecialNet.

Cost: Standard telephone charges in addition to subscription to SpecialNet.

Helpful Reference Works

Bowen, C., & Peyton, D. *How to get the most out of CompuServe.* New York: Bantam On-line Services Library.

Bowen, C., & Peyton, D. *The complete electronic bulletin board starter kit with RBBS-PC software.* New York: Bantam Electronic Publishing. $39.95.

Center for Special Education Technology. (1990). *Directory of assistive technology data sources.* Reston, VA: Author.

Glossbrenner, A. *The complete handbook of personal computer communications: Everything you need to know to go on-line with the world.* New York: St. Martin' s Press.

Moore, J. (1989). On-line telecommunications demystified. *Exceptional Parent, 19*(7), 42–46, 69–70.

Index